Unified Protocols
for Transdiagnostic Treatment
of Emotional Disorders
in Children and Adolescents

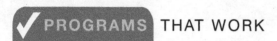 PROGRAMS THAT WORK

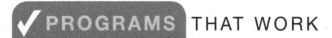
Unified Protocols for Transdiagnostic Treatment of Emotional Disorders in Children and Adolescents

THERAPIST GUIDE

JILL EHRENREICH-MAY
SARAH M. KENNEDY
JAMIE A. SHERMAN
EMILY L. BILEK
BRIAN A. BUZZELLA
SHANNON M. BENNETT
DAVID H. BARLOW

OXFORD
UNIVERSITY PRESS

OXFORD
UNIVERSITY PRESS

Oxford University Press is a department of the University of Oxford. It furthers
the University's objective of excellence in research, scholarship, and education
by publishing worldwide. Oxford is a registered trade mark of Oxford University
Press in the UK and certain other countries.

Published in the United States of America by Oxford University Press
198 Madison Avenue, New York, NY 10016, United States of America.

© Oxford University Press 2018

CIP data is on file at the Library of Congress
ISBN 978–0–19–934098–9

11

Printed by Marquis, Canada

Stunning developments in healthcare have taken place over the last several years, but many of our widely accepted interventions and strategies in mental health and behavioral medicine have been brought into question by research evidence as not only lacking benefit, but perhaps, inducing harm (Barlow, 2010). Other strategies have been proven effective using the best current standards of evidence, resulting in broad-based recommendations to make these practices more available to the public (McHugh & Barlow, 2012). Several recent developments are behind this revolution. First, we have arrived at a much deeper understanding of pathology, both psychological and physical, which has led to the development of new, more precisely targeted interventions. Second, our research methodologies have improved substantially, such that we have reduced threats to internal and external validity, making the outcomes more directly applicable to clinical situations. Third, governments around the world and healthcare systems and policymakers have decided that the quality of care should improve, that it should be evidence based, and that it is in the public's interest to ensure that this happens (Barlow, 2004; Institute of Medicine, 2001, 2015; Weisz & Kazdin, 2017).

Of course, the major stumbling block for clinicians everywhere is the accessibility of newly developed evidence-based psychological interventions. Workshops and books can go only so far in acquainting responsible and conscientious practitioners with the latest behavioral healthcare practices and their applicability to individual patients. This new series, ProgramsThatWork™, is devoted to communicating these exciting new interventions for children and adolescents to clinicians on the frontlines of practice.

The manuals and workbooks in this series contain step-by-step detailed procedures for assessing and treating specific problems and diagnoses. But this series also goes beyond the books and manuals by providing ancillary materials that will approximate the supervisory process in assisting practitioners in the implementation of these procedures in their practice.

In our emerging healthcare system, the growing consensus is that evidence-based practice offers the most responsible course of action for the mental health professional. All behavioral healthcare clinicians deeply desire to provide the best possible care for their patients. In this series, our aim is to close the dissemination and information gap and make that possible.

This volume, *Unified Protocols for Transdiagnostic Treatment of Emotional Disorders in Children and Adolescents*, inaugurates a new collection of books published as part of the Treatments That Work series, TTW: Transdiagnostic Programs, established to reflect and respond to the growing acknowledgement in our field of the importance of the spectrum approach to mental health treatment. This Therapist Guide presents a transdiagnostic approach to the treatment of emotional disorders in young people. These disorders include a range of anxiety disorders and depressive disorders; however, the treatment can also be applied to trauma and stress-related disorders, somatic symptom disorders, and obsessive-compulsive disorders – among many others. This manual is intended for use with any child or adolescent whose area of concern is an emotional disorder and for whom reducing problematic emotional behaviors is the primary treatment target. This *Therapist Guide* is meant to be used in conjunction with one of two companion workbooks, *Unified Protocol for Transdiagnostic Treatment of Emotional Disorders in Children: Workbook* or *Unified Protocol for Transdiagnostic Treatment of Emotional Disorders in Adolescents: Workbook*.

Anne Marie Albano, Editor-in-Chief
David H. Barlow, Editor-in-Chief
Programs *That Work*

References

Barlow, D. H. (2004). Psychological treatments. American Psychologist, *59*, 869–878.

Barlow, D. H. (2010). Negative effects from psychological treatments: A perspective. American Psychologist, *65*(2), 13–20.

Institute of Medicine. (2001). Crossing the quality chasm: A new health system for the 21st century. Washington, DC: National Academy Press.

Institute of Medicine. (2015). Psychosocial interventions for mental and substance use disorders: a framework for establishing evidence-based standards. Washington, DC: National Academy Press

McHugh, R. K., & Barlow, D. H. (2012). Dissemination and implementation of evidence-based psychological interventions. Oxford: Oxford University Press.

Weisz, J. R., & Kazdin, A. E. (2017). Evidence-based psychotherapies for children and adolescents (3rd ed.). New York: Guilford.

All forms and worksheets from books in the PTW series are made available digitally shortly following print publication. You may download, print, save, and digitally complete them as PDFs. To access the forms and worksheets, please visit http://www.oup.com/us/ttw.

Contents

Acknowledgments *xi*

Introduction *xiii*

Part One   Adolescents (UP-A)

Chapter 1   Core Module 1: Building and Keeping Motivation   *3*

Chapter 2   Core Module 2: Getting to Know Your Emotions and Behaviors   *33*

Chapter 3   Core Module 3: Introduction to Emotion-Focused Behavioral Experiments   *53*

Chapter 4   Core Module 4: Awareness of Physical Sensations   *69*

Chapter 5   Core Module 5: Being Flexible in Your Thinking   *81*

Chapter 6   Core Module 6: Awareness of Emotional Experiences   *103*

Chapter 7   Core Module 7: Situational Emotion Exposure   *119*

Chapter 8   Core Module 8: Reviewing Accomplishments and Looking Ahead   *135*

Chapter 9   Module-P: Parenting the Emotional Adolescent   *145*

Part Two   Children (UP-C)

Chapter 10   Introduction to the *Unified Protocol for Transdiagnostic Treatment of Emotional Disorders in Children* (UP-C)— Structural and Pragmatic Considerations in Using the UP-C   *171*

Chapter 11   UP-C Session 1: Introduction to the *Unified Protocol for the Transdiagnostic Treatment of Emotional Disorders in Children*—C Skill: Consider How I Feel   *181*

Chapter 12   UP-C Session 2: Getting to Know Your Emotions—
              C Skill: Consider How I Feel   *207*

Chapter 13   UP-C Session 3: Using Science Experiments to Change
              Our Emotions and Behavior—C Skill: Consider How
              I Feel   *225*

Chapter 14   UP-C Session 4: Our Body Clues—C Skill: Consider
              How I Feel   *243*

Chapter 15   UP-C Session 5: Look at My Thoughts—L Skill: Look
              at My Thoughts   *259*

Chapter 16   UP-C Session 6: Use Detective Thinking—U Skill: Use
              Detective Thinking and Problem Solving   *275*

Chapter 17   UP-C Session 7: Problem Solving and Conflict
              Management—U Skill: Use Detective Thinking and
              Problem Solving   *293*

Chapter 18   UP-C Session 8: Awareness of Emotional Experiences—
              E Skill: Experience My Emotions   *309*

Chapter 19   UP-C Session 9: Introduction to Emotion Exposure—
              E Skill: Experience My Emotions   *329*

Chapter 20   UP-C Session 10: Facing Our Emotions—Part 1—
              E Skill: Experience My Emotions   *347*

Chapter 21   UP-C Sessions 11 Through 14: Facing Our
              Emotions—Part 2—E Skill: Experience My
              Emotions   *365*

Chapter 22   UP-C Session 15: Wrap-up and Relapse Prevention—
              S Skill: Stay Healthy and Happy   *379*

Part Three   Variations and Adaptations

Chapter 23   UP-A Group and UP-C Individual Therapy Variations,
              Other Adaptations—Considerations for Adapting UP-A
              and UP-C for Use with Different Populations   *397*

References   *409*

About the Authors   *413*

Acknowledgments

The UP-C and UP-A are products of collaboration. Their genesis lies in the support of *David H. Barlow, Ph.D.* and colleagues at the Center for Anxiety and Related Disorders at Boston University, particularly the mentorship received via an initial funded award from the National Institute of Mental Health to the first-author (K23 MH073946) that paved the way for the early development and evaluation of the UP-A. Over time, the support, creativity and input of numerous graduate students and staff at both Boston University and the University of Miami's Child and Adolescent Mood and Anxiety Treatment Program have further shaped and defined the UP-C and UP-A. *Stefania Pinto* made a particularly notable contribution to these volumes in terms of creating all illustrations and many of the forms, worksheets and handouts available throughout the UP-C and UP-A. *Monica Nanda, Ph.D.* made a notable written contribution to Module 6 of the UP-A. *Julie Lesser, M.D.* also kindly contributed a conceptualization of the "Double Before/During/After" framework that has been adapted and incorporated into this draft for parents of youth in UP-C or UP-A treatment.

It is important to note that many of the ideas that helped shape the UP-C and UP-A are a product of being avid students of youth psychotherapy ourselves and the ideas that blossomed from observing the great work of colleagues working in similar or related domains of treatment over the years and hearing their critical feedback of our approach. Overall, the scope of student and colleague contributions to these volumes is extensive, with the specific number of people contributing being too long to list. The contributions of each and every one of these students and colleagues are heartily acknowledged.

General Introduction to the *Unified Protocol for Transdiagnostic Treatment of Emotional Disorders in Children* and the *Unified Protocol for Transdiagnostic Treatment of Emotional Disorders in Adolescents*

The therapy manuals included in this volume—the *Unified Protocols for Transdiagnostic Treatment of Emotional Disorders in Children and Adolescents*—may be unlike others you have previously used with youth exhibiting anxiety, obsessive-compulsive, depressive, and/or stress-related disorders. However, there are similarities between these manuals and other clinical training materials you may have used in the past:

- The UP-C and UP-A **DO** include evidence-based treatment strategies to help you in assisting your child and adolescent clients to function better in their lives.
- The UP-C and UP-A **DO** include specific guidelines for treatment delivery.
- The UP-C and UP-A **DO** contain information about how to include parents in treatment and introduce parent-directed strategies to help promote long-term uptake of youth-directed therapy skills.

Similar to the *Unified Protocol for Transdiagnostic Treatment of Emotional Disorders* (UP; Barlow et al., 2013), this guide for youth is also unique in that the evidence-based treatment skills presented may be applied by you, the therapist, to children and adolescents with a wide variety of emotional disorders. In fact, the UP-C and UP-A Therapist Guide and companion workbook materials actually **do not focus on any one specific emotional disorder**, but rather present evidence-based intervention strategies using general emotion-focused language whenever possible, and use examples that reference the experiences of fear, worry, sadness, and anger. In other words, this treatment guide takes a *transdiagnostic* approach to the treatment of the emotional disorders. Some of the disorders that may be targeted with the UP-C or UP-A include—but are not limited to—anxiety disorders (e.g., generalized anxiety disorder, social anxiety disorder, separation anxiety disorder, specific phobias, panic disorder, illness anxiety disorder, agoraphobia) and depressive disorders (e.g., persistent depressive disorder, major depressive disorder). However, this treatment is also flexible enough for use with some trauma and stress-related disorders (including adjustment disorders), somatic symptom disorders, tic disorders, and obsessive-compulsive disorders. In fact, the transdiagnostic presentation of evidence-based intervention techniques within these treatments may be particularly useful for children and adolescents presenting with multiple emotional disorders or mixed/subclinical symptoms of several emotional disorders. Overall, this manual is intended for use with any child or adolescent whose area of primary concern—as identified by you and the family—is an emotional disorder and for whom reducing the frequency and intensity of problematic emotional behaviors is the primary treatment target.

Applications of the Unified Protocols

We have discovered through research on the Unified Protocols for adults, adolescents, and children that a transdiagnostic approach to the treatment of emotional disorders may also be useful with clients struggling with other types of disorders predominated by frequent and intense experience of certain emotions, as well as difficulty effectively regulating those emotions. These include eating disorder symptoms; non-suicidal self-injury; mood regulation difficulties more typical of developing borderline personality features or some bipolar disorder presentations; and some disruptive behavior problems, like oppositional defiant disorder, when they co-occur with other emotional disorders. However, these applications are ideally attempted once you are familiar with or experienced in using the Unified Protocols, as they are still currently under investigation and/or may involve integrating the skills in the UP-C or the UP-A with other evidence-based treatment approaches. Therefore, such applications are not discussed at length in this Therapist Guide. However, readers interested in advanced applications of the UP may also wish to review a publication on the use of the adult UP with an array of clinical populations (Farchione & Barlow, 2017).

Materials Found in This Introduction

In the remainder of this introduction, you will find an overview of the rationale for the use of the UP-C and the UP-A, as well as a summary of the current evidence base for the Unified Protocols. In the concluding sections of this introduction, we also provide a general overview of just the UP-A and a brief guide for delivering this treatment. *You will find a detailed introduction and guide to using the UP-C, more specifically, in Chapter 10 of this book.* Chapters 1 through 9 of this Therapist Guide detail the application of each section of the UP-A. Parent handouts summarizing chapter content are provided at the end of each of these UP-A chapters to facilitate communication between adolescent clients and their parents about session content. Chapters 11 through 22 of this Therapist Guide then detail the session-by-session application of the UP-C. Chapter 23, the final chapter of this Therapist Guide, contains guidelines for adapting and implementing these treatments in different formats and for children and adolescents with varying emotional disorder symptom profiles that include obsessive-compulsive, tic, and trauma/stress-related concerns. Together, we hope that these materials will help you think flexibly about delivering these treatments to children and adolescents with diverse symptom presentations.

Rationale for the UP-C or UP-A for Your Child and Adolescent Clients

The Unified Protocols Provide a Means for Targeting Commonalities Among Emotional Disorders

One reason to implement a unified or transdiagnostic approach with your child and/or adolescent clients is that the techniques that make up this approach target core dysfunctions that may underlie emotional disorders (Marchette & Weisz, 2017). Anxiety and depressive disorders, in particular, share common genetic, neurobiological, and environmental risk factors (Boomsma, Van Beijsterveldt, & Hudziak, 2005; Eley et al., 2003; Middledorp, Cath, Van Dyck, & Boomsma, 2005; Wilamowska et al., 2010). Emotional disorders such as anxiety and depression also tend to co-occur at high rates, both concurrently and sequentially. That is, a child who exhibits one emotional disorder is more likely than not to experience one or more additional emotional disorders (Angold, Costello, & Erkanli, 1999; Leyfer, Gallo, Cooper-Vince, & Pincus, 2013), and children who experience early anxiety symptoms are at comparatively higher risk for both future anxiety disorders and other related emotional disorders, such as depression (Brady & Kendall, 1992; Cummings, Caporino, & Kendall, 2014; Keenan & Hipwell, 2005).

Barlow and colleagues (2014b) have argued that the reason for this high co-occurrence between emotional disorders is that such disorders share a core dysfunction known as ***neuroticism***. Neuroticism is considered a temperament style, or a pattern of approaching the world in relatively stable, characteristic ways that is present from an early age (Barlow, Ellard, Sauer-Zavala, Bullis, & Carl, 2014; Barlow & Kennedy, 2016). Children, adolescents, and adults high in neuroticism often demonstrate *high levels of negative affect*, whereby they experience strong emotions such as fear, anxiety, sadness, and/or anger more frequently than others do. In response to these strong or intense emotions, individuals high in neuroticism become *distressed, anxious, and uncomfortable*. Although a child may not necessarily articulate this distress, his or her actions or emotional expressions may communicate that such emotional experiences are very difficult for him or her to endure. In order to relieve this distress, individuals typically *take actions to suppress, avoid, escape, distract from, or otherwise control these uncomfortable feelings*. These behaviors are *negatively reinforced* over time because when the individual avoids or escapes strong emotions and the situations that elicit them, the discomfort does go away! Unfortunately, over the long term, engaging in these types of avoidant strategies to relieve distress prevents that individual from learning more helpful or effective ways to cope with strong emotions. Children or adolescents high in neuroticism may demonstrate this pattern of behavior across a variety of triggers in their environments and a range of emotion states, placing them at risk for any one of a number of emotional disorders.

When you are considering whether your child or adolescent client is appropriate for the Unified Protocols, please note that the overall goal here is not to eliminate strong or intense emotions! That is not only an impossible goal, but it also misunderstands our purpose in the Unified Protocols. The goals in the UP-C and UP-A are to, in fact, allow the youth to experience their strong or intense emotions with less distress and better usage of more helpful and less avoidant actions to manage such experiences.

The Unified Protocols Address Parenting Practices and Behaviors Associated with Multiple Emotional Disorders

In addition to youth-specific risk and vulnerability factors for emotional disorders, parents of youth with emotional disorders may fall into patterns of behavior or patterns of responding that, over time, inadvertently reinforce the youth's intense experience of strong emotion and use of ineffective coping strategies (Ginsburg, Siqueland, Masia-Warner, & Hedtke,

2004; Drake & Ginsburg, 2012). Specifically, parents of children with various emotional disorder symptoms may struggle to effectively manage their child's or adolescent's emotional distress, may become impatient or critical when their child or adolescent has difficulty with strong emotions, and may practice unhelpful or ineffective ways of managing their *own* distress in front of their child. Therefore, core *emotional parenting behaviors* (e.g., criticism, overcontrol/overprotection, modeling of avoidance, and inconsistency) that typically exacerbate or maintain child and adolescent emotional disorder symptoms are also targeted in the UP-C and UP-A. However, it is important to keep in mind that these treatments are primarily child- and adolescent-focused, and it may be necessary to discuss the possibility of referring parents to their own treatment should parent psychopathology interfere with achieving the child's or adolescent's treatment goals.

The Unified Protocols Bring Together Evidence-Based Change Principles in a Single Treatment

Because emotional problems or disorders have so much in common, they may respond to similar intervention strategies like those delivered in the Unified Protocols. In fact, many of the existing cognitive-behavioral therapy (CBT) manuals for emotional disorders in youth share a common set of treatment components, including emotion education, cognitive restructuring techniques, and behavior change strategies. One difference between these manuals and the Unified Protocols is that most existing CBT manuals describe the application of such skills to one specific problem area, like depression, anxiety, or obsessive-compulsive disorders, as opposed to emotional disorders more generally. The Unified Protocols apply CBT and other evidence-based treatment techniques, such as awareness and mindfulness skills, in a flexible manner that allows the therapist to personalize and tailor strategies to almost any emotion and to the types of problems a youth is experiencing currently. In fact, each UP-A module or UP-C session is explicitly designed to target the mechanisms maintaining the emotional disorders described above (e.g., reducing distress or avoidant responses to intense emotion). Another unique feature specific to the adult UP and UP-A (as described further below) is its modular presentation structure, which provides you with the options of delivering the treatment as a whole or streamlining it to further personalize the intervention.

Evidence Supporting the Adult UP

The adult UP (Barlow et al., 2011) is a treatment that works for adults with anxiety and co-occurring emotional disorders. Support for the efficacy of the UP can be observed across randomized controlled trials (RCTs), along with several ancillary studies. In an initial RCT of the UP, investigators found a large effect size for reductions in the severity of both primary and co-occurring emotional disorders at post-treatment (Farchione et al., 2012). In addition to improvements reported immediately post-treatment, adults who had undergone treatment with the UP generally maintained treatment gains at a six-month follow-up point (Bullis et al., 2014). A five-year, federally funded clinical trial of the UP suggests that this approach may be similarly effective when compared to outcomes from evidence-based treatments that target single emotional disorders, and may promote lesser dropout or attrition from treatment as compared to manuals targeting single disorders (Barlow et al., 2017). UP researchers are also studying several broad, cross-cutting features of neuroticism theoretically underlying emotional disorders that are targeted in the UP. Evidence thus far suggests that changes in underlying factors theoretically linked to the presence of emotional disorders, including maladaptive emotion regulation strategies, negative affect, fear of negative emotions, and anxiety sensitivity, are significantly related to changes in symptoms of emotional disorders during treatment (Conklin et al., 2015; Farchione et al., 2012; Sauer-Zavala et al., 2012). One study suggests that changes in theoretical cross-cutting features of emotional disorders (i.e., mindfulness and reappraisal) as well as in anxiety and depressive symptoms come after the implementation of certain core treatment components of the UP (i.e., mindfulness changes following use of emotional awareness techniques and reappraisal changes coming after use of cognitive flexibility/cognitive reappraisal skills) in an adult with several emotional disorder symptoms (Boswell, Anderson, & Barlow, 2014). The potential efficacy of the UP for individuals with a larger variety of core emotional problems, including those with borderline personality disorder or bipolar disorder, is emerging (Ammerman et al., 2012; Ellard, Deckersbach, Sylvia, Nierenberg, & Barlow, 2012; Lopez et al., 2015). The UP was also viewed as satisfactory and acceptable as an adjunct treatment for suicidal inpatients with a variety of emotional concerns (Bentley, 2017; Bentley et al., 2017). Preliminary work has also suggested that the UP is efficacious whether delivered in its more typical individual therapy format or in a group therapy format (Bullis et al., 2015).

Evidence Supporting the UP-A

The UP-A has also been shown to help adolescents with emotional disorders such as anxiety and depression across multiple baseline, open-trial, and RCT investigations (Ehrenreich, Goldstein, Wright, & Barlow, 2009; Ehrenreich-May et al., 2017; Queen, Barlow, & Ehrenreich-May, 2014). In our initial multiple baseline and open-trial studies of the UP-A, adolescents with an anxiety or depressive disorder experienced significant improvements in these symptoms from pre- to post-treatment (Ehrenreich et al., 2009; Trosper, Buzzella, Bennett, & Ehrenreich, 2009). Results from a waitlist-controlled RCT (Ehrenreich-May et al., 2017) provided evidence that the UP-A works as a treatment for adolescents exhibiting a range of emotional disorders. Adolescent participants in the RCT experienced significant reductions in anxiety and depression symptoms and in overall global severity from pre- to post-treatment and continued to make gains through a six-month follow-up point, albeit at a slower pace (Ehrenreich-May et al., 2017; Queen, Barlow, & Ehrenreich-May, 2014). In addition to ongoing efficacy trials of the UP-A, several current investigations of the UP-A are under way in non-research settings such as community mental health centers and children's hospitals. Applications of the UP-A are also being studied as a universal prevention program for emotional disorders and for intervention purposes in several countries.

Evidence Supporting the UP-C

The UP-C was initially developed as a universal anxiety and depression prevention program for younger children (Ehrenreich-May & Bilek, 2011). After showing promise as a group prevention approach, Ehrenreich-May and Bilek (2012) adapted the program into an engaging and developmentally sensitive group treatment for youth with emotional disorders and their parents and investigated its initial efficacy in an open trial with a small group of children between the ages of 7 and 12. Results from this initial investigation again supported improvement in symptoms of anxiety, depression, and related disorders from pre- to post-treatment

(Ehrenreich-May & Bilek, 2012). Kennedy, Bilek, & Ehrenreich-May (under review) completed a RCT comparing the UP-C to an established group anxiety-focused CBT treatment for children with anxiety disorders. The 47 children who participated in this trial were also between the ages of 7 and 12 and had a variety of emotional disorders, including anxiety, depression, and obsessive-compulsive disorders. No differences in anxiety symptoms were observed between the UP-C and the more traditional, anxiety-focused CBT treatment arm, with both treatments conveying significant improvements in child- and parent-reported anxiety symptoms and the majority of principal diagnoses remitting by the end of treatment. Interestingly, parent reports of child depressive symptoms were significantly lower within the UP-C condition as compared to the anxiety-focused CBT condition at post-treatment, which may underscore the value of the transdiagnostic focus of the UP-C. The UP-C (as compared to anxiety-focused CBT program) also conferred greater improvement in sadness dysregulation and cognitive reappraisal over the course of treatment (Kennedy, Bilek, & Ehrenreich-May, under review). The authors of this trial interpreted the equivalence of these approaches for anxiety as important for inspiring confidence in users that adoption of a child UP does not mean sacrificing the good effects of more typical child CBT for anxiety disorders in youth and may add benefits for other emotional disorder symptoms.

Structural and Pragmatic Overview of the UP-A

Introduction to the UP-A

The UP-A is a transdiagnostic approach to treating adolescents (ages 13–18) with emotional disorders. Depending upon developmental level, individuals just outside this age range may also be appropriate for this treatment, although you may wish to consider using the UP-C (included in this volume) or the adult version of the UP as options for those just below or above these age thresholds or cognitive ability levels. The UP-A is presented in this volume as a **modularized, individual therapy–based approach** for treating emotional disorders, although suggested modifications for delivering this treatment in a group setting are provided in Chapter 23 of this Therapist Guide. The following sections summarize the general content of this treatment, its modular structure, and important considerations for therapists delivering this treatment to adolescents and their families.

> **Therapist Note**
>
> *If you wish to use the UP-C at this time, please consult Chapter 10 for a more thorough overview of important structural and pragmatic considerations for delivering that treatment.*

Description of UP-A Treatment Modules

The UP-A is unique in its use of a *flexible and modular* approach. There are eight **core** or primary modules of varying length in this treatment and one additional parent module, as outlined in Table I.1 (UP-A Overview). Note that we specify a range for the recommended number of sessions for most modules. These are only recommendations, but following these will allow for application of the UP-A in 12 to 21 sessions (average in our prior research trials is about 16 sessions). You are **encouraged to use all core modules in the order they are provided (e.g., 1–8)** and to draw upon the optional parent module when needed. You may also employ a fully modularized application of the treatment (e.g., in which any treatment module may be selected in any order), although you are encouraged to do so only after applying the core modules in the order specified to at least one full case, as there is a logical flow and build to the materials over time. Given the degree of flexibility this treatment allows, it is imperative that a therapist is versed in the basics of its structure and points of flexibility before beginning with an initial adolescent.

Information about the adolescent client (e.g., cognitive level, emotional awareness, motivation), data gleaned from weekly ratings of the client's top problems (described in the sections below and in Chapter 1 of this Therapist Guide), and/or any other data-based tools for weekly symptom monitoring and home learning assignments may help you to determine the length of any given module. Throughout each module, you will notice boxes identifying and describing potential home learning assignments you may wish to assign. For modules that may take several sessions to deliver, you can use the locations of these boxes as guidelines for natural stopping points. In general, we encourage you to assign home learning assignments at the end of each session following the first module, even if modular material needs to be moved.

Parent Involvement in Treatment

Module-P: Parenting the Emotional Adolescent sessions may be used as *parent-only sessions* or may be used for *parent-only time in a given*

Table I.1 UP-A Overview

Module	Title	Recommended # of Sessions	Module Content
1	Building and Keeping Motivation [Chapter 1 in this Therapist Guide]	1 or 2	▪ Build rapport with your adolescent client. ▪ Discuss key problems and set goals. ▪ Determine what motivates the adolescent to change.
2	Getting to Know Your Emotions and Behaviors [Chapter 2 in this Therapist Guide]	2 or 3	▪ Provide psychoeducation about different emotions. ▪ Discuss the purpose of emotions. ▪ Introduce the three parts of an emotion. ▪ Introduce the cycle of avoidance and other emotional behaviors.
3	Introduction to Emotion-Focused Behavioral Experiments [Chapter 3 in this Therapist Guide]	1 or 2	▪ Introduce the concepts of opposite action and emotion-focused behavioral experiments. ▪ Teach the adolescent how to track emotion and activity levels. ▪ Engage the adolescent in emotion-focused behavioral experiments for sadness (and potentially other emotions).
4	Awareness of Physical Sensations [Ch. 4 in this Therapist Guide]	1 or 2	▪ Review the connection between physical feelings and strong emotions. ▪ Develop the adolescent's awareness of his or her physical feelings. ▪ Conduct sensational exposure exercises to help the adolescent learn to tolerate uncomfortable physical feelings.
5	Being Flexible in Your Thinking [Chapter 5 in this Therapist Guide]	2 or 3	▪ Develop the adolescent's ability to think flexibly about emotional situations. ▪ Introduce some common "thinking traps" (i.e., cognitive distortions). ▪ Link thoughts to actions by teaching Detective Thinking and Problem Solving skills.
6	Awareness of Emotional Experiences [Chapter 6 in this Therapist Guide]	1 or 2	▪ Introduce and practice present-moment awareness. ▪ Introduce and practice nonjudgmental awareness. ▪ Conduct generalized emotion exposures by asking the adolescent to practice awareness skills when exposed to general emotional triggers.

Table I.1 Continued

Module	Title	Recommended # of Sessions	Module Content
7	Situational Emotion Exposure [Ch. 7 in this Therapist Guide]	2+	▪ Review skills the adolescent has learned in treatment so far. ▪ Discuss the rationale for situational emotion exposures, introduced to the adolescent as another type of behavioral experiment. ▪ Conduct situational emotion exposures in session and assign additional exposures for home learning.
8	Reviewing Accomplishments and Looking Ahead [Chapter 8 in this Therapist Guide]	1	▪ Review skills and progress toward goals. ▪ Create a relapse prevention plan.
P	Parenting the Emotional Adolescent [Chapter 9 in this Therapist Guide]	1–3	▪ Build parent awareness of responding to the adolescent's distress. ▪ Introduce four common emotional parenting behaviors and their opposite actions (opposite parenting behaviors).

adolescent-focused session and thus may be incorporated into any session when needed. Parent-directed time or whole sessions **may be useful for any parent** but are particularly important in cases where parent behaviors and attitudes are obviously contributing to an adolescent's symptoms or interfering with his or her ability to fully engage with therapy sessions or implement therapeutic strategies at home. Such situations may include high levels of parent accommodation of emotional disorder symptoms, overcontrolling or overprotective behaviors that limit the adolescent's autonomy, lack of positive reinforcement of appropriate adolescent behavior, mild difficulty with adolescent behavior management, dismissiveness of the adolescent's feelings or progress, and lack of understanding of treatment objectives. In our experience with the UP-A, *at least one parent-directed session or session with significant parent-directed time is useful* to engage support for planning and execution of emotion-focused behavioral experiments and/or situational emotion exposures, particularly if the parent is needed to help arrange these or if the parent has a history of aiding in youth emotional behaviors. In addition, you may include parents at the end of each session (if they are available) to review content. In the beginning of Core Module 1, you and the adolescent should discuss how best to include parents in treatment.

Structure of UP-A Treatment Sessions

Following your first session with the adolescent (as described in Core Module 1), most sessions should follow the same general structure:

1. **Obtain a weekly rating of top problems**. Weekly top problem ratings may be easily and quickly obtained from the adolescent at the beginning of each session and entered on the *Weekly Top Problems Tracking Form* (see Chapter 1 for further instructions). You may obtain top problem ratings from the parent before the session begins, at the end of the session when the parent is brought back into the room, or at any other appropriate point of interaction with the parent. As long as top problems are completed at EACH session, you have conducted this activity correctly.

2. **Briefly engage the adolescent in rapport-building by asking about an activity or an event, or so forth, that might be relevant to the adolescent**. Be cautious, however, not to spend too much time engaging in the discussion of less relevant familial or personal stressors or events (e.g., disagreement with a friend, conflict with a parent or romantic partner) that seem only momentarily problematic. Often, discussion of these common events in an adolescent's life can be quickly framed in terms of the UP-A goals for a given session. In these cases, a good strategy is to note the crisis or current problem and let the adolescent (or parents) know you will return to discussing this with them. It can then be used as an example later in the session when teaching a module concept or skill. The same is true of indications about a pattern of symptom change or a new behavior or emotional difficulty. Summarize the concern presented and suggest management of the difficulty with skills to be presented in the module, as appropriate. Clearly, there are times when a new crisis or emergency will need to be the focus of a given session, but if this is occurring on a regular basis or completely limiting the ability to continue in the UP-A manual, you may wish to consider whether this is because the youth's problems no longer fit well with the UP or if it is because of difficulty refocusing the youth or parents on UP skills in session. Whatever the cause, you should attempt to promptly and directly address the issue with the adolescent and parent.

3. **Review home learning assignments the adolescent has completed to acknowledge and reinforce the adolescent's effort with these tasks.** If the adolescent does not complete home learning assignments independently, generate emotionally evocative events and interactions from the week (use the parents as a resource if the adolescent isn't offering necessary information) and use these events to help the adolescent complete home learning assignments in session. You may also wish to guide the adolescent in using problem-solving skills (UP-A Module 5) to identify and address barriers to home learning assignment completion. While it is not ideal to spend a significant amount of time in session addressing and making up incomplete home learning assignments, you should assist the adolescent with completing at least some part of the home learning assignment in session so as not to reinforce avoidance and/or noncompliance with this task. Module 1 contains further information about steps to take if weekly home learning assignment completion is problematic. When you review these assignments, assist the adolescent with understanding the functional relationships between his or her emotions, reactions, and consequences using examples from the "Before, During, and After" homework sheet (see UP-A Module 2). Make sure to use specific labeled praise as you note adolescent understanding and application of treatment concepts to encourage related behaviors outside of sessions.

4. **Introduce new skills.** The amount of time spent on introducing or reviewing a skill varies depending on the module. For example, UP-A Module 2 includes a great deal of educational material about emotions and behaviors, potentially requiring a more didactic presentation, while later modules involve more hands-on practice of skills.

5. **Practice new skills in session, using a neutral or hypothetical example that does not directly apply to the adolescent's emotions and behaviors.** Discussing one's own emotional experiences is often more difficult than speaking about the experiences of others. Wherever possible in the UP-A, we suggest introducing a new skill with an activity or enjoyable example to engage the adolescent's focus and improve understanding of that technique or concept. For adolescents who have more limited emotional awareness, high interpersonal sensitivity, or cognitive challenges, it can be useful to also illustrate a concept or use a more generalized context when teaching a new skill (*"Some teenagers who have strong angry feelings might use Problem Solving to help work through potential solutions that can help.*

Let me give you an example . . ") before moving on to more sensitive or personal examples appropriate to skill practice.

6. **Practice the new skill in session, applying it to the adolescent's own emotional experiences.** Once the skill is fully introduced and understood, an adolescent can more easily apply the concept to his or her own experiences. Using as many personally relevant examples and activities to reinforce skill knowledge, including the liberal evocation of emotion in session, is highly preferred. Notably, there may be some modules where such personalized practice occurs in a separate session from skill introduction.

7. **Assign home learning assignment(s).** Home learning assignments should relate as directly as possible to session content. Practicing skills at home allows adolescents to apply concepts to real-life experiences outside of the therapy context, which helps generalize skills. The expectation is that the adolescent will be able to use and apply skills learned in therapy to his or her own life. Additionally, several monitoring forms (i.e., *Before, During, and After* form and *Weekly Activity Tracking* form) may be given as home learning assignments consistently throughout therapy to maintain the adolescent's focus on emotional experiences and approach behaviors.

Materials Needed for Sessions

Materials necessary for given module sessions may vary depending on the content or emotion exposure exercises planned for that session. However, you should have tools available for didactic material explication in every session (e.g., something to visually present material on, such as a whiteboard, paper, and markers or pens, and/or the UP-A workbook). Generally speaking, access to a desktop computer or laptop and internet/Wi-Fi connection is helpful in certain modules for generating emotion exposure ideas or for practicing emotion exposures in session. A television, tablet, or other media playback device may also be useful, if a computer or internet access is not available. You may also wish to carefully consider your ability to conduct emotion-focused behavioral experiments and situational exposure sessions offsite before such sessions and consider local resources (e.g., school, train stations, shopping malls, bookstores) that may be helpful in conducting situational exposures, if possible and appropriate for your adolescent client (see UP-A Modules 3 and 7).

The *Unified Protocol for Transdiagnostic Treatment of Emotional Disorders in Adolescents: Workbook* materials will foster adolescent understanding of the concepts in this treatment. This workbook contains didactic explanations and examples of skills, core module worksheets, and forms and worksheets for home learning assignments. Therapists preparing to use this Therapist Guide should also review workbook materials in advance to optimize use of specific forms, worksheets, and other materials provided in them during sessions. You can give this workbook to your adolescent client and have him or her review it independently, but you may prefer to review the workbook materials in smaller chunks each session with your adolescent client and go over home learning assignments carefully in person to ensure understanding and minimize burden. Summary forms for the UP-A modules are also available for parents; they appear at the end of each UP-A module in this Therapist Guide. These pages should be distributed during the course of each core module to promote parent empathy and awareness of UP-A skills.

The Importance of Home Learning Assignments

The handling of home learning assignments in this treatment is unusual in that it is tied to its modular design. Because sessions within a given module may vary in length and the number of module goals covered, individual home learning assignments are assigned following completion of a given module *goal* regardless of which session this goal is met in. Therefore, following the presentation of treatment material associated with each goal, a suggested homework practice is listed. Be attentive to issues of adolescent burden in assigning these homework assignments, especially for those adolescents who complete a large number of goals in a given weekly session, and modify or combine assignments when necessary. One exception to these rules is the *Before, During, and After* form, which is given at each session from the end of Core Module 2 onward, to help monitor emotion awareness and opposite action practice throughout treatment. Additionally, tracking of activities using the *Weekly Activity Tracking Form* is given at each session starting at the end of Core Module 3 onward, for those engaging in ongoing emotion-focused behavioral experiments. Overall, on a weekly basis, pay careful attention to which home learning assignments are most appropriate for a given adolescent, in light of his or her motivation, preparation, and particular emotional disorder challenges.

General Considerations in Using the UP-A

Due to the transdiagnostic nature of this treatment, some of the terminology in this Therapist Guide may be unfamiliar to you or may be used differently from how you have encountered this terminology before in other evidence-based treatment manuals. Below, we provide some additional notes about how to frame certain treatment concepts and about terms we wish you to consider as you prepare to use this treatment.

1. You should generally refrain from using the term "negative" to describe an adolescent's emotions or emotional states, although it is often difficult to refrain from doing so. For descriptive purposes, we do so in this Therapist Guide too. Instead, as you will note throughout, we typically encourage use of the terms "intense," "strong," or "uncomfortable" to describe such emotions or states. The main point here is that you should endeavor to avoid stigmatizing the adolescent's emotional experience as particularly negative or labeling it as overly positive. Rather, we encourage reference to the intensity and comfort levels associated with the emotions experienced, regardless of the type of emotion discussed.

2. Similarly, when referring to the physiological component of a given emotion, we encourage the use of terms such as "feelings in my body," "body clues," or "physical sensations," as the term "feelings" is too easily confused with broader emotion concepts.

3. We use the term "parent" to describe the caregiver(s) attending treatment with the adolescent throughout this Therapist Guide. We freely acknowledge the large variety of parental figures (e.g., grandparents, stepparents, guardians, other relatives, older siblings) who may be a given adolescent's primary caregiver and the wide array of family compositions you may observe in your practice, including the possibility of multiple primary caregivers. We simply use the term "parent" here as shorthand to reference the primary caregiver (or caregivers) attending treatment with an adolescent.

4. The gender of the adolescent client referred to throughout this manual is purposely switched between male and female from one module to the next. We recognize that some adolescents may identify their gender in ways other than female or male and encourage you to use pronouns and gender identity references appropriate to your adolescent client.

5. There are references to numerous forms, worksheets, and figures in this manual. Generally, the term "form" refers to something that is

intended to be filled out by the adolescent on several or more occasions during treatment. A "worksheet" refers to material that is intended to be completed in its entirety on a single occasion or for a single home learning assignment. "Figures" are images, diagrams, or example forms/worksheets that appear in the workbook to help illustrate specific concepts or skills. You may find it helpful at times to instruct the adolescent to turn to the relevant figure during session as you introduce and explain various concepts and skills.

Ending the UP-A Well

One particular challenge to a flexible, modular approach to treatment like this one is deciding when to end treatment. Although this challenge presents itself with many treatment formats, the flexible nature of each UP-A module, particularly Module 7, can complicate decision making about the timing of termination. Readiness for termination can be assessed in a number of ways, but we provide several suggestions to guide your decision making. Reduction of *Top Problems* ratings to the low to medium range for each problem (e.g., "0–3") may signal that the original presenting problems are no longer substantially interfering or distressing, and movement toward termination may be advisable. This is particularly true if an adolescent has completed all or the majority of items on the *Emotional Behavior Form*, and ratings for all or most items have reduced substantially. It is important to note that not *all* items on the *Emotional Behavior Form* need to be completed before termination, and Module 8 contains materials to assist the adolescent and you in planning exposures or other skills that the adolescent can use at home after treatment ends.

At a minimum, we suggest proceeding through each UP-A module before initiating termination and adhering to the recommended number of sessions for each module outlined in Table I.1 of this introduction. Of course, some families decide to terminate treatment earlier than recommended due to life stress, financial constraints, or other factors. In these cases, we would certainly recommend use of Problem Solving (Module 5) to address any potential barriers to treatment, as well as use of motivational enhancement strategies (Module 1) to reinvigorate motivation for treatment. If the adolescent or family continues to indicate an intention to terminate treatment, we strongly suggest scheduling a termination session to discuss Module 8 materials, regardless of the stopping point for treatment overall.

Time to Get Started

Thank you for taking the time to learn more about the UP-C and UP-A! While learning any new treatment approach can be overwhelming, we sincerely hope these treatments provide you with a set of flexible and widely applicable tools that may be of use to any child or adolescent client struggling with emotional disorders. We know that the flexibility of these materials and their application is a benefit, and we also recognize that it can take time to feel comfortable with both the core principles of change presented in each module of the UP-A or session of the UP-C and learn how to integrate those ideas with the particulars of the client and family you are endeavoring to help. To that end, at the start of every UP-A chapter, you will find a section that helps orient you to not only the practical materials and goals for that module, but also the overarching theoretical purpose of that module and its applicability to an array of emotional disorder presentations. By reviewing the key purpose of each module as you go along and keeping this in mind, you will soon learn how to be adept at using the Unified Protocol materials both flexibly and faithfully to produce excellent effects for a large number of your child and adolescent clients.

PART ONE

Adolescents (UP-A)

CHAPTER 1

Core Module 1: Building and Keeping Motivation

(Recommended Length: 1 or 2 Sessions)

MATERIALS NEEDED FOR THE MODULE

- Module 1: Building and Keeping Motivation—Workbook Materials:
  1. *Defining the Main Problems* (Worksheet 1.1)
  2. *Weighing My Options* (Worksheet 1.2)
- *Defining the Main Problems—Parent* (Appendix 1.2 at the end of this chapter)
- *Weekly Top Problems Tracking Form* (Appendix 1.3 at the end of this chapter)
- A parent module summary form is provided at the end of this chapter to help support review of module materials with the parent(s) of your adolescent client. You may also use materials from Chapter 9 (Module-P) to help support these discussions.

Overall Core Module 1 Goals

During Core Module 1, you will describe the purpose and structure of treatment, and together with the adolescent and parent, determine the parent's involvement in treatment. Using Worksheet 1.1: *Defining the Main Problems* from the adolescent workbook and Appendix 1.2: *Defining the Main Problems—Parent* at the end of this chapter, *both the adolescent and parent should be asked to identify and rate the severity of three top problems* they would like to address over the course of treatment, and these top problems should be used to assess and build motivation for change. Motivational enhancement strategies are introduced in this module as the primary means of building both the adolescent's and the parent's motivation for change, but these may be used more or less in session depending on the adolescent's baseline readiness for change and family investment in therapy. The ideas and concepts presented in this module (also see Appendix 1.1: *Additional Motivational Enhancement Topics*) may also be utilized throughout treatment **and can be returned to throughout the course of therapy as needed**, but are especially useful when first developing rapport and whenever the adolescent is struggling to remain engaged and move forward in the UP-A. In addition to providing an introduction to the basic structure of treatment and discussing confidentiality and agency/practice procedures, *the goals of this module are as follows:*

- **Goal 1:** Orient the adolescent and family to treatment concepts and structure (including level of parent involvement).
- **Goal 2:** Obtain three top problems from the adolescent, as well as severity ratings for each top problem. Identify "SMART" goals related to top problems.
- **Goal 3:** Strengthen the adolescent's motivation for change by identifying initial steps to achieve SMART goals, by using motivational enhancement techniques, and by using the decisional balance exercise. Secure adolescent commitment to treatment. (This goal is optional and may be used if time permits or if motivation is low for change.)
- **Goal 4:** Discuss parent's motivation for treatment; obtain parent ratings of adolescent top problems and explore any barriers to regular and continued engagement with treatment; and strengthen the parent's motivation for change using the motivational enhancement techniques described in this module (motivational elements to be used as needed). Secure parent commitment to treatment.

Therapist Note—Unified Protocol Theory

*At the beginning of each UP-A module, there will be a **Therapist Note** that serves as a brief reminder about how that module's content links to the overall theory and case conceptualization model of the Unified Protocols. In Module 1, you will be doing several tasks for which it will be vital to keep the Unified Protocol theory and case conceptualization model in mind, as described in the Introduction. First, you will be engaging your adolescent client in a discussion about the **function** of strong emotions in her life as* *you build initial rapport and motivation. In other words, what things has she been doing in response to her strong emotions? What has worked for her? What has not? Second, as you establish top problems and SMART goals in this module with both the adolescent and parent(s), it will be vital to consider how these problems and goals fit within the framework of the Unified Protocol. Would we expect such a problem to change with this specific intervention? If so, how? Can you use language or modify problems or goals to better fit with the prevailing theory or case conceptualization model of this approach? If so, you are encouraged to do so.*

Adolescent Motivational Enhancement in the UP-A—A Primer[1]

Before we describe specific module content, a basic understanding of the motivational enhancement techniques to be used in the UP-A may provide a useful framework for understanding how to build and support motivation within this module and throughout treatment. This module describes a number of motivational enhancement techniques that can be used to help increase the adolescent's and the parent's motivation to change and commitment to engage in the treatment process. Motivational enhancement is a therapeutic technique than can decrease an adolescent's ambivalence about and resistance to changing problematic or interfering behaviors. It is important to emphasize that motivational enhancement techniques are not skills to be taught to the client per se (although worksheets such as those in the UP-A that promote goal setting and treatment commitment are often utilized); generally, it is a *conversational style* that should be used not only in this initial module but throughout treatment *whenever ambivalence is encountered.* The main enhancement strategy described here is **motivational interviewing**, which gives the therapist a way of offering choices to the adolescent and encouraging evaluation of the adolescent's choices without force or judgment. Motivational interviewing also helps resolve ambivalence by increasing discrepancy between the adolescent's current behaviors and the desired goals while simultaneously minimizing resistance. There are also techniques discussed that

---

[1] The motivational interviewing techniques described in this module are not original to the UP-A. They are derived from Miller and Rollnick (2002) and Sobell and Sobell (2003). Techniques discussing how to address therapy homework non-compliance and emotional avoidance at the end of this module are also described in Leahy (2003).

more specifically target **emotional avoidance** and **home learning assignment compliance**, which may be used primarily as references for you to support adolescent involvement during subsequent modules.

Motivational enhancement is important in the UP-A because adolescents are often conflicted about wanting to change or are hesitant about engaging in therapy. This is understandable from a developmental perspective given that adolescents do not often think about their behavior, including the types of avoidance behaviors and strong emotions we target in the UP-A, from a long-term perspective. It is also common that an adolescent is not referring herself to therapy. Many clients are persuaded by someone else (parents and teachers, for example) to engage in treatment. Additionally, this treatment asks a lot of the client and family, and many adolescents or their parent(s) might not be ready initially to work toward changing their behavior.

Emotional disorder symptoms typically go hand in hand with treatment ambivalence. In particular, adolescents suffering from symptoms of depression may be lacking motivation for many activities, including therapy. In addition, the emotional avoidance and ensuing avoidance behaviors that typically accompany anxiety and depressive disorders can also lead to treatment ambivalence, as these behaviors may feel needed or beneficial to the adolescent in the short term. It is imperative that you keep the adolescent's perspective in mind and learn what is important enough to her to motivate continued engagement. It is important that the therapist not use techniques that increase resistance, some of which are described at the end of this module, as this will increase the adolescent's opposition to the therapy process and decrease the potential for therapeutic change.

A change in the adolescent's motivation may take time. That doesn't mean you need to stay on this module for more than one or two sessions at this time, but rather you may simply need to be more attentive to such issues in future sessions. Motivation may wax and wane throughout the adolescent's time in treatment. It is common for therapists to encounter some ambivalence during emotion-focused behavioral experiments (especially for adolescents experiencing significant depression), during the situational emotion exposure module, and with home learning assignments throughout the modules (for all adolescents). Any treatment material may spark some resistance or, in all likelihood, outside life stressors or family issues may promote resistance at times in treatment.

Ambivalence can be obvious, such as a client being chronically late for sessions, arguing with the therapist, or refusing to try a new technique in session, or more subtle, such as avoiding discussions that cause distress by switching to another topic or interrupting the therapist. If this occurs, you should use data-based monitoring tools and top problem ratings within and between modules to help you most effectively refocus treatment on presenting problems and better understand factors delaying progress. It is also important for you to recognize if or when you are beginning to feel frustrated with the adolescent, which is a common response to a client's ambivalence about therapy. If you begin to feel helpless in efforts to move the adolescent forward or feel as if you are doing all of the hard work, this can lead you to label the adolescent as "unmotivated" or "resistant," which can impact your relationship profoundly. Therefore, not only are the techniques described below helpful for decreasing adolescent ambivalence, *they are also there to reduce your feelings of helplessness and frustration.*

Essential Components of Motivational Interviewing

1. *Express empathy:* This is seen as the cornerstone of motivational enhancement and relates to any experiences conveyed by the client. It is marked by the underlying attitude of *acceptance* in an effort to understand the client's feelings and perspectives without judging, criticizing, or blaming. Ambivalence is not viewed as psychopathology. Instead, it is accepted as a normal part of human experience, and a normal part of the therapeutic process.

2. *Develop discrepancy:* The adolescent's awareness of the consequences of her behavior is important. A discrepancy between present behavior and future goals will motivate change. By pointing out the discrepancy in a nonjudgmental manner, you lead the adolescent to present her own arguments for change. Discrepancy is explicitly developed in Module 1 using the decisional balance exercise in Goal 3 (below).

3. *Avoid arguments:* Arguments are easy to fall into but can be counterproductive to change. When you defend your position, it breeds defensiveness in the client.

4. *Roll with resistance:* The therapist invites the client to see a new perspective, but this perspective is not imposed. If the adolescent is ambivalent about the new perspective, do not enforce it.

5. *Support self-efficacy:* Belief in the possibility of change is an important motivator. The client is responsible for choosing and carrying out personal change.

Empathy

High levels of empathy during treatment have been shown to be associated with positive treatment outcomes across different types of psychotherapy. As a therapist, you are familiar with empathy or compassion and how it can be expressed. Here are a few reminders about what empathy looks like in session:

- Listen in a supportive, reflective manner that demonstrates your understanding of your adolescent client's concerns and feelings.
- Give sharp attention to each new client statement.
- Continually use *reflective listening*—listening actively through a series of verbal (e.g., "I understand") and nonverbal (e.g., nodding) behaviors while also working to clarify what the adolescent is saying and making sure there is mutual understanding.
- Communicate respect for and acceptance of the client and her feelings.
- Establish a safe environment for the client where you listen rather than tell.

Additional motivational enhancement techniques are provided in Appendix 1.1 at the end of this module. These include the following:

- A definition of resistance and techniques for decreasing resistance
- Strategies that are useful when encountering resistance
- Avoidance as a particular source of resistance in the UP-A
- Methods for addressing struggles around home learning assignments/skills practice

Core Module 1 Content (Divided by Goals)

Goal 1

Orient the adolescent and family to treatment concepts and structure (including level of parent involvement).

Introduction to UP-A Structure and Purpose

Welcome the adolescent and parent to this first session of the UP-A. As you initially orient the adolescent and parent to the structure and purpose of the UP-A, several elements should be emphasized. You may start by describing the UP-A broadly:

> *"The UP-A contains strategies that have been shown in research to help adolescents cope more effectively with strong emotions and the situations in which they often have strong emotions."*

You can then note that this treatment is not designed to get rid of strong emotions. Rather, this treatment is designed to help the adolescent *learn new ways to manage her emotions* so that these strong emotions do not mess up her life. You may briefly explore, while the parent is still in the room, how strong emotions have impacted the adolescent's life, or wait on further discussion of this topic until after the parent leaves the room. As the adolescent is the expert on her own emotional experience, emphasize that you will serve as a kind of coach, but the adolescent will be the one to practice the strategies she learns. Indicate that together you and the adolescent will be talking about many different emotions, but that the emotions she experiences most *frequently* and *intensely* are the ones you will be talking about most often. You should indicate that you will return to this topic and discuss strong emotions and related emotional behaviors later in this session and more in subsequent sessions.

The Role of Out-of-Session Practice

Attending sessions and listening to the concepts will only set the stage for change. Practice of the concepts in "real life" is what will result in noticeable, lasting changes. Every week, the adolescent will be given home learning assignments from the UP-A workbook to aid in the process of practicing the skills learned in session. These workbook materials should be filled out at home and brought to the following session to remind the adolescent of the work she did over the past week, as well as to remind her of any problems, setbacks, or obstacles that may have occurred.

Course of Treatment

The length of the UP-A is not specifically dictated ahead of time, but on average, treatment lasts approximately 16 weeks. Sessions are typically conducted weekly but may occur more frequently if necessary to ensure the adolescent's safety (as appropriate to your treatment setting).

Use of Workbook Materials

During each session you will be covering a fair amount of material. The workbook has been designed to supplement and support Therapist Guide materials in order to ensure that all information is learned and practiced in and out of session.

Discuss Parental Involvement in Treatment and Rapport Building

At this point, you may excuse the parent from session. You may choose to give the parent a copy of the *Parent Summary Form for Core Module 1: Building and Keeping Motivation* and *Defining the Main Problems—Parent* (Appendix 1.2 in this chapter) to complete while the parent is waiting for you to finish the remaining adolescent portion of this first session. These parent materials can be found at the end of this chapter. The problems endorsed by the parent out of session can then be discussed and confirmed as the parent-rated top three problems when the parent returns to session. *Alternatively, you can wait and have the parent and adolescent complete their respective versions of the Defining the Main Problems worksheet together at the end of this first session to promote collaboration and consistency across adolescent and parent problems to be rated weekly.*

Once alone, remind the adolescent that this treatment will be most successful if all members of the team are aware of the skills being taught and of the concepts being learned. Inform the adolescent that you will be checking in with the parent regularly and may have some sessions with just the parent(s), but that you would like to do so in a way that is comfortable for the adolescent. You should discuss with the adolescent what parental check-in format would make her most comfortable. Parental check-ins will be required for this treatment; therefore, the adolescent should not be given the option of denying parent check-ins.[2] Some suggestions are below:

- 5- to 10-minute check-in with parent at the end of session with adolescent in the room

---

[2] The exception to this would be in the case of a strong negative parental influence on treatment (e.g., interfering levels of parental psychopathology, history of abuse or extreme conflict).

- 5- to 10-minute check-in with parent at the end of session with adolescent out of the room
- Up to three partial or full sessions with parent to help him or her support the adolescent even more (i.e., Module-P sessions), plus 5- to 10-minute check-ins

Ask the adolescent what she is most comfortable with and try to use this as a guideline for parent involvement. However, it may be good to indicate to the adolescent that you may need to return to this discussion later (for example, if she requested no Module-P sessions, but you feel it would be helpful to have one or more later).

Next, you *may* spend a bit of time getting to know the adolescent by asking non-intimidating questions about her interests and life (e.g., family, friends, and school), particularly if the adolescent appears reluctant or hesitant about therapy. Techniques of motivational enhancement should be interwoven into the conversation in order to assess and enhance the adolescent's motivation for treatment. Remember—it's okay if this module is more than one session, if that's appropriate to secure the adolescent's motivation for therapy. It's also okay to just "dive right in" to top problems next.

Goal 2

Obtain three top problems from the adolescent, as well as severity ratings for each top problem. Identify "SMART" goals related to top problems.

Therapist Note
Some adolescents may naturally identify goals before top problems. In these instances it may be appropriate to switch the order of discussion.

Identifying Top Problems

In order to elicit top problems (Weisz et al., 2011), begin a brief discussion about why the adolescent believes she is in treatment and what she sees as her main problems (at least three for tracking on the *Weekly Top Problems Tracking Form* in Appendix 1.3) currently.

First, refer to Worksheet 1.1: *Defining the Main Problems* to guide this discussion. Allow the adolescent to state whatever problems come to mind. If she generates problems that are clearly outside the scope of this intervention, first be sure to fully understand the problems she is describing, allowing her the opportunity to correct any misunderstandings (e.g., by reflecting back what is heard). In addition, it may be useful to review any pretreatment assessment materials with the adolescent to help prompt identification of her more impairing concerns. This can be a useful time to remind the adolescent that this treatment is designed to help her *learn new skills to manage her strong emotions* so that they do not keep her from doing things she would like to be able to do. One way to generate top problems consistent with the UP-A model in this section is to ask the adolescent:

"What are some situations in which you typically feel MOST overwhelmed or distressed? What situations do you find you are avoiding? Do you find yourself doing other things, like distracting yourself, to feel better in any situations? Are you avoiding, distracting yourself, or doing other things to feel better because of intense emotions or bothersome situations?"

Therapist Note

It is common for adolescents to note difficulties in social or romantic relationships as top problems. These concerns can be addressed in the UP-A. For example, if the adolescent says, "I want to have more friends," assess what she thinks is keeping her from having more friends. If it's her tendency to avoid situations with new people because she feels uncomfortable in these situations, offer hope that this can be addressed within the protocol.

If the adolescent says only that her parent is forcing her to come to treatment, ask her to identify what her parent perceives to be the main problems. If the adolescent is unsure or unwilling to provide examples, you may need to reference material discussed during the adolescent's intake assessment (if applicable) or you may need to encourage a discussion between the parent and the adolescent about the parental rationale for seeking treatment at this time.

Therapist Note

Negotiating top problems if the adolescent feels coerced into receiving treatment can be tricky. Try your best to empathize with the adolescent's perspective if this is the case. Starting this discussion by focusing on SMART goals rather than top problems may help to engage a more wary adolescent.

Here are some questions that might help get the conversation started:

"Whose idea was it that you come here?"
"Why do you think you are here?"

"What makes _____ think that you need to come here?"
"What will convince _____ that you don't need to come here?"
"What does _____ think is the reason that you have (name of the behavior)?"
"What does _____ say you need to do differently?"
"Are you happy with the way things have been going in your life lately?"
"Is there anything you would like to see change in your life?"

Top problems are a central tool for ongoing progress monitoring in the UP-A. Thus, they should be scored weekly on the *Weekly Top Problems Tracking Form* (see Appendix 1.3). Progress along the three adolescent and parent top problems (whether identified as the same three problems or two different sets of problems) can be presented back to clients and families weekly, as such data may be useful for maintaining treatment motivation over time.

Identifying SMART Goals

The second half of Worksheet 1.1: *Defining the Main Problems* involves goal setting. The main aim of this exercise is to increase the adolescent's self-efficacy. It is important to discuss and normalize the fact that adolescents can sometimes feel overwhelmed at the outset of treatment—both about the potential to go from how distressed they are now to substantial relief from their conditions *and* all the things that need to happen to get there! To a certain extent, an initial focus on top problems versus goals may also feel overly negative in tone. To help address this state of feeling overwhelmed and keep a hopeful outlook, we use a goal-setting exercise to create a set of manageable goals from the client's top problems. We introduce this exercise by explaining to the adolescent that one factor that predicts success in treatment is setting manageable, concrete goals early on (Weisz et al., 2011).

We are going to refer to these as SMART goals—goals that are *S*pecific, *M*easurable, *A*ttainable, *R*elevant, and *T*ime-Bound:

- Specific goals are well defined and refer to the aspect of behavior change that is most relevant for the adolescent (e.g., "improving my grades in school" versus "doing better at school").
- Measurable goals allow for some observation of improvement over time (e.g., "making three new friends" versus "making friends").
- Attainable goals are those that allow for the possibility of achievement during the course of treatment.
- Relevant goals are those most central to the adolescent's top problems and the UP-A treatment model.

■ Time-bound goals are those that have some specified timeframe in which measurable change will occur (e.g., "getting out of bed on time each day for the next month").

However, in the UP-A, goals can be a variety of short-term, long-term, or ongoing targets. For example, some goals could be achieved in a few hours (such as "Go to the gym today") whereas others might be things the adolescent is always working toward (such as "Feeling more comfortable talking to peers"). Although we encourage clients to discuss any goals they may have (regardless of type), it's important to make any larger, more abstract goals as concrete and specific as possible using the SMART framework, when time permits or as may be relevant to motivational enhancement. A good question to ask yourself as a therapist here is this: Can this adolescent achieve her SMART goal in the time we have allotted for therapy using the UP-A? If so, you have likely achieved a set of goals that you can use for ongoing motivational enhancement throughout treatment to come.

Optional Goal 3

Strengthen the adolescent's motivation for change by identifying initial steps to achieve SMART goals, by using motivational enhancement techniques, and by using the decisional balance exercise. Secure adolescent commitment to treatment. (This goal is optional and may be used if time permits or if motivation is low for change.)

Identifying Steps to Achieve SMART Goals

Adolescents who *need additional motivational enhancement* may benefit from taking the three SMART goals identified from Worksheet 1.1: *Defining the Main Problems* and identifying actionable "baby steps" that may be helpful in achieving these goals. The purpose of this exercise is to encourage the adolescent (a) to understand that change is possible and (b) to build self-efficacy by identifying avenues for encouraging *approach*-oriented (versus avoidance-oriented) solutions to her problems. When identifying these approach-oriented steps, it's important to recognize that the adolescent may not be ready to take larger steps toward these goals at this time; however, she may find that smaller, approach-oriented steps are possible.

Strategies for Evoking Change Talk

Clients are generally much more willing to change when they come up with their own reasons for doing so as opposed to being told to by someone else. This is certainly important to consider when treating adolescents given the strong developmental needs for autonomy in this age group. Once you have elicited a list of three top problems and SMART goals from the adolescent, the following strategies are useful in encouraging the *client to discuss the importance of change* (i.e., to engage in "change talk"):

1. Ask evocative and open-ended questions.
   "What do you make of that?"
   "Can you tell me more?"
   "What do you think you might do?"

2. Explore the pros and cons of change, first asking about the benefits of keeping the status quo, then asking about possible risks of having things stay the same.
   "What do you like about how things are going now?"
   "Is there anything about what's going on that bothers you?"
   "Tell me more about that."

3. Ask for elaboration when change talk emerges.
   "In what ways?"
   "Could you tell me why that was a concern?"

4. Ask for specific examples to strengthen change talk when it emerges.
   "When was the last time that happened?"
   "Give me an example."
   "What else?"

5. Use the past to help the adolescent make decisions about the future by exploring times when current behaviors weren't a concern.
   "You said things used to be better for you. What has changed?"
   "What were things like before you started [insert behavior]?"

6. Look forward to the future to help the adolescent discover whether current behaviors are helping her achieve what she wants out of life.
   "If you were 100 percent successful in making the changes you want, what would be different?"
   "How would you like your life to be five years from now?"
   "If you didn't try to make changes, what might happen?"

Conduct Decisional Balance Exercise and Secure Commitment to Return to Therapy

If the adolescent continues to struggle with motivation and commitment to therapy, work to build a discrepancy between her current actions and her desired future outcomes as they relate to treatment. Try to clarify the costs that the adolescent views as associated with making therapy-related changes in her behavior at this time. Use Worksheet 1.2: *Weighing My Options* in the workbook to reinforce this idea and, ideally, secure commitment to coming to therapy for at least the next several sessions to see if benefits/pros can outweigh the cons identified. You can also more simply ask:

"What are the worst things that might happen if you don't make this change?"
"What are the best things that might happen if you do make this change?"

Goal 4

Discuss parent's motivation for treatment; obtain parent ratings of adolescent top problems and explore any barriers to regular and continued engagement with treatment; and strengthen the parent's motivation for change using the motivational enhancement techniques described in this module (motivational elements to be used as needed). Secure parent commitment to treatment.

Obtain Parent Ratings of Their Adolescent's Top Problems

At the end of the first session, make sure that you save enough time to bring the parent back into the room. This can be with or without the adolescent also present depending on the adolescent's preference and your clinical judgment of whether it would make sense to have both the parent and adolescent in the room together. Once the parent is present, review and assess the appropriateness of the parent's top problem list, take the parent ratings of top problem intensity, and begin assessing the parent's motivation to participate as necessary in the adolescent's treatment and potential barriers that might interfere with full engagement with the treatment process. Again, it is ideal to have the adolescent and parent collaborate and agree on three problems that will be rated by both each week. However, if agreement seems hard to achieve at this time, you can proceed with three separate problems for each informant. It is possible that the adolescent may be upset or angry with the parent for identifying a problem the adolescent did not bring up. Normalize this concern and reiterate that all opinions are valuable in this treatment.

Discussing and Building Parent Motivation

You are strongly encouraged, in this module or at later time points, to use motivational enhancement techniques when interacting with the parent. Sometimes lack of motivation for treatment on the part of a parent can strongly impact treatment progress. Parent motivation should be assessed during initial sessions and monitored throughout treatment if issues arise (e.g., problems with attendance, issues with parents helping enforce skills with younger adolescents). The purpose of using motivational enhancement strategies with the parent during this initial session is twofold:

1. To build the parent's motivation to engage in treatment (i.e., by consistently bringing the adolescent to session, participating in sessions when asked, assisting the adolescent with home learning assignments, and providing an environment that supports the adolescent's ability to change)
2. To identify potential barriers that will prevent the adolescent and parent from fully engaging in treatment, and to work to overcome these barriers. Barriers can include but are certainly not limited to difficulty affording the cost of treatment, difficulty arranging transportation to and from treatment, work or family commitments that get in the way of treatment attendance, driving distance from home/work to the clinic, significant resistance from the adolescent, fatigue, or simply trying to fit treatment into a hectic schedule.

It is important to discuss both parent motivation and potential barriers early in treatment. Problems with engagement and attendance may be the result of low parent and/or adolescent motivation to change, significant barriers standing in the way of treatment progress, or both. Use motivational enhancement strategies to build parent motivation for change if you perceive that parent motivation is low. On the other hand, where significant barriers to treatment exist, you may find it useful to employ problem-solving techniques from Module 5 (Chapter 5 in this Therapist Guide) to generate solutions to foreseeable barriers.

> **Therapist Note**
>
> *Although there is no explicit home learning assigned for Module 1, you might find this to be a good opportunity to reinforce the importance of home learning assignments to this treatment, discuss upcoming home learning assignments, and work on overcoming anticipated barriers to their completion as specified below. You may also choose to return to this section of Module 1 later in treatment to troubleshoot noncompliance with home learning assignments if it arises.*

The client's completion of home learning assignments is an essential component of this protocol for increased understanding of treatment concepts, utilization of learned techniques, generalization of learned adaptive behaviors to multiple settings, and increased comfort with uncomfortable emotions and/or sensations. Completing the home learning is essential for maximum therapeutic gain.

Many clients will resist completing their home learning assignments for a variety of reasons. It is important for you to underscore the importance of compliance with home learning assignments and to reinforce completed home learning in every session until the benefits of home practice are self-reinforcing this behavior.

Function of Noncompliance with Home Learning Assignments

When an adolescent is consistently coming in without having practiced skills during the week, your first task is to find out *why*. The reason behind a client's not completing the assigned tasks will not only help to solve this issue but will likely provide clues for therapy overall. Below are common reasons why people do not follow through with home learning assignments and strategies to address them:

1. *"I don't think it will help."* This might be a clue that the client does not believe in the therapeutic rationale. It will be important to link home learning to the client's stated goals. Don't assign something to practice unless the adolescent has expressed an understanding of and agreement to the assignment. Doing so might lead to more resistance and less openness to change.

2. *"I wasn't sure how to complete it."* This could simply mean the home learning assignment is too vague. It will be important to explain when, where, with whom, for how long, and with what materials the assignment should be completed. Often there is an underlying perfectionism in clients causing them to assume that home learning assignments need to be done "perfectly." Address this black-and-white thinking in session and assure the client that there is not a right or wrong way to complete an assignment.

3. *"I forgot."* In this case, prompts might be necessary, particularly for clients who live in chaotic environments or who have too much to do throughout the day. Help the client create reminders around her home or at school, or call the client midweek if you have the time.

4. *"It was too difficult."* This might imply a deeper fear of failure when doing the assignments or a fear of the emotional dysregulation that could come from the assignment, or it might simply be that the task was too great. As a rule, it is best to start with behaviors that the client is already doing some of the time. Anticipate possible difficulties and develop backup plans. Have the client practice in session and ensure that she experiences success in the session.

5. *"It didn't seem important."* You should reinforce the importance of home learning assignments by using language that implies their importance. You should also consistently review the past week's home learning assignment at the beginning of each session. If the client tries to bring up an important issue, express your intention to discuss it *after* home learning assignment review. This should be less of an issue if the adolescent contributes to choosing an assignment, so strive for this in each session.

Parent Summary Form for Core Module 1:
Building and Keeping Motivation

Core Module 1 is designed to help you and your teen identify problems and build motivation for treatment. You and your teen will each identify goals for his or her treatment, reasons for wanting to accomplish these goals, the steps you can each take to meet these goals, potential barriers that may make it difficult to reach these goals, and signs that will let you know that your teen is achieving these goals. You and your teen will also each identify three **Top Problems** or issues you would like to be addressed in treatment, and these issues will be rated at every session in order to make sure that the treatment is working to target and reduce problems that both you and your teen would like to address.

In addition to identifying the things that may be going "wrong" for your teen right now because of the strong emotions he or she is having, it is helpful to think about the goals your teen wants to achieve in order to address these issues. In this treatment, we are asking you to identify a type of goal that allows you and your teen to both build motivation for treatment tasks to come by noting how your teen's life could be improved through working on his or her top problems. We refer to these goals using the acronym "SMART." A **SMART goal** is:

- Specific: Specific goals are ones that are clear, concrete, and well defined. An example of a goal that is not specific is "doing better at school." A better, more specific goal is "my teen raising her Algebra grade from a 'C' to a 'B.'"
- Measurable: Measurable goals are goals that can be observed and tracked over time so that you can see how much progress your teen is making. An example of a goal that is not measurable is "making friends," because it is difficult to know whether someone is making progress toward this goal. Did your teen achieve the goal if he made one new friend, or must he make more? A better, more measurable goal is "making three new friends."
- Attainable: A goal that is attainable means a goal that your teen can achieve, or that is within his or her reach. Some goals are not attainable because they are very unlikely or because only a very, very small number of people could possibly reach them (for example, "become the Queen of England"). Other goals are not attainable because they would take a very long time to achieve, much longer than the amount of time your teen will be in treatment (for example, "get into a good college" if your teen is only 14). A better, more attainable goal is "my teen raising her GPA from last semester to ___ this semester."
- Relevant: A goal that is relevant is one that is meaningful to your teen and one that has something to do with the emotions that your teen will be focusing on in this treatment, such as fear, sadness, or anger. A goal that is not likely to be relevant to your teen's treatment is "save enough babysitting money to buy a car" or "clean my room every day." Although these may very well be great goals, they may not have much to do with the emotions we will be focusing on in treatment. A better goal is "raise my hand in every class, no matter how nervous I feel."

- Time-bound goals are goals that are very specific about when and how often you would like something to occur. A goal that is not time-bound is "get out of bed in the morning." A better, more time-bound goal is "get out of bed when my alarm goes off each day for the next month."

Goals and top problems may differ between parents and teens. That's okay! You and your teen's therapist will work together to finalize your top problems in session and will help you and your teen to rate these weekly going forward.

Identifying Potential Barriers

It is also important to discuss with your teen's therapist any potential barriers that may limit your or your teen's ability to work toward these goals. Examples of barriers include difficulty affording the cost of treatment, difficulty arranging transportation to and from treatment, work or family commitments that may get in the way of treatment attendance, driving distance from home/work to the clinic, significant resistance from the teen, fatigue, or simply trying to fit treatment into a hectic schedule. It is important to identify these barriers early in treatment, so that you, your teen, and the therapist can work together to identify potential solutions.

What can I do to support my teen by building and keeping motivation for treatment?

✓ Attend every session with your teen.
✓ Identify the value and benefits of treatment.
✓ Listen to your teen's concerns (if any) and review your teen's goals, purpose, and motivation for seeking therapy.
✓ Help your teen overcome any barriers to treatment.
✓ Have confidence in your teen's ability to reach his or her therapy goals!

Maintaining Motivation

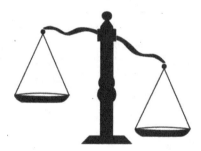

One way to maintain motivation for treatment is to look at the anticipated benefits and costs of engaging in treatment and changing behaviors by using skills learned in therapy. If the benefits of changing outweigh the costs, then teens are more likely to stay in treatment!

Appendix 1.1: Additional Motivational Enhancement Topics

What About Resistance?

Change is difficult for anyone. Every therapist reading this manual has set a goal before (e.g., going to the gym more often, eating more nutritious meals) and not followed through with it. Changing behaviors that stem from symptoms of anxiety and depression is just as difficult, if not more so. It is imperative to understand that resistance does not necessarily reflect the adolescent's "true" character. It is a response, certainly, but it is not necessarily oppositional in nature. Instead, it may signal a disconnect between where the therapist is and where the adolescent is. This may include differing treatment goals, low readiness to change, and differing views about the role of the therapist. As a therapist, you directly influence levels of resistance and should remain aware of where the resistance is stemming from as it will be important to address this if change is to occur. Often it is just as important to know what *not* to say as it is to know what *to* say. Below are examples of language that can create "traps" for you and the client, in which resistance is increased, motivation is challenged, and progress is stalled.

Question/Answer Trap

In this "trap," the therapist and client fall into a pattern of question/answer, question/answer, and so on. Although seemingly benign, and often necessary due to a need for further information from the adolescent, this pattern tends to elicit only passive responses and closes off access to deeper conversation. Therefore, clients are not encouraged to explore issues in depth. It also cuts short the adolescent's chances to explore motivation and offer reasons for changing. The optimal pattern is to ask open-ended questions continually, with reflective listening as the primary response to answers.

Therapist: *You're here because you're anxious in school?*

Client: *Yeah.*

Therapist: *Are you afraid of taking tests?*

Client: *Yeah.*

Therapist: *Are you afraid of the students?*

Client: *Yeah.*

Therapist: *How many friends do you have?*

versus

Therapist: *So, what brings you here?*

Client: *I don't know.*

Therapist: *You're not sure why you're here.*

Client: *Yeah.*

Therapist: *How are things going for you at home?*

Client: *Not so good.*

Therapist: *Not so good, huh. Tell me more about that.*

Confrontation/Denial Trap

Most therapists have had the experience of meeting with an adolescent who is not yet ready to change, and who provides a reasonable argument in response to every statement the therapist makes about why change should happen. The therapist and client then engage in an argumentative back-and-forth in which the client counters each argument for change with an argument for remaining the same. The more the therapist defends his position, the more the adolescent defends her position, until she is more convinced to keep the status quo than she was before the session. If you leave your client with no other option than to argue with you, that is what you will get.

Therapist: *Well, your parents tell me you're depressed and won't leave your room.*	**Therapist:** *So, your parents brought you here because they say you're depressed. Is that true?*
Client: *I'm not depressed.*	**Client:** *No.*
Therapist: *Well, you meet the criteria.*	**Therapist:** *So you feel pretty okay?*
Client: *A lot of my friends are bummed out like me.*	**Client:** *Well, sometimes. Sometimes I feel good, but lately that's been less and less.*
Therapist: *Being sad is different than being depressed.*	**Therapist:** *What's that like?*
Client: *I'm not depressed. I feel fine.*	**Client:** *It's awful. I used to see my friends all the time.*
	Therapist: *That sounds really hard.*

(the word **versus** appears between the two columns)

Expert Trap

Therapists can sometimes provide direction to the adolescent without first helping her determine her own goals, direction and plans. The problem with this approach is that clients may tend to passively accept the therapist's suggestions and may only halfheartedly commit to the difficult work involved in changing. A therapist using motivational interviewing is nondirective, only offering suggestions for change when the client's motivation is high, after initial exploration of multiple pathways to change, or upon the adolescent's request.

Client: I'm not sure the awareness exercises work for me.

Therapist: Well, research shows that this is helpful. You should give it a try.

Client: But I did try it, and it didn't help.

Therapist: Try it a little longer. It'll work eventually if you really give it a shot.

versus

Client: I'm not sure if these awareness exercises work for me.

Therapist: No? In what way?

Client: I can't concentrate on my breath for that long! It's stupid.

Therapist: I wonder if there are other ways of doing it that will feel more helpful to you?

Labeling Trap

Labels are commonly used in psychology, and this pattern can filter into session. However, as Miller and Rollnick state, "because such labels often carry a certain stigma in the public mind, it is not surprising that people with reasonable self-esteem resist them" (2002, p. 68). Some education about a client's disorder might prove beneficial, but the emphasis should be on her ability to change behavior, not on the label that has been given to her group of symptoms.

Client: So people have said I'm depressed. I hate that word.

Therapist: You do meet the criteria for depression.

Client: So you're saying I am depressed?

Therapist: It's just a word. I wouldn't let it get to you.

versus

Client: So people call me "depressed." I hate that word.

Therapist: You don't like being called depressed?

Client: No, it's a stupid label. People say they're depressed if they're sad for, like, a day.

Therapist: And things feel worse than that for you?

Client: Yeah.

Premature Focus Trap

Although the premise of motivational interviewing does not mean that therapists simply follow the client's lead—as is done in Rogerian or person-centered therapy—you are cautioned against focusing too quickly on a specific problem or aspect of a problem. This can be trickier if the parents have identified what they feel is an issue. It is important to draw on the adolescent's perspective of the problem.

Therapist: Well, I talked to your parents, and it sounds like school is a big issue for you.

Client: Yeah, the kids are so mean there.

Therapist: They also said that you don't turn in homework. How long has that been going on?

versus

Therapist: Well, you know that I met with your parents earlier. I have an idea of what's on their mind, but now I want to hear what's on your mind.

Client: I can't stand the kids at school.

Therapist: Really? Tell me why.

Client: They're so mean to me.

Blaming Trap

Clients may wish to blame others for their problems. Therapists may feel compelled to help the adolescent take responsibility for difficulties that might have arisen. Neither of these urges is useful. Blame is irrelevant to treatment gain. Miller and Rollnick (2002) suggest establishing a "no-fault" policy when counseling a person.

Client: I can't stand my parents. If they hadn't grounded me, then I wouldn't have snuck out of the house.

Therapist: Well, rules are rules. And this isn't the first time you've snuck out.

Client: But they don't even get it!

Therapist: You're old enough to know better, though.

versus

Client: I can't stand my parents. If they hadn't grounded me then I wouldn't have snuck out of the house.

Therapist: I know it was frustrating. How did things go when you snuck out?

Client: It was fun at first, but getting in trouble with the cops was scary.

Therapist: It sounds like that part really troubled you.

Useful Strategies When Encountering Resistance

The therapist's style can either increase or decrease a resistance to change, and it is of utmost importance that you use strategies that will reduce the likelihood of defensiveness in the adolescent. These strategies have often been referred to overall as *rolling with resistance*. It is important to restate that resistance is not considered opposition by the client but a signal of dissonance in the therapeutic relationship. The techniques described in Table 1.1 are simply to help reduce this dissonance.

Table 1.1 Techniques to Help Reduce Dissonance

Technique	Description	Examples
Simple Reflection	One way to reduce resistance is simply to repeat or rephrase what the client has said. This communicates that you have heard the person, and that it is not your intention to get into an argument with the person.	*Client:* But I can't join that club. I mean, I don't know anyone! *Therapist:* Joining that club seems nearly impossible because staying home feels safer. *Client:* Right, although maybe I could see what it would take to join.
Amplified Reflection	This is similar to a simple reflection, only the therapist amplifies or exaggerates to the point where the client may disavow or disagree with it. It is important that you not overdo it, because if the client feels mocked or patronized, she is likely to respond with anger.	*Client:* But I can't join that club. I mean, I don't know anyone! *Therapist:* Oh, I see. So you really couldn't join that club because everyone would make fun of you. *Client:* Well, it might not be as bad as all that. But it would still be hard.
Double-sided Reflection	With a double-sided reflection, you reflect both the current, resistant statement, and a previous, contradictory statement that the client has made.	*Client:* But I can't join that club. I mean, I don't know anyone! *Therapist:* You can't imagine how you could join a new club, and at the same time you're worried about not having many friends.
Shifting Focus	Another way to reduce resistance is simply to shift topics. It is often not motivational to address resistant or counter-motivational statements, and counseling goals are better achieved by simply not responding to the resistant statement.	*Client:* But I can't join that club. I mean, I don't know anyone! *Therapist:* You're getting way ahead of things here. I'm not talking about your joining that club today, and I don't think you should get stuck on that concern right now. Let's just stay with what we're doing here—talking through the pros and cons—and later on we can worry about what, if anything, you want to do about it.
Rolling with Resistance, or Coming Alongside	Resistance can also be met by rolling with it instead of opposing it. There is a paradoxical element in this, which often will bring the client back to a balanced or opposite perspective. This strategy can be particularly useful with clients who present in a highly oppositional manner and who seem to reject every idea or suggestion.	*Client:* But I can't join that club. I mean, I don't know anyone! *Therapist:* And it may very well be that when we're through, you'll decide that it's worth it to keep to yourself and stay in your room most of the day. That will be up to you. It might be worth not trying.
Reframing	Reframing is a strategy in which you invite clients to examine their perceptions in a new light or in a reorganized form. In this way, new meaning is given to what has been said.	*Client:* My mom keeps telling me that I need to deal with my problems, go to therapy, clean my room. She's such a nag! I'm tired of her telling me what to do. *Therapist:* Your mom must care a lot about you to tell you something she feels is important for you, knowing that you will likely get angry with her.

Table 1.1 Continued

Technique	Description	Examples
Agreeing with a Twist	This is a lesser way of rolling with resistance. You initially agree with the client's claim but with a slight change in direction. This offers you a way of influencing the direction of the conversation without creating a therapeutic disruption.	*Client: But I can't join that club. I mean, I don't know anyone!* *Therapist: You've got a good point. And even if it means making some new friends, I wouldn't want you to feel uncomfortable.*
Emphasizing Personal Choice	People tend to assert themselves more if they think their independence is on the attack. A response that will squelch this reaction is to assure the person that in the end, she has the ultimate say in what she does.	*Client: But I can't join that club. I mean, I don't know anyone!* *Therapist: It was just a suggestion. What you do with it is completely up to you. No one can force you to walk in and sign up.*

Avoidance as a Source of Resistance

The cornerstone of this treatment is decreasing emotional behaviors, and yet this is an area in which many adolescents are highly resistant as it involves purposely experiencing feelings of fear and intense discomfort. In addition to the motivational enhancement techniques discussed, here are some additional ways to approach resistance to the intentional experiencing of emotions, whether in the form of exposure or emotion-focused behavioral experiments:

1. Elicit from the adolescent short-term and long-term consequences of continuing her current emotional responses.

2. Most clients will ask, "Why should I try to feel bad on purpose?" When this happens, use cognitive reappraisal and Socratic questioning techniques to explore their maladaptive beliefs (e.g., "I won't be able to stop crying") about emotional avoidance and ensuing emotional behaviors. It is important to understand the adolescent's thoughts behind the emotion. Is it fear that the emotion will never go away? Is the belief that being successful at facing emotions will lead to feeling better and therefore more responsibility? Help clients track the consequences of changing or keeping emotionally driven behaviors in and between sessions. Ask clients to test their prediction that something awful might happen. Be open to ways and times that emotional avoidance and behaviors can be adaptive for the client. For example, if the adolescent shows emotions when she is bullied, this might lead to more teasing and is therefore a maladaptive use of expressing emotion.

3. For some clients, it might be necessary to teach coping skills (e.g., cognitive reappraisal, problem solving) before asking them to confront emotions. This would require some modification of the module order to maximize treatment benefits.

4. Help the client recognize and change maladaptive ways of avoiding emotion little by little. Begin with small steps and work upward for clients having great difficulty. For example, for a client who avoids the experience of sadness, you can first block subtle moves, such as hiding tears or changing the subject when a distressing topic arises. Work up from there.

Appendix 1.2: Defining the Main Problems—Parent

In this space, write down the main reasons for coming to treatment. Include things that you think bother your teen and/or things that you or other people in your teen's life think are a problem. These things could include feelings of intense sadness, anxiety, or anger experienced by your teen. Problems could also include attitudes or behaviors that lead to your teen getting in trouble, or things your teen does that might be harmful to your teen or others. *After identifying three "top problems," try to identify a SMART goal for treatment related to each problem or concern.* Your teenager will be filling out a very similar form with his or her top problems and SMART goals in the course of his or her treatment.

1. _____

What is my goal? _____

2. _____

What is my goal? _____

3. _____

What is my goal? _____

Appendix 1.3: Weekly Top Problems Tracking Form

Weekly Top Problems Tracking Form	
ADOLESCENT:	PARENT:
1.	1.
2.	2.
3.	3.

Not at All a Problem			Somewhat a Problem			Very Much a Problem		
0	1	2	3	4	5	6	7	8

	Adolescent Ratings	**Parent Ratings**	
	1._____	1._____	What worked well this week?
Week 1	2._____	2._____	
	3._____	3._____	
	1._____	1._____	What worked well this week?
Week 2	2._____	2._____	
	3._____	3._____	
	1._____	1._____	What worked well this week?
Week 3	2._____	2._____	
	3._____	3._____	
	1._____	1._____	What worked well this week?
Week 4	2._____	2._____	
	3._____	3._____	
	1._____	1._____	What worked well this week?
Week 5	2._____	2._____	
	3._____	3._____	
	1._____	1._____	What worked well this week?
Week 6	2._____	2._____	
	3._____	3._____	

	1._____	1._____	What worked well this week?
Week 7	2._____	2._____	
	3._____	3._____	
	1._____	1._____	What worked well this week?
Week 8	2._____	2._____	
	3._____	3._____	
	1._____	1._____	What worked well this week?
Week 9	2._____	2._____	
	3._____	3._____	
	1._____	1._____	What worked well this week?
Week 10	2._____	2._____	
	3._____	3._____	
	1._____	1._____	What worked well this week?
Week 11	2._____	2._____	
	3._____	3._____	
	1._____	1._____	What worked well this week?
Week 12	2._____	2._____	
	3._____	3._____	
	1._____	1._____	What worked well this week?
Week 13	2._____	2._____	
	3._____	3._____	
	1._____	1._____	What worked well this week?
Week 14	2._____	2._____	
	3._____	3._____	
	1._____	1._____	What worked well this week?
Week 15	2._____	2._____	
	3._____	3._____	
	1._____	1._____	What worked well this week?
Week 16	2._____	2._____	
	3._____	3._____	

CHAPTER 2

Core Module 2: Getting to Know Your Emotions and Behaviors

(Recommended Length: 2 or 3 Sessions)

MATERIALS NEEDED FOR THE MODULE

- Module 2: Getting to Know Your Emotions and Behaviors—Workbook Materials:
  1. *Emotions I Have* (Worksheet 2.1)
  2. *Emotion Identification Practice* (Worksheet 2.2)
  3. *Breaking Down My Emotions* (Worksheet 2.3)
  4. *Tracking the Before, During, and After* (Form 2.1)
- *Therapist Key to the Emotions I Have Worksheet* (Appendix 2.1 at the end of this chapter)
- A parent module summary form is provided at the end of this chapter to help support review of module materials with the parent(s) of your adolescent client. You may also use materials from Chapter 9 (Module-P) to help support these discussions.

Assessments to Be Given at *Every* Session:

- Parent and Adolescent Ratings: *Weekly Top Problems Tracking Form* (Appendix 1.3 at the end of Chapter 1 in this Therapist Guide)

During Core Module 2, education regarding the nature of several key emotions will be provided, which will include a discussion of the structure and function of these emotions. With the adolescent, you will begin to map out his emotional experiences in an attempt to teach him to understand the course of his emotional experiences, examining what happens *Before, During, and After* a given emotion. The role of avoidance or other relevant emotional behaviors in the development and maintenance of emotion cycles should also be taught. Wherever possible, you should root the discussion of treatment concepts in the emotions and behaviors most frequently experienced by the adolescent. Specific goals for this module include:

■ **Goal 1:** Begin learning emotion identification skills.
■ **Goal 2:** Provide education about emotions, their function, and their impact on behavior.
■ **Goal 3:** Introduce the three parts of an emotional experience.
■ **Goal 4:** Discuss reinforcement and the maintenance of learned behavior.
■ **Goal 5:** Teach the adolescent to break down his emotional experience—determining the "Before, During, and After" of the identified experience.

Therapist Note—Unified Protocol Theory

Core Module 2 sets the stage in many ways for both the "transdiagnostic" focus and the focus on problematic emotional behaviors in the UP-A. By encouraging knowledge about the structure and function of a range of emotions (and not just those that seem most impairing at present to you, as the therapist), you are allowing the adolescent to personalize and invest in his understanding of relevant, intense emotion states. Moreover, this module includes an important focus on WHY emotional behaviors, like avoidance or aggression, are problematic for the adolescent to engage in during an intense emotion state; this is a key point for the adolescent and his parent to understand if they are to start engaging in new or "opposite" actions, as will be introduced beginning in Core Module 3. Finally, the introduction of Tracking the Before, During, and After home learning assignment (Form 2.1) at the end of this module is vital to aid the therapist and adolescent in conducting functional assessments of the adolescent's responses to intense emotions and other relevant triggers in his environment, particularly as the adolescent adds new skills to respond more adaptively to such triggers during the course of the UP-A.

This module is very didactic in tone but includes essential treatment concepts. Therefore, you are encouraged not to rush through the material, but to take the time necessary to ensure the client understands the material being presented. Remember the flow of this manual: first use examples and illustrate the concept in as engaging a manner as possible, and then personalize it. It's okay to make some of the examples silly, funny, or otherwise exciting to further engage your adolescent client.

Core Module 2 Content (Divided by Goals)

> **Therapist Note**
> - *Don't forget to start each session re-rating top problems with the adolescent and parent.*
> - *Don't forget to give parents the Core Module 2 summary form to aid in their understanding of this module's important material and spend some time in one session during this module to review this form with them.*

Goal 1
Begin learning emotion identification skills.

Emotion Identification

This section is designed to assess the adolescent's knowledge of various emotion words and will lay the groundwork for the adolescent's understanding of the treatment model. Those adolescents with high levels of emotion awareness or cognitive ability may be able to complete this section rather quickly, but for *all adolescents* this is a valuable time to assess the full range of emotions they are experiencing.

Emotion Words

At the beginning of this section, refer the adolescent to the *Emotions I Have* worksheet (Worksheet 2.1). As you can see, this worksheet includes a list of common emotion words. In reviewing this list with the adolescent, ask him about his understanding of, and experience with, the emotions listed. For instance, you might say:

"Now I'd like us to think about emotions that many people experience. You may have heard these words before or they may be brand new to you. First, I'd like us to just read through the list together."

After reading through the list, you should assess the adolescent's understanding of these emotional states. If he appears to be having difficulty identifying what these emotion words refer to, it may be helpful to ask him a series of questions (as exemplified below) about the emotions he is having difficulty identifying. Refer to Appendix 2.1 at the end of this module for the *Therapist Key to the Emotions I Have Worksheet* for useful definitions of each emotion. Assuming the adolescent is able to correctly identify all of the emotions listed by providing an appropriate description, move on to the next section. Otherwise, spend some time familiarizing the adolescent with these emotion words.

"Now that we've read through the list, I'd like to ask you a few questions about some of these emotions. The first emotion is anger. *What do you think it means to feel* anger *or be* angry? *Have you ever felt this way? How did you know you were feeling* angry?*" [adolescent's reply] "Excellent. Let's talk about a few others."*

For an adolescent who is having difficulty, try to focus your efforts on helping him identify at least one or two components of the three parts of an emotional experience (i.e., thoughts, physical sensations, or behaviors). This will help prepare him for the discussion to come.

Suggested Home Learning Assignment: Emotion Identification Practice

Ask the adolescent to turn to *Emotion Identification Practice* (Worksheet 2.2) in the workbook. Explain that this is work to be done at home between this session and the next. Let the adolescent know he can refer to *Emotions I Have* (Worksheet 2.1) while completing the home learning.

Goal 2
Provide education about emotions, their function, and their impact on behavior.

Emotion Education

Once you understand the adolescent's level of basic emotion identification skills and have provided guidance in identifying emotions, you will begin to provide him with information about emotions more generally and how intense emotions lead to actions that may be causing some challenges for him, more specifically. If the adolescent shows great difficulty with emotion identification, present the following material slowly and concretely, using as many examples as feasible and asking him to help you summarize points throughout.

Under normal circumstances, emotions (e.g., fear, anxiety, sadness, and anger) are powerful responses to things going on in our lives—they are telling us something about what is going on around us and how we might respond. When emotions are uncomfortable, they feel that way because the emotion wants us to **do something**—take action, get away, get help—whatever we need to do to make that emotion less intense. (The emotion does not want to be ignored because it is trying to tell us something important.) When emotions make us feel good or are enjoyable, they are also telling us something—they are encouraging us to keep doing the things that resulted in our feeling that way. When things are enjoyable we want to do them more; when they are uncomfortable we may want to avoid them.

Emotional Behaviors

For simplicity, we will call any behavior that is motivated by an emotional experience an **emotional behavior** or an **emotionally driven behavior** (use whichever term seems more appropriate for the developmental level of the adolescent). This doesn't mean that all emotional behaviors are bad or harmful. However, emotional behaviors are hard to resist (or change). *This makes sense*; remember, our emotions are meant to *motivate some helpful action*. Sometimes emotions may even be important to our survival (like in the case of fear) because they motivate action in a truly dangerous situation, so it seems natural that they may be hard to resist.

Therapist Note

As you select emotions to focus on, keep in mind that some emotions feel more like they drive emotional behaviors in the present moment (e.g., fear, anger), while others drive more future-oriented emotional behaviors (e.g., anxiety). Discuss this difference between present-oriented and future-oriented emotional behaviors as needed/appropriate for the adolescent's cognitive level and problem set.

Examples of Common Emotions and Emotional Behaviors

Tell your client that now you are going to give him an example of a situation and that you will ask him to identify what the emotion is AND what the emotional behavior is in the example.

Fear

Use the following example, or something similar, to illustrate the discussion:

> *"Imagine you are walking to school and hear tires screeching. You're startled by the noise and look around to see what is making the noise. You see that a car is speeding toward you and the sound is the driver slamming on the breaks in an attempt to stop the car. You immediately feel afraid and quickly jump out of the way."*

Ask the adolescent to identify what the emotion is *and* what the emotional behavior is in the above example.

Have the adolescent describe his understanding of, and experience with, fear before offering the following definition. When presenting the definition below, try to use the adolescent's language, if at all possible:

> *"This is an example of a time when the emotion of fear was helpful or useful. Fear is like nature's alarm system—it is a response to your belief that there is danger. It signals the need for immediate action and/or attention. When you feel afraid you probably feel as though you need to keep an eye on whatever or wherever you think the threat may be (or may come from). Fear is also completely* normal, natural, *and useful in keeping us safe—at least it's useful if there is actually something* truly *dangerous around."*

Emphasize how adaptive the emotional behavior in the above example is. In this situation, it is clear that fear motivated escape from the situation more quickly than would have been possible if you had to stop to think about what was going on before reacting.

Make sure the adolescent understands that part of what makes fear such a powerful motivator is the discomfort we feel when we're afraid. It's natural to want to decrease that discomfort, and many times the quickest way to do that is to get away from whatever we believe is making us afraid. This response is completely natural and may happen outside of awareness. However, there are other ways to deal with our fear—when avoiding the things we're afraid of is keeping us from doing things we'd like to do, then exploring some of these other options may be really useful.

Sadness

Use the following example, or something similar, to illustrate the discussion:

"Let's pretend your best friend moved away and it's been several weeks since you last spoke with him. You start to think he's forgotten about you and that you'll never see him again. You might be incredibly sad for a while and you might feel like nothing else matters. You may sometimes feel as if you have no energy or that you won't be able to have fun without your best friend, so there is no point in even trying. After you've spent some time thinking about what you've lost, you'll likely start to feel better."

Ask the adolescent to identify what the emotion *and* the emotional behavior is in the above example.

Have the adolescent describe his experience with and/or his understanding of sadness before offering the following definition. When presenting the definition below, try to use the adolescent's language, if at all possible:

"Sadness is a natural response to some perceived disappointment or loss. It is a basic response to the perceived loss of an idea, object, person, privilege, or thing. When feeling sad, many people want to withdraw from the outside world or at least engage in less activity. It can be useful to take the time to mourn what was lost and the many ways this may impact your life."

Explain that our emotions are telling us something about our situation and are helping us to do something useful. They are letting us know that something we valued is no longer a part of our lives and we need to take a period of time to "come to grips" with the loss, usually with the help of friends and family, and reassess our own, very changed situation.

Anxiety

Use the following example, or something similar, to illustrate the discussion:

"Imagine that you are getting ready for a big test. Rather than studying you decide to watch some television. Halfway through a favorite show you start to think that you haven't studied enough and worry that you will not do very well. You notice your shoulders are getting tight. After a while, you also feel a stomachache. You're really getting worried. You decide to turn off the TV and make a list of all the things you need to study tonight."

Ask the adolescent to identify what the emotion *and* the emotional behavior are in the above example.

Have the adolescent describe his experience with and/or his understanding of anxiety before offering the following definition. When presenting the definition below, try to use the adolescent's language, if at all possible:

> *"Anxiety is an emotion focused on future possibilities and is sometimes referred to as worry. When we experience anxiety or worry, we often reduce our activity and focus our minds on possible sources of future threat or danger (like an upcoming test, an illness, or a more global threat, like to the environment). Ideally, this focus on a potential threat or danger will help us reach a solution. However, when we are unable to identify a solution, we may get stuck and feel unable to draw our focus away from the identified threat. It's at these times that we may need to make an extra effort to think of ways to solve the problem at hand or, if the problem cannot be solved, to think about it in a different way so that it bothers us less."*

Explain that our emotions are telling us something about our situation and trying to help us to do something to reduce an uncomfortable emotion. In this case, feeling anxious is probably a result of feeling ill prepared for a coming exam. Making a list of study activities is an attempt to reduce the worry and the discomfort that comes with it.

Anger

Use the following example, or something similar, to illustrate the discussion:

> *"Someone tells you that a person you felt was your close friend has been saying awful things about you. The next day at school, you feel like you have to do something. You decide to tell other people an embarrassing secret about the person you thought was your close friend. When you see that person, you give her a 'mean look' and then walk away."*

Therapist Note

For some adolescents, an example of physical aggression, rather than relational aggression (as in the example above), may be more appropriate.

Ask the adolescent to identify what the emotion *and* the emotional behavior is in the above example.

Have the adolescent describe his experience with and/or his understanding of anger before offering the following definition. When presenting the definition below, try to use the adolescent's language, if at all possible:

"Anger is a natural response to the belief that you have been hurt or mistreated. Anger is also normal if you believe that something you care about is being hurt, mistreated, or devalued, and this includes ideas, things, dreams, values, and people you care about. Anger motivates us to take action to defend ourselves or the things we care about. Anger is often directed at the person or thing that we believe is threatening the object, person, or thing we care about."

Explain that our emotions are telling us something about our situation. Our emotions are trying to motivate us to do something that may reduce the uncomfortable emotion, which may or may not be an action that resolves the situation. In this example, giving the friend a "mean look" and then walking away may or may not solve the problem, but it was probably done as a way to reduce, or at least vent, one's anger.

Therapist Note

The material above focused on intense "negative" emotions. For adolescents with depression or other concerns that include low positive emotion or anhedonia, it may be particularly important to review the definition and function of "positive" emotions like joy or happiness in this section before moving on.

Suggested Home Learning Assignment: Purpose of Emotions

Ask the adolescent to turn to the *Purpose of Emotions* section in Chapter 2 of the workbook. Explain that this material should be reviewed at home between this session and the next.

Goal 3
Introduce the three parts of an emotional experience.

Three Parts of an Emotional Experience

Emotion Twister

To begin to illustrate the idea of the three parts of an emotional experience and how the parts may blend together to cause strong and uncomfortable emotional experiences, you should describe the concept of an *Emotion Twister* (Albano, Clarke, Heimberg, & Kendall, 1998). Refer to Figure 2.1: *Emotion Twister* in the *Three Parts of an Emotion* section in the workbook, where you will see "Thoughts," "Physical Sensations," and "Behaviors" whirling around the twister. Let the adolescent know that together, these are the three core components of an emotional experience. However, emotions often build quickly and get quite intense, so the individual parts of these emotions may start to blur together. Remembering and identifying the separate parts will help us figure out which skills are going to be most useful in reducing and dealing with those emotion twisters.

Use the *Emotion Twister* model to encourage the adolescent to share a story about a time or times when he experienced a strong or overwhelming emotion and felt that his thoughts, physical sensations, and behaviors became all "twisted" together. Encourage him to describe a single experience as fully as possible. Introduce the idea that every emotion is preceded by a **trigger**, or cue. Suggest that one way to better understand our emotional experiences is to try to break down our emotional experiences into parts.

> *"Before an emotional experience occurs, every emotion is preceded by a trigger, or something that sets the emotional experience in motion. This could be a situation, hearing some news, seeing something, a comment from a friend or family member, or interacting with someone. It can also be a physical sensation or thinking about certain things. There's a trigger for every emotion, even though sometimes the specific trigger may be hard to identify."*

Work with the adolescent to identify a potential **trigger** for the strong emotional experience discussed above, solely for the purpose of trying to help him identify the parts of his emotional experience: the thinking part, the feelings (physical sensations) part, and the doing (behavioral) part. To do this, you might ask the following:

"What were you thinking?"
"How did your body feel?"
"What did you do?"

Use Worksheet 2.3: *Breaking Down My Emotions* to illustrate the interaction of the three parts, identifying how each part can affect the others and may make the emotional experience feel that much more intense. If the first emotion chosen by the adolescent for discussion is not one that makes him uncomfortable, you may ask him to repeat the exercise with one of the emotions circled that do cause discomfort. You may choose to use the script below (adapted from Albano, Clarke, Heimberg, & Kendall, 1998) as an example for introducing the interaction among the three parts.

"These three parts of an emotion, the thoughts, physical sensations, and behaviors, all interact and feed upon one another. These parts may build up slowly or really, really, quickly. Remember—there is always a trigger! For example, if you know that you have a big paper due next Monday, you may start thinking about it over the weekend (this may be the trigger). If you're thinking that you're not going to be able to get it done because you don't even know how to do it (these are your thoughts), you may start to feel your muscles and stomach tense up (these are your physical sensations). In an effort to make these feelings go away, you may decide to watch some TV to get your mind of the paper (which is an emotional behavior). This is one example of what might happen when you know about an event that's going to occur and you're anticipating what it will be like.

Unlike in that example, sometimes the emotion can build up really quickly. For instance, if you go to the dentist for a regular checkup and he tells you 'I have to pull your tooth, and I can do it now,' your feelings might build up REALLY fast. Your thoughts might be 'Oh no, this is going to hurt; I don't want to do this.' You may even notice your hands getting sweaty and your stomach turning over and over (your physical sensations). You might look for your mom or tell the dentist you don't have time to do it right now and will have to schedule it another time (this is the emotional behavior).

In both cases, all three parts of the emotion were active. The more you focus on any one of these parts, the more likely they will build on and intensify the others."

Work through another example of a time when the adolescent experienced a strong emotion, helping him to identify the trigger and break the emotion down into the thoughts, physical sensations, and behaviors. If the adolescent has difficulty generating an example, refer back to the *Emotions I Have* worksheet in the workbook to remind him of the emotions that he experiences most often. You may also find it useful to ask the adolescent to circle at least one emotion that makes him feel uncomfortable or to work through an example using an emotion he finds enjoyable first and then a more uncomfortable emotion.

Suggested Home Learning Assignment: Breaking Down Emotions Practice

Ask the adolescent to turn to the *Breaking Down My Emotions* worksheet (Worksheet 2.3) in the workbook. Explain that the adolescent should use this form to identify thoughts, physical sensations, and behaviors during one emotional experience this week. (This home learning assignment should be considered *optional* if you *also* plan to complete the *Before, During, and After* content in the same session.)

Goal 4

Discuss reinforcement and the maintenance of learned behavior.

Learned Behavior—Principles of Reinforcement

> **Therapist Note**
> *The notion that we repeat certain emotional behaviors because they have been reinforced over time by our own avoidance, escape, or other emotional behaviors in the face of strong or distressing emotions (i.e., getting away from what causes us to experience uncomfortable emotions feels better than experiencing them, so we continue doing this) may be challenging for some adolescents to comprehend.*

Cycle of Avoidance

The discussion of the three parts of an emotional experience can be used to suggest that certain emotional behaviors (particularly behaviors allowing us to avoid or escape from uncomfortable emotions) may act to maintain the difficulties that the adolescent is experiencing. These may include behaviors or thoughts. Emphasize that the adolescent always chooses to *do something* to try to manage his emotional symptoms, but that not all choices will have the same result. Some strategies may work in the *short term*, but with the adolescent you will be exploring whether they work in the *long term*. For instance, is the way the adolescent is coping actually helping to manage the uncomfortable emotion, or does the emotion tend to come back again and again?

Suggest that avoidance of triggers that bring about uncomfortable emotions may make the adolescent feel better in the short term. However, it is probably not possible to avoid all the triggers that may bring about uncomfortable feelings. Even if it were possible, trying to do so would probably be exhausting!

> **Therapist Note**
> *In some cases, avoidance, escape, withdrawal, or other safety behaviors will not be obvious to the therapist. Other behaviors that may be serving to quickly reduce distress, like aggression or angry behaviors, are more obvious in the course of the adolescent's "emotion twister." In the case of aggression, the adolescent is taking a different, more approach-oriented action to reduce his distress. But, in the long term, his distress will return in the face*

of similar triggers (e.g., someone he doesn't like at school, parent–child conflict) and he will return to an emotional behavior like aggression because he may not have experience with how else he can cope. If this is the case with your client, you can use the term "cycle of aggression" or "cycle of angry behaviors" instead of "cycle of avoidance" to illustrate that concept here.

Gently introduce the idea that engaging in avoidant (or other relevant emotional behavior) strategies (including obvious and subtle avoidance, aggression, cognitive avoidance, escape behaviors, rituals, withdrawal behaviors, and so forth) actually may maintain some of these uncomfortable emotions in the long term. This is because avoiding something that makes us feel uncomfortable immediately *makes us feel better*. We quickly learn to use the avoidant strategy again the next time we have a similar, uncomfortable emotion because it seemed to make us feel better last time. This is the **cycle of avoidance**. You may choose to use the following example (or a similar one) to illustrate this concept:

"Imagine that you're worried about going to a friend's party. You know a few people are coming from school, but most of the people who will be at the party are going to be people you don't know. You start worrying a little bit when you get the invitation, thinking about the fact that you won't know most of the people there. By the time the party arrives you're kind of freaked out. Your stomach is in knots. You decide that you're not going to go after all. After making this decision you feel a huge sense of relief. Sure, you kind of wish you were going, but you tell yourself there'll be another party to go to and so missing this one isn't so bad.

The next time you get an invitation to a party, you start to worry again about the people who will be there, expecting that you may not know very many people and that you wouldn't know what to say to them. You decide there is no point in going and that you would just embarrass yourself. You decide not to go. Again, you feel a huge sense of relief.

After relying on the same coping strategy again and again our minds begin to automatically jump to the same way of feeling better: doing the same thing you did last time, even if it only meant you felt better for a short time. After using this strategy for a while, you may not feel there are other options worth your attention and that this is the only strategy that will work. Getting even a little relief from avoiding what you're uncomfortable with can result in a powerful cycle. We're going to call that the 'cycle of avoidance.'"

Engage the adolescent in a discussion of the long-term consequences of using avoidant strategies to manage emotions, drawing from examples that are relevant to his own emotional experiences. Make sure to emphasize the ideas that (1) using avoidant strategies prevents us from facing the emotion and realizing that it is not as scary or upsetting as we think and (2) using avoidant strategies may have a negative impact on our social life, grades, or other areas because such strategies stop us from doing things that may be important or enjoyable.

It is important to make sure the adolescent understands how it is possible that his behaviors (and his responses to his uncomfortable emotions) may be maintaining the symptoms of his disorder/presenting complaint(s). It is *not* important for the adolescent to recall the specific experience that marked the beginning of the disorder/presenting complaint(s), although some may be able to remember.

Therapist Note

*Even if specific situations are not escaped from or avoided, check whether the adolescent carries things with him (e.g., cell phone) to try and feel better or if he seeks reassurance from others. People often do things such as this because they feel they would not be able to handle the situation or the emotion associated with a given situation if they didn't have those objects or get that reassurance. In time you will be asking the adolescent to remove these **safety behaviors**, but for now it is important only to be aware of the issue of safety/avoidance behaviors.*

Goal 5

Teach the adolescent to break down his emotional experience—determining the "Before, During, and After" of the identified experience.

Before, During, and After

Therapist Note

In the Unified Protocol for adults (Barlow et al., 2011), the Before, During, and After assessment and home learning assignment are referred to using the acronym "ARC"—Antecedent, Response, Consequence. As you consider the material below and its centrality to the UP-A model, remember that what we are looking for on every Before, During, and After assignment is increasing the adolescent's understanding of the ARC model as it relates to emotionally intense situations in his life and the contingencies maintaining behavioral choices in emotionally intense scenarios.

As noted in the information above, the choices we make in response to an emotion (i.e., emotional behaviors) can influence and/or maintain uncomfortable emotional experiences. In order to change these cycles, we must first be able to identify them. We call these cycles the Before, During, and After of an emotional experience and will spend some time learning to identify them now.

> "We have begun talking about your emotional experiences, some of which may feel overwhelming or uncomfortable for you. The first step toward making these experiences less uncomfortable and more manageable is to gain a better understanding of when, where, and why they are occurring and to do this on an ongoing basis. This means starting to look more closely at your experiences, monitoring what is happening when they occur, as well as taking note of what happened before and what comes after.
>
> Let's walk through an example so that we can practice identifying the Before (the trigger or cue), the During (our emotional response to the trigger), and the After (the consequences of our emotional responses)."

Walk through an example that is relevant to the adolescent's own experiences or an example that is relevant to you (if appropriate), if the adolescent struggles to come up with a personally relevant idea here.

> "It is important to note that the 'Before' that triggers our emotional experience can be something that has just happened or something that happened in the past. It can be a situation or a thing that triggers our emotions, or it may be a thought, a feeling in our body, or a memory of a past event."

Use the adolescent's own experiences and his understanding of the three parts of an emotional experience to illustrate the possibilities for his *emotional response* to the trigger. Emphasize that not all parts of the emotion (thoughts, physical sensations, and behavior) need to be completed here, just the relevant components that describe his response to that trigger.

With regard to the "After" component, help the adolescent to identify things that have occurred as a result of his indicated emotional response to the trigger, both more immediately and over the longer term. Some consequences here may seem positive initially (e.g., in the case of avoidance or a compulsive behavior, where the adolescent felt better at first), but the consequences are actually not helping him out in the long term, during which strong emotions may increase as a result of certain emotional behaviors. Short- and long-term consequences such as these may be noted in the "After" column of the *Tracking the Before, During, and After* form (Form 2.1) in the workbook.

Try to help the adolescent describe the Before, During, and After associated with at least one emotionally intense situation. Remind him that you know he has at least some strategies that are already working. The goal of this treatment is to *learn new skills to manage his emotions* so that they do not interfere with, or mess up, his life, and thus the more honest and forthcoming he can be on the Before, During, and After assignment, the better you will know how to help him.

A big part of the motivational work at this stage will be to help the adolescent understand that he can change what isn't working to achieve the outcomes he desires.

Suggested Home Learning Assignment: Tracking the Before, During, and After of Emotional Experiences

Ask the adolescent to turn to the *Tracking the Before, During and After* form (Form 2.1) in the workbook. Explain that filling out this form is work to be done at home between this session and the next. Ask the client to report (on the form) how he copes with emotionally intense situations. Indicate that the adolescent should write down these situations as close to the time they occur as possible to ensure greater accuracy.

Therapist Note

This home learning assignment will repeat weekly from this point on in treatment. Each week, you should work with the adolescent to identify and experience increasingly intense and personal emotions as he works toward applying treatment skills in increasingly challenging situations. You may want to bring extra copies of this form to each session, as the adolescent will likely complete several forms over the full course of treatment.

Parent Summary Form for Core Module 2:
Getting to Know Your Emotions and Behaviors

Why Do We Have Emotions?

*Emotions are **normal, natural, and necessary** for survival! Your teen's emotions guide how he or she acts in different situations and help him or her respond to things that happen. Many times your teen's emotions direct his or her behavior automatically so your teen doesn't have to spend time thinking about what to do; this is known as an **emotional behavior**. Most of the time these behaviors are helpful, but they may not always be.*

Core Module 2 is designed to help your teen identify different emotional states, why we need emotions, and how emotional experiences can be broken down into thoughts, behaviors, and physical sensations. This information is essential to understanding why strong emotions are sometimes hard to deal with!

When Emotions Get in the Way

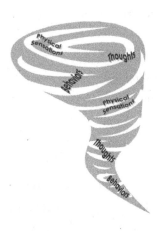

Emotions often build quickly and get quite intense—we call this overwhelming sensation an *Emotion Twister*. Sometimes your teen's emotions tell him or her to act in ways that aren't helpful. Anxiety may lead your teen to avoid situations, worry, seek reassurance from others, or rely on safety signals. Depression may lead your teen to withdraw from activities or interactions. Anger may lead your teen to behave in aggressive or confrontational ways. These strong emotional experiences tell your teen to do things that help him or her avoid such emotions and thus feel better in the *short term*. Your teen then repeats these emotional behaviors because he or she learns that these behaviors are able to quickly get rid of strong emotions! However, this avoidance ends up making him or her feel worse in the *long term*, so the strong emotions return, and your teen attempts to get rid of those emotions again using unhelpful emotional behaviors. This is known as the *Cycle of Avoidance*.

Three Parts of an Emotional Experience

By becoming more aware of unhelpful emotional behaviors, your teen can begin to change the way he or she acts in response to strong emotions. First, your teen will learn to identify the triggers of his or her emotional experiences and the three parts of emotions: *the thoughts one has, physical sensations, and emotional behaviors.*

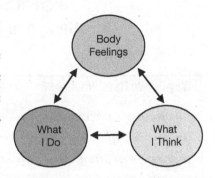

Tracking the Before, During, and After

What Can I Do to Support My Teen in Understanding the Link Between His or Her Emotions and Behaviors?

✓ Use emotion words at home. If you're feeling happy, say it out loud and state why (for example: "I am feeling happy because we're having a family movie night").

✓ We all need emotions! Instead of trying to get rid of, challenge, or dismiss your teen's intense emotions, help him or her identify the emotion, the trigger, and the reaction—the thoughts, behaviors, and physical sensations associated with that trigger. This will make it easier to understand and get through an emotion twister!

✓ Listen to your teen if he or she talks about emotions. Show concern for and interest in your teen's feelings, but make sure not to be too intrusive!

✓ Encourage and support your teen's non-avoidant behavior.

✓ Model helpful emotional behaviors, especially when you are feeling stressed, frustrated, or anxious (for example: "I am scared that this blood test will hurt, but I am going to get it anyway and prove to myself that I can do it and be okay").

✓ Find a balance between paying attention to your teen and giving him or her space.

To help your teen become more aware of triggers that may be associated with strong emotions, his or her reactions to those triggers, and the consequences of actions he or she takes, your teen's therapist will ask him or her to track these parts of the emotional experience on a *weekly basis.* In order for your teen to change his or her emotional experiences, it is important that he or she keeps tracking this information as he or she tries new strategies to help.

Appendix 2.1: Therapist Key to the Emotions I Have Worksheet

All of these emotions are normal and natural responses that can often be helpful.

Anger: A strong feeling of displeasure or madness aroused by the belief that we have been hurt, that we are being mistreated, or that someone or something we want or care about is being hurt or mistreated

Happiness: Characterized by feelings of enjoyment or satisfaction

Anxiety: Concern about a future threat or uncertainty (sometimes referred to as worry)

Sadness: Feeling down or upset due to the loss of a goal, a thing, or a person

Joy: Great delight, pleasure, or happiness

Fear: Response to danger; known as nature's alarm system

Boredom: A result of disinterest or when you are no longer interested in something

Embarrassment: Feeling self-conscious or ashamed about something you may have said, done, or thought or witnessed someone else doing

Excitement: Feeling stirred up about something or looking forward to something in the future

Hopelessness: Lacking optimism about a situation, feeling down, or despairing that there is no solution or chance of things improving

Pride: Taking pleasure or satisfaction for something you have accomplished or done well; having a high opinion of your abilities

Shame: Feeling guilty or worthless because you believe you have done something dishonorable, improper, or ridiculous

Surprise: Feeling astonishment or wonder because of something unexpected; feeling shocked about something you had not anticipated

Jealousy: Feeling envious or resentful of what another has or does; desiring something you do not have that others do

Irritation: Feeling annoyed, impatient, or bothered by someone or something

CHAPTER 3

Core Module 3: Introduction to Emotion-Focused Behavioral Experiments

(Recommended Length: 1 or 2 Sessions)

MATERIALS NEEDED FOR THE MODULE

- Module 3: Introduction to Emotion-Focused Behavioral Experiments—Workbook Materials:
  1. *List of Commonly Enjoyed Activities* (Worksheet 3.1)
  2. *My Enjoyable Activities List* (Worksheet 3.2)
  3. *Kate's Emotion and Activity Diary* (Figure 3.1)
  4. *Kate's Emotion and Activity Graph* (Figure 3.2)
  5. *Emotion and Activity Diary* (Worksheet 3.3)
  6. *Emotion and Activity Graph* (Worksheet 3.4)
  7. *Weekly Activity Planner* (Form 3.1)
  8. *Tracking the Before, During, and After* (Form 3.2)
- A parent module summary form is provided at the end of this chapter to help support review of module materials with the parent(s) of your adolescent client. You may also use materials from Chapter 9 (Module-P) to help support these discussions.

Assessments to Be Given at *Every* Session:

- Parent and Adolescent Ratings: *Weekly Top Problems Tracking Form* (Appendix 1.3 at the end of Chapter 1 in this Therapist Guide)

This core module has two overarching purposes: (1) to introduce the idea of taking "opposite" or different actions from those that have been maladaptive during intense emotional states in the past and (2) to reinforce this concept by engaging in a series of "behavioral experiments" to demonstrate the tolerability of such opposite actions, focusing initially on opposite actions for sadness, withdrawal, and depression. These goals are brought to life by conducting a "behavioral experiment" with your adolescent client to demonstrate the relationship between activity levels and emotional experiences and to help your client incorporate additional enjoyable activities into her daily life. This module may be considered a "preventive intervention" even for adolescents with high activity levels currently and/or no notable problems with anhedonia or low positive affect. *We feel that at least one session to introduce these concepts is important for any client with emotional disorder concerns.* However, some clients will require ongoing behavioral experiments for several weeks beyond the introduction of this concept. Often such clients will have depression or be at strong risk for depression. Goal 4 is particularly directed at clients who require ongoing behavioral experiments and may not be appropriate for other clients. You may choose to spend an additional session conducting emotion-focused behavioral experiments for other emotions, including anger or guilt. There will also be further opportunities to conduct such behavioral experiments later in the UP-A (i.e., Modules 4, 6, and 7).

- **Goal 1:** Introduce the concepts of opposite action and emotion-focused behavioral experiments.
- **Goal 2:** Identify activities that the adolescent enjoys and can engage in during emotion-focused behavioral experiments.
- **Goal 3:** Introduce the idea of tracking emotion and activity levels, and encourage the adolescent to conduct a behavioral experiment for sadness/withdrawal.
- **Goal 4:** Set the stage for ongoing behavioral experiments during future treatment sessions.

> **Therapist Note—Unified Protocol Theory**
> *Core Module 3 expands upon a point you, as the therapist, started to make in Core Module 2: some actions taken during the height of intense emotional experiences, such as avoidance, withdrawal, or aggression, are unhelpful in the long term, even though they are distress-relieving in the*

short term. In this module, you are building on the client's growing aware-ness of her responses to emotion-related triggers by encouraging a series of "experiments" to explore whether utilizing differing or opposite actions from those that maintain emotional disorder symptoms can eventually lessen the intensity of such symptoms. In other words, in this module we are beginning to encourage adaptive and approach-oriented behaviors that can reduce impairment for your adolescent client. We focus on sadness and withdrawal here to show that, by engaging in more enjoyable types of activ-ities, in more frequent activity, or in activities that promote daily self-care, adolescents can observe whether such actions reduce sadness and related symptoms over the longer term. Although this module focuses primarily on opposite action and behavioral experiments for sadness and related emo-tions, it also serves the purpose of introducing terms like "opposite action" and "behavioral experiment" that you can use when encouraging a range of more adaptive behavioral choices by your adolescent client.

Core Module 3 Content (Divided by Goals)

Therapist Note
- *Don't forget to start each session re-rating top problems with the adoles-cent and parent.*
- *Don't forget to give the parent the Core Module 3 summary form to aid in his or her understanding of this module's important material. Spend some time in one session during this module to review this form with the parent.*

Goal 1

Introduce the concepts of opposite action and emotion-focused behavioral experiments.

Introducing Opposite Action

The first goal of this module is to introduce a few new terms to your adolescent client that you may then reference throughout the remainder of the UP-A. The first of these terms is "opposite action," or the idea of acting opposite or differently from an emotion's predominant action-related urges. The concept of opposite action can be introduced using the

Table 3.1 Common Emotional Behaviors and Their Opposite Actions

Emotion	Emotional Behaviors	Opposite Action
Anger, frustration	Yell, express anger, use physical aggression (e.g., hitting, kicking)	Speak in a calm voice; apologize; put yourself in the other person's shoes; go for a walk instead of acting on aggression
Anxiety	Behavioral avoidance, emotional avoidance, distraction	Approach-oriented behaviors
Guilt	Avoid the person or situation that is causing the guilt	Apologize and admit the wrong (if guilt is justified)
Shame	Hide the thing that is causing shame	Talk about what is causing the shame and try not to hide it

example of avoidance behaviors associated with fear. If you feel afraid of talking in front of your teacher, your emotionally driven behaviors might include looking down or staying quiet, even when you know the answer to a question asked by your teacher. The opposite actions in this case would be looking at your teacher and responding to a question asked in class. As the therapist, you can easily build a bridge from Module 2 or from review of the client's Top Problems to this concept. For example, review of the Before, During, and After form home learning assignment may quite naturally lead to a discussion of possible opposite actions that may be more useful or adaptive responses when the adolescent feels overwhelmed. You might also discuss with your adolescent client some opposite actions she could take in the course of feeling other intense emotions. To guide this discussion, we have provided some examples in Table 3.1, but feel free to solicit additional examples from the adolescent.

Emotion-Focused Behavioral Experiments

We introduced the concept of opposite action at the beginning of this module because we are going to ask the adolescent and her family to start engaging in these types of new or different actions. But change is hard and may be a difficult "sell" to an adolescent who has been engaging in avoidance or withdrawal behaviors for some time or to a family that has gotten in the habit of reinforcing such avoidance (see Chapter 9 [Module-P] for a discussion of how to monitor and counter such emotional parenting behaviors). Thus, we want to suggest to the adolescent and her parent that we will start moving toward such opposite action first by conducting a series of "behavioral experiments." A behavioral experiment in this case refers to an information-gathering exercise that can be used to test whether one's thoughts or beliefs are true, and/or provide an opportunity to gain new information. In Core Module 3, the new information we would like the adolescent to acquire is related to engaging in opposite actions for sadness. Specifically, instead of engaging in emotionally driven behaviors associated with sadness (such as lying down, taking a nap, or decreasing activity levels), the adolescent is asked to try to incorporate new or greater levels of enjoyable or personally important activities into her schedule to see if doing so improves how she is feeling and decreases her emotional experience of sadness. Eventually we may ask the adolescent to engage in other new actions or behavioral experiments as treatment progresses. This is just one of our first steps toward feeling better over the long term.

Conducting a Behavioral Experiment for Sadness and Related Symptoms

There are two primary reasons an adolescent might wish to use activity as a means to change her emotional experiences:

1. She is feeling kind of "down" or "sad" at times and her body may feel as though it doesn't want to do things it previously enjoyed.
2. She is not necessarily feeling sad or blue on a regular basis, but might benefit from re-evaluating whether her current activities are consistent with her values or what she wishes to be doing with her time. While not every adolescent has the ability to alter her activity schedule extensively (e.g., she needs to take piano lessons because her parent values the activity more than she does), this module is an opportunity to "take stock" and think about ways to make sure her overall activity scheme is one that builds a positive "sense of self" or self-efficacy for the future.

Returning to the three parts of an emotional experience, remind the adolescent that together you have examined the impact of her thoughts/interpretations and physical sensations on her emotional experiences. You should state that, just as thoughts and feelings can cause emotional behaviors, changing behaviors can also impact thoughts, feelings, and so forth. Explain that now you would like to turn your attention to the impact of her behaviors on her emotional experience. To do this, you will be asking her to conduct a behavioral experiment in which she will monitor both the types of activities she regularly engages in and her emotional experiences each day. Explain to the adolescent that, the closer her emotion level comes to approaching the higher numbers on the scale, the more energetic, relaxed, excited, and/or happy she is feeling. Inform the adolescent that for most people, the types of activities we engage in impact our emotional experiences. Knowing this allows us to choose activities to reduce uncomfortable emotional states (e.g., anger, anxiety, fear, sadness). You may choose to use an example to illustrate the point that being more active and/or doing more pleasurable activities can make thoughts, feelings, and the entire emotional experience more pleasant (e.g., you may ask your client how she feels when she is sitting inside and watching a movie on a rainy day versus going out with friends/family).

Therapist Note

You can also illustrate the idea of a behavioral experiment and the potential relationship between emotion and activity in this initial session of Core Module 3 by demonstration. You can choose to create an impromptu "dance party" in session by playing a popular, upbeat song that you, the client, and even the parent dance to and rate how each person's emotional experience changed from before the activity to after, using a 0-to-8 scale. You can also engage your adolescent client in other activities, such as dribbling a ball, playing a game, or even doing a favor for a clinic assistant/receptionist.

Goal 2

Identify activities that the adolescent enjoys and can engage in during emotion-focused behavioral experiments.

Suggest that this week, you would like the adolescent to practice monitoring her emotional experiences and trying, **at least twice**, to alter the emotional state she is experiencing by engaging in an activity that is associated with a different emotional experience and that is consistent with her values. If the adolescent does not believe this is possible, do not try to argue with her. Rather, suggest that she try it out and see.

Therapist Note

There are some commercially available apps for electronic devices that allow adolescents to track their mood and activity. These are not required applications but may be useful for engaging the more "tech-savvy" teen.

Commonly Enjoyed Activities

Increasing activity levels—whether through physical activity, social inter-actions, or other types of activities—can increase pleasant emotions such as happiness or joy and decrease unpleasant emotions such as sadness or anger. This idea is at the heart of the emotion-focused behavioral experi-ment you will be introducing to your adolescent client during this ses-sion. Some adolescents will require a more basic idea of this experiment to start—such as getting out of bed on time for school or self-care behaviors. However, these can easily be incorporated along with other more obvi-ously pleasant activities in this module (see Optional Activity below). To this end, work with the adolescent to generate a list of activities that she currently engages in OR activities that she believes she would enjoy if she participated in them. Tuning into potentially enjoyable activities will help her monitor such activities. Adolescents who are currently very sad or anhedonic may have difficulty generating a list of enjoyable activities. You may refer to Worksheet 3.1: *List of Commonly Enjoyed Activities* and point it out to the adolescent. You can also suggest that the adolescent consider options from one of five categories of efficacy-building or enjoy-able activity:

- **Service activities**—Doing something directly for others or to improve the conditions of other people
- **Fun activities**—Spending time doing things that she enjoys, either by herself or with other people
- **Social activities**—Spending time with other people who are positive and fun
- **Mastery activities**—Doing something to learn a skill, working toward mastery
- **Physical activities**—Getting up and doing some activity or playing a game

"Think about the activities you do in a typical day. Are there things that you do because they make you feel good or because they are very important to you? Can you think of a few activities that can sometimes change your emotional experience and help you to feel better? If you are having a hard time thinking of some activities, Worksheet 3.1 contains a list that might be helpful. On Worksheet 3.2: My Enjoyable Activities List, write down two or three activities that you would enjoy, or that you think would be personally meaningful to you, as well as those that you would be able to engage in and keep track of over the next week. You can always add more to this list later if you want."

Optional Activity: If the adolescent is having trouble selecting interesting, personally meaningful, and/or fun activities, suggest that she imagines that she has a day off from school with nothing scheduled. What would she do to enjoy herself with no limits placed on her? Use this scenario to brainstorm activities. Then, considering whether such plans are (a) realistic, (b) can occur regularly, and (c) are positive, legal activities, use this to help generate a list of activities the adolescent could possibly do to act opposite to how sadness makes her want to act and change her emotional experience at these times. Write this list down on Worksheet 3.2: *My Enjoyable Activities List*. Again, some adolescents may first need to focus on more "instrumental" or basic self-care behaviors before they can focus on fun or other important activities per se, and these can be listed on the back of the enjoyable activities list as well.

It is important to help the adolescent identify enjoyable activities that she can do by herself as well as with other people so that she has multiple options depending on whether there are people available to spend time with or not. It is also important to point out that successful activities are not the same thing as being "perfect" or "the best." If the adolescent is having difficulty coming up with activities, provide a few examples of realistic activities, such as taking a walk or run, painting, playing music, taking photographs, watching a movie with a friend, playing a game of catch or one-on-one basketball with a friend or family member, finishing homework early on a Monday night, helping a peer at school with a project, and so forth.

Therapist Note

Remember—this is a behavioral experiment and should be continually framed as such for the adolescent. We are going to track her activity and emotional experiences, as specified below, to see if this "experiment" helps her to feel good this week or to set the stage for feeling good in the future.

Therapist Note

In discussing activities the adolescent finds personally enjoyable, conflicts between parent and adolescent may emerge that require some negotiation and further discussion. For example, the adolescent may indicate that she no longer wants to play an instrument because she does not find this to be enjoyable. However, it may be important to her parent's values and beliefs that the adolescent continue practicing and playing the instrument. Such conflicts between adolescent and parent values with regard to daily activities can be a target for discussion during joint time with the parent at the end of this session and while reviewing potential home learning assignments.

Goal 3

Introduce the idea of tracking emotion and activity levels, and encourage the adolescent to conduct a behavioral experiment for sadness/withdrawal.

Keeping Track of Enjoyable Activities

In order to determine whether doing these enjoyed activities actually changes the intensity of the adolescent's emotional experience of sadness and/or helps the adolescent feel better, she will monitor her emotional experiences along with the activities she engages in. Begin the discussion of monitoring by reviewing an example with the adolescent (see Figure 3.1: *Kate's Emotion and Activity Diary* in the workbook). Looking at Kate's diary and Figure 3.2: *Kate's Emotion and Activity Graph,* note that the dashed line is her daily emotion level on a 0-to-8 scale, with 8 corresponding to feeling extremely energetic, happy, and/or relaxed and 0 corresponding to feeling neutral, "blah," or not happy at all. The solid line is the daily total of relevant activities. In reviewing this material with your adolescent client, you will want to explore the connections between Kate's activities and her emotional experiences. It is important to emphasize that it is not only the *number* of activities the adolescent engages in that is related to her emotional experiences, but also the *quality* of these activities and how consistent they are with her values and what she personally finds enjoyable.

As can be seen, the lines tracking Kate's emotions and activities tend to move up and down together, suggesting that one is probably related to the other. Suggest to the adolescent that for most people, the type and/or intensity of emotions they experience and the number and/or quality of enjoyable activities are usually closely related.

You can introduce the idea of your client doing her own Emotion and Activity Diary experiment using the following explanation:

> *"Part of your assignment for this session is to keep track of your emotion level each day, and how many fun activities you do each day. You will do this using your own Emotion and Activity Diary (Worksheet 3.3), which looks just like Kate's. This is how you do it: Each day, look at the list we generated on Worksheet 3.2:* My Enjoyable Activities List *or other activities from Worksheet 3.1:* List of Commonly Enjoyed Activities. *Count up how many of these activities you did that day, and write that total number in the box marked 'Number of Activities' for that day.*

For example, if you listened to music and then talked to a friend on the phone, you would write the number 2 in the 'Number of Activities' box for that day. At the end of each day, just sit down and think through the day, and get a total of all of the enjoyable activities you did. Try to write down which activities you did in the notes section, as well. Think about what time of day would be good for you to fill this out. What do you think?

At the same time, you should also fill out your 'Emotion Level' boxes on Worksheet 3.3: Emotion and Activity Diary. *If you notice any patterns or reasons for doing more or fewer activities, write some notes about this in the notes section of the Diary. You can choose to chart these the way we did for Kate, as well, using Worksheet 3.4:* Emotion and Activity Graph.

Try to record your activities as best you can. The goals are for you to learn something about yourself and to see how your activity level is related to the type of emotions you experience and how strong they are."

If ending your session at this point in Core Module 3, you will likely want to assign the suggested home learning referenced below (Tracking Emotion and Activity Levels). In order to do so, you will need to come to a consensus with the adolescent about one to three activities she would be willing to engage in during the subsequent week. When facilitating a discussion about the selection of such activities, you can certainly reference tools such as Worksheet 3.2: *My Enjoyable Activities List.* However, it's important to "meet your client where she's at" with regard to her activity type and level at present, particularly when it is low in the context of depression or when certain activities may be particularly anxiety-provoking beyond what you are prepared to have her engage in at this stage of treatment.

Ultimately, when producing the activity or activities to focus on here, the therapist should think about the idea of *shaping* this new opposite action. Shaping refers to the reinforcement of behaviors that approximate or come close to the desired new behavior. In other words, it's okay to start with a behavior that just approaches the goal activity, rather than achieves it immediately. So, if the adolescent is interested in photography, for example, but is engaging in relatively little activity outside the home because of depression and social anxiety, you could start with having her simply walk around her room or house taking photos, then move to eventually having her take photos outside her home or in increasingly socially relevant situations.

- It can be helpful to conduct a brief, functional assessment with the adolescent and/or the parent in order to plan out certain times when behavioral experiments would be most impactful (e.g., adolescent often becomes bored and sad when home alone after school).

Observing the Relationship Between Emotions and Activity

If you assign Worksheets 3.3: *Emotion and Activity Diary* and 3.4: *Emotion and Activity Graph* for home learning, in the subsequent session you should briefly work with the adolescent to analyze the pattern of her emotions and activity, with an overarching goal of promoting better self-awareness of different emotion states and the co-occurrence of activity with such states. You should also discuss any behavioral experiments the adolescent engaged in during the week and ask her to reflect upon any resulting changes in her emotional experience.

For some adolescents, activity levels and emotion levels may BOTH have been at appropriate or high levels throughout the week. If this is the case, ask the adolescent to identify how she was feeling during various activities. Also ask if these activities were more often service, fun, social, mastery, or physical activities (or some combination of these) and how her emotions differed (if at all) across these types of activities.

For other adolescents, their emotional levels and activities may have been at generally consistent or appropriate levels, but there may have been a temporary interruption of activity and reductions in emotion level due to uncomfortable emotional experiences or other outside events. If this is the case, it is important to help the adolescent become more aware of such patterns and that withdrawal from activity may not be a very helpful emotional behavior in such cases, as it can lead to feeling worse (if appropriate to circumstances).

Generate and discuss times when feelings of sadness, anxiety, irritability, and/or stressors may have led the adolescent to limit her engagement in enjoyable activities, either currently or in the past (e.g., lots of school assignments or a fight with friends or parents resulting in a desire to avoid other activities, eventually culminating in the adolescent feeling worse). Indicate that brief periods of withdrawal from activity may be helpful or adaptive in allowing us to think through things in our life and move forward. However, when such avoidant behaviors or other withdrawal strategies become consistent, it is important to act opposite of what the emotion is telling us to do in order to get back to a healthier state. We can do this by increasing our service, fun, social, mastery, and physical activities, or by engaging in a single enjoyable activity more often.

Goal 4

Set the stage for ongoing behavioral experiments during future treatment sessions.

Ongoing Behavioral Experiments in the UP-A

For some adolescents with persistent sadness, anhedonia, or very low activity levels, it is possible that you will wish to continue doing these types of sadness- or withdrawal-related behavioral experiments weekly or even for the remainder of treatment! That doesn't mean you need to stay in Core Module 3 for the rest of treatment, but rather you can use Form 3.1: *Weekly Activity Planner* to plan future pleasant or instrumental, self-care behaviors for experiments each week. It may be important to pointedly discuss the need for a focus on self-care or instrumental behaviors (versus enjoyable activities alone) with the adolescent and/or the parent before scheduling such assignments, as these assignments may involve sensitive topics or vary in their frequency (e.g., adolescent brushes teeth some days, but not others; goes to school generally on time, but falls asleep in class). You should be as precise as possible in scheduling experiments for such activities.

Like other exposure activities to intense emotions, these types of behavioral experiments may be met with initial resistance or refusal by adolescents with more significant depression symptoms if they are perceived to be "too big" or "too much" for the adolescent to handle effectively at the moment. Therefore, approach weekly behavioral experiments such as these with the concept of *baby steps* in mind. In the "baby steps" analogy, one needs to learn to roll over, then scoot, then crawl, and then stand before actually learning to walk. Thus, instrumental or self-care experiments may need to start small and build in intensity or frequency over time.

You should meet any positive actions that increase activity—both instrumental and enjoyable—with enthusiasm. You should meet resistance or refusal with attempts to re-evaluate the baby step proposed. *What were the barriers that kept the adolescent from trying this baby step? How can they be altered or surmounted with a future assignment?* Non-completion of behavioral experiment activities doesn't necessarily mean removing them altogether from future home learning assignments. In fact, refusal or reluctance *could* indicate stronger needs for such experiments or interfering levels of another emotion like anxiety. Thus, you may need to work more closely with the adolescent and parent to structure such experiments and ensure that the adolescent's environment adequately supports them.

Alternatively, you may be working with an adolescent who does not struggle with persistent sadness or anhedonia but engages in frequent and maladaptive behaviors in response to other emotions. *If this is the case, it may be useful to spend an additional session in this module focusing on emotion-focused behavioral experiments for other emotions.* You could begin such a session by encouraging the adolescent to identify opposite actions for the emotional behaviors with which she is struggling (e.g., guilt-related behaviors, anger-related behaviors, etc.) and then together designing a behavioral experiment or two around these emotions to be completed in session and/or for home learning. For adolescents with obsessive-compulsive and related disorders or for whom it seems indicated to begin situational emotion exposures (see Therapist Note below), this may also be a good opportunity to introduce and practice the idea of acting opposite to what obsessive-compulsive disorder (or their urges) or fear is telling them to do.

> **Therapist Note**
> *Note that there are important skills to come in the UP-A Core Modules 4 through 6 that will support the conduct of further and more challenging behavioral experiments, including exposure work. We will focus more on behavioral experiments as they relate to fear, anxiety, and avoidance*

behavior specifically in Core Module 7. Therefore, while one can definitely choose to focus on exposure activities starting at this point in treatment versus sadness-related experiments or following sadness-related experiments, and alternative home learning suggestions are provided below if you wish to do so, please consider adolescent and family readiness for exposure before you move in this direction. For example, if you find that time is short for additional sessions with your adolescent client or your adolescent client has mostly straightforward fear and anxiety, you could incorporate materials to introduce situational emotion exposure from Core Module 7 at the end of Core Module 3 here and proceed by including some type of situational emotion exposure in the last 15 to 20 minutes of each subsequent session or ahead of presenting Core Modules 4 through 6 altogether. For these adolescents, introduce Form 7.1: Emotional Behavior Form in session or for home learning to help the adolescent and/or the parents identify targets for ongoing exposure as another type of emotion-focused behavioral experiment in subsequent sessions. Other content from Core Module 7 may also be useful here as well to ensure adolescent/parent understanding of why exposure techniques support ongoing opposite action experiments. Otherwise, the standard approach to treatment would be to wait until after you present Core Modules 4 through 6 in their entirety to proceed with situational emotion exposures.

Suggested Home Learning Assignment: Ongoing Behavioral Experiments

Use Form 3.1: *Weekly Activity Planner* as often as needed in this module or future modules to promote ongoing behavior change. This home learning form can be presented along with Form 3.2: *Tracking the Before, During, and After,* as the goals of both forms are different and complementary. If two such home learning assignments seem excessive to the client, consider which of these two forms is more important for your adolescent client to complete this week.

Parent Summary Form for Core Module 3:
Introduction to Emotion-Focused Behavioral Experiments

Core Module 3 is designed to help your teen begin learning new, more helpful behaviors that he or she can engage in when experiencing strong emotions.

Opposite Action and Emotion-Focused Behavioral Experiments

First, your teen will learn about taking an **opposite action** when an emotion is making your teen want to act in ways that may not make him or her feel better in the long run (e.g., avoiding when anxious or going to sleep when sad). Your teen will learn to start doing what we call **emotion-focused behavioral experiments**, or practicing differing or opposite actions when feeling strong emotions. We use the example of sadness in order to introduce this concept of acting differently from how the emotion is making your teen want to act. Since the emotional behaviors commonly associated with sadness include wanting to do nothing, lay down, take a nap, and avoid activity, we will be challenging your teen to identify activities he or she can engage in regularly to feel better. Just as thoughts and feelings can cause emotional behaviors, changing behaviors can change thoughts, feelings, and the entire emotional experience. This means that choosing to engage in activities when sad or down can actually change the way your teen is feeling. Your teen will learn the direct relationship between emotions and the number and type of enjoyable activities he or she engages in per day.

Learning How to Have Fun . . . Even When We're Feeling Down

What Can I Do to Support My Teen with Behavioral Activation?

✓ Don't overdo it! If your teen is not used to being active, gradually increase the level of activity into his or her daily schedule. Remember, **brief** periods of withdrawal may be helpful in allowing your teen to think through things and move forward.

✓ Find out what activities are fun for your teen, and let your teen decide on activities.

✓ Plan family activities or outings. Doing new activities together is also a good way to get a reluctant teen to try new things. Behavioral activation can be fun for the entire family!

✓ Encourage your teen to join an extracurricular activity at school.

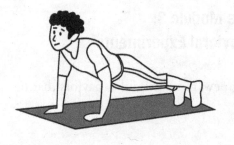

The types or amount of activities your teen engages in impacts his or her emotional experiences. It can be helpful for your teen to identify times when he or she often becomes bored or sad and to plan pleasant activities during those times. For some teens experiencing high levels of sadness or irritability, doing activities may be challenging at first. For these teens, starting out slowly with simple activities such as taking a walk is a great start! For such teens, the idea of participating in pleasant activities will likely be discussed and planned for weekly.

CHAPTER 4 — Core Module 4: Awareness of Physical Sensations

(Recommended Length: 1 or 2 Sessions)

MATERIALS NEEDED FOR THE MODULE

- Module 4: Sensational Awareness—Workbook Materials:
  1. *Body Drawing* (Worksheet 4.1)
  2. *Monitoring How My Body Feels* (Worksheet 4.2)
  3. *Tracking the Before, During, and After* (Form 4.1)
- A parent module summary form is provided at the end of this chapter to help support review of module materials with the parent(s) of your adolescent client. You may also use materials from Chapter 9 (Module-P) to help support these discussions.

Assessments to Be Given at *Every* Session:

- Parent and Adolescent Ratings: *Weekly Top Problems Tracking Form* (Appendix 1.3 at the end of Chapter 1 in this Therapist Guide)

Overall Core Module 4 Goals

The overarching purpose of Core Module 4 is to give the adolescent client a greater awareness of his body's reactions to intense and/or distressing emotion states and to introduce principles of interoceptive or "sensational" exposure as a means to cope with or "stick with" strong physical sensations (when not associated with any genuine, immediate threat) until his body returns to a less distressed state. Taking this approach and an acceptance-oriented stance toward uncomfortable physical sensations may be incompatible with taking actions to avoid or suppress these sensations prematurely. The interoceptive exposure techniques in this module were originally developed with panic disorder symptoms in mind, although the body drawings and body scanning techniques are broadly applicable to a range of concerns and especially relevant for adolescents with poor distress tolerance or high reactivity to sensations in their bodies. You may wish to consider using Goal 1 and 2 techniques specified below for all adolescents and use some or all sensational exposures depending on the needs of the individual client. However, it should be noted that interoceptive or sensational exposures also provide a good avenue for introducing exposure and its effects to adolescents and may be a safer and easier experiment for the adolescent to engage in while learning more about his body's response to exposure techniques.

- **Goal 1:** Describe the concept of physiological or body sensations and their relationship to intense emotions.
- **Goal 2:** Work with the adolescent to identify the feelings he has during emotional experiences using the body drawing and body scanning exercises.
- **Goal 3:** Conduct sensational exposures with the client to promote awareness of body feelings.

Therapist Note—Unified Protocol Theory

In Core Module 3, your adolescent client learned about opposite action and how to conduct an emotion-focused behavioral experiment while feeling sad, blue, or irritable. In Core Module 4, we continue the theme of emotion-focused behavioral experiments, but this time in the context of the action tendencies we feel when our bodies produce a particularly strong sensation. Just as importantly, in this Core Module, we also introduce the concept of becoming more aware of our body state while experiencing a strong or intense emotion through didactic teaching, experiential exercise, and practice of attending and awareness skills while invoking uncomfortable feelings in one's body.

Goal 1

Describe the concept of physiological or body sensations and their relationship to intense emotions.

Therapist Note

- *Don't forget to start each session re-rating top problems with the adolescent and parent.*
- *Don't forget to give the parent the Core Module 4 summary form to aid in understanding of this module's important material and to spend some time in one session during this module reviewing this form with him or her.*

Becoming Aware of Our Physical Sensations

Adolescents may benefit from an initial, concrete discussion of how to become more aware of individual parts of one's emotional experiences. You should re-introduce Worksheet 2.3: *Breaking Down My Emotions*, as needed, emphasizing the three parts of an emotional experience. You should circle the "feelings" portion of the form and explain that becoming aware of physical sensations or "feelings" that occur during emotional experiences can help adolescents consider how best to respond to these body sensations. If we recall the information from Core Module 2, there are times body sensations (or, as they are referred to in the adolescent workbook, **body clues**) associated with a range of emotions can feel very intense—such as when we experience fear or anger and our body is giving us very strong signals to take action. The purpose of Core Module 4 is to take a "deeper dive" into our understanding of such sensations and learn how to manage these effectively when they feel particularly strong or uncomfortable.

For some adolescents, it will be helpful to review the **fight-or-flight response** here. The fight-or-flight response is a physiological reaction that occurs when we perceive that a harmful event, attack, or threat to survival is imminent. When we experience this response or reaction, our brain activates our sympathetic nervous system and releases a large amount of hormone into our bodies very suddenly to allow us to fight off this attack or flee the threat we perceive quickly.

Some of the reactions our bodies have when we experience a fight-or-flight response include the following:

- Acceleration of heart and lung functions
- Flushing or paling
- A slowdown in digestion
- Constriction of the blood vessels in some parts of the body and dilation in those blood vessels associated with muscle action
- Inhibition of tear production and salivation
- Shaking
- Tunnel vision and/or pupil dilation

A sample script for describing how the fight-or-flight response can contribute to uncomfortable emotional experiences in adolescents with emotional disorders is this:

"The purpose of your body taking these quick actions is (1) to increase blood flow to muscles and away from other parts of your body that don't need it as much; (2) to supply the body with extra energy; and (3) to give you extra speed and strength—all to run away or fight off an attacker! The human body is pretty amazing in this way."

However, some individuals may be experiencing sensations or body clues associated with a fight-or-flight response even when their body isn't clearly in danger. As you might imagine, these feelings can be super uncomfortable, so it would be natural if you then turned your attention outward and looked for another source of this potential threat or harmful event. Part of our purpose today is to learn how YOUR body reacts to such feelings of threat or concerns about harm and what to do if we perceive these things when we are not truly in danger."

Some adolescents may have poor awareness of their body clues and may require your assistance in identifying them. Commonly, adolescents will confuse thoughts or emotion words with the physical sensations themselves. In order to further emphasize body awareness, you can use the body drawing and body scanning techniques below to improve clarity. However, if the adolescent insists that he does not experience somatic sensations of distress following these activities, roll with this resistance and consider working on identifying such experiences as they come up more naturally in future generalized emotion exposures and situational emotion exposures.

Goal 2

Work with the adolescent to identify the feelings he has during emotional experiences using the body drawing and body scanning exercises.

Identifying Common Physical Sensations—Body Drawing

Using Worksheet 4.1: *Body Drawing*, ask the adolescent to identify specific parts of his body where he experiences body clues of distress, and have him mark his body drawing with examples. To make this activity more fun, the adolescent can also name the figure or give his own examples of bodily sensations experienced. As noted above, sensations associated with anger and fear similar to those noted as part of the fight-or-flight response may be easiest to identify with this figure.

You can use this figure in a multitude of ways to elicit personalized accounts of where in his body the adolescent perceives distress. You can start by generating more generalized ideas of triggers that might typically produce body clues (e.g., *You are about to give a big presentation. Where do you feel nervous? Maybe excited?*) and then further personalize your questions to get a better sense of sensations experienced. You may find it useful to also personalize this figure by type of trigger (e.g., social versus physical threats) or type of emotion (e.g., sadness versus joy). Some therapists have their clients "color code" their responses to different triggers or emotions on their body drawing (e.g., blue for body clues related to sadness and red for anger).

Reinterpreting the Feelings in Our Bodies—Body Scanning

Body scanning is a type of present-moment awareness skill similar to those we will be reviewing during Core Module 6. However, this skill can be introduced in the current module for purposes of encouraging the adolescent to "stick with" and approach, rather than avoid, sensations of bodily distress when there is no active threat or harmful event occurring, such as during the sensational exposure practice provided in Goal 3 below. Like other present-moment awareness skills, a primary goal of body scanning is to "*notice it, say something about it, and experience it*" regarding any sensations that are occurring and to stay present while "watching" such sensations over time. This framework for practicing present-moment awareness is adapted from Linehan's (2015) description of the "what" skills of mindfulness. Often, such sensations will reduce naturally as the body returns to its resting state or *homeostasis*, although the amount of time until the adolescent feels less distressed may vary from person to person. More about body scanning in the context of sensational exposure is provided below. And a worksheet describing the "*notice it, say something about it, and experience it*" skill associated with body scanning may also be found in Chapter 6 of the adolescent workbook (Worksheet 6.1). However, a good plan for body scanning is to have the adolescent do the following:

- Scan his body for any signs of discomfort or distress
- Observe the sensations occurring in his body and rate these on a 0-to-8 intensity scale
- Use self-talk to describe the sensations occurring to himself (or out loud to you)
- Participate by staying in the present moment and "watching" the sensations and how they change over time
- Discontinue exposure practice when sensations are manageable enough for the adolescent to proceed with the next task

Goal 3

Conduct sensational exposures with the client to promote awareness of body feelings.

Reinterpreting the Feelings in Our Bodies—Sensational Exposure

You will be asking the adolescent to engage in a series of behavioral experiments meant to help him better understand his body clues and work toward experiencing them without making overt attempts to change, minimize, or escape them via emotional behaviors. This will be done through the use of **sensational exposures**, or exposures to one's internal or physical sensations. Referencing the three parts of an emotional experience, point out that the physical sensations he experiences will influence his thoughts, behaviors, and emotions. When we view our body feelings as harmful, in the absence of any genuine threat, we are likely to engage in emotional thinking or emotional behaviors to escape them. Engaging in sensational exposures will help the adolescent learn if emotional behaviors are strongly influenced by the presence of uncomfortable physical sensations, and if so, how to break these cycles. During sensational exposure it should be emphasized that any physical sensations he experiences are a normal, natural part of his emotional experience and that it will be helpful for him to work toward awareness of these sensations when they are present.

In order to help the adolescent learn that these physical sensations can be experienced without taking actions to lessen them (e.g., when I'm feeling short of breath, I have to get away as soon as possible; when my body feels heavy, I can't do anything else; when my face is really hot, I have to vent my anger at whoever I'm mad at), you will be asking him to practice several exercises. When choosing these exercises, you should consider which exercises will result in him feeling these same physical sensations he experiences when in the height of strong emotions. Use Worksheet 4.2: *Monitoring How My Body Feels* to track what physical sensations arise, and ask the adolescent to notice how intense these sensations are during this in-session behavioral experiment. Use the body scanning technique following the evocation of intense sensations to develop the adolescent's awareness of these experiences and how they may change over time. A sample script for introducing sensational exposures follows:

> *"Sometimes uncomfortable body feelings can become linked with emotional thoughts or behaviors, like thinking something bad is going to happen or that we need to leave some place because we feel uncomfortable in our bodies. As we've discussed, sometimes these feelings in our bodies happen because there is something truly dangerous happening, but often these sensations occur out of the blue, without anything truly dangerous occurring. Even though nothing bad is going to happen to us in these situations, we still may want to get away or think something is going to go wrong at these times. In order to help with this, you will be working on experiencing strong body feelings that you purposely make happen and watching as your body naturally recovers from these experiences. In order to do this, we're going to conduct another behavioral experiment and practice experiencing these physical sensations while we're here in the office. Hopefully, this will start to show you that just experiencing these physical sensations does not mean that there is definitely something dangerous going on around you."*

You may choose to do all or a subset of the sensational exposures listed in Box 4.1, but it is strongly suggested that you do at least two or three different types of these tasks with your client. An example is described below, although you do not need to use this hyperventilation example; any of the examples in Box 4.1 can provide a good place to start.

If you choose to start with hyperventilation, ask the client to take three or four deep breaths and exhale very hard (at about three times the normal rate); the goal is to feel as if one is hyperventilating, as if trying to blow

Box 4.1 Sensational Exposure Options

- Shake head from side to side (does not need to be done quickly) for 30 seconds
- Place head between knees for 30 seconds, then lift head (to an upright position) quickly
- Run in place for 1 minute
- Hold breath for 30 seconds
- Tense the muscles throughout the body for 1 minute or hold a pushup position for as long as possible
- Spin in a chair (relatively quickly) for 1 minute
- Hyperventilate for 45 seconds (see exercise described in the text)
- Breathe through a thin straw (e.g., a coffee stirrer or cocktail straw) for 1 to 2 minutes while holding nostrils closed
- Stare at a bright light for 1 minute and then read a short paragraph immediately after
- Stare at a single point on one's hand for 3 minutes

up a balloon. If the client is reluctant, you might model this activity first and then ask the adolescent to repeat the behavior after you. Ask him to continue this until you let him know it is time to stop (try not to tell him how long the exercise will last; after all, when these physical sensations are occurring in the context of an intense emotion, the adolescent has no idea how long these physical symptoms will last and so he should learn to be aware of them regardless of how long they may last). Be sure that he maintains an adequate speed and depth of breathing. If you model sensational exposures or practice them along with the adolescent, it would be ideal to make sure at least some practices are done just by the adolescent himself so that he does not associate you as a "safety person" in such exposures.

Continue the exercise for approximately 45 seconds. When finished, ask the adolescent to use body scanning to look for the source of the discomfort or intense feelings in his body. Once he has observed these, ask him to describe these sensations to himself or aloud, then focus on the sensations in the present moment and watch them to notice what happens to their intensity. Use Worksheet 4.2: *Monitoring How My Body Feels* to facilitate completion of this exercise.

Once the adolescent has participated in one sensational exposure and understands the rationale for these exercises, utilize additional sensational exposures to further illustrate treatment concepts. For an adolescent who regularly experiences uncomfortable physical sensations, you may wish to also identify further sensational exposures that are similar to his usual experiences, in addition to the standard tasks listed in Box 4.1.

Suggested Home Learning Assignment: "Sensational Awareness"

For all youth, assign Form 4.1: *Tracking the Before, During, and After*. You may also assign practice of two or three sensational exposures for further practice as home learning. Choose those sensational exposures that were experienced most intensely in session for home learning to further illustrate that evoking such sensations is harmless and will likely become easier with practice. Each of the assigned sensational exposures should be completed at least three times during the week. The adolescent may track his experiences using another copy of Worksheet 4.2: *Monitoring How My Body Feels*. For simplicity sake, the adolescent's practices could also be tracked on the *Before, During, and After* form and reviewed at the next session.

Parent Summary Form for Core Module 4: Awareness of Physical Sensations

Core Module 4 is designed to help your teen increase his or her awareness of emotion-related body feelings. Physical sensations are a normal, natural part of our emotional experiences. Our bodies typically give us clues to let us know how we are feeling. For example, when feeling anxious, some individuals get stomachaches or headaches, shake, sweat, or have an increased heart rate. We sometimes refer to these physical reactions as part of the body's "fight-or-flight" response. When these sensations occur, some teens may interpret them as harmful. When teens begin to identify and link their physical sensations with their emotions, they can begin to reinterpret these sensations as natural and harmless and practice behaviors to manage these more effectively.

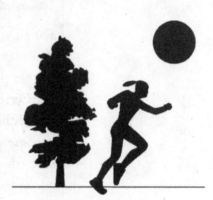

Sensational Exposures

Your teen may engage in sensational exposures with his or her therapist and related practice at home during this module. The purpose of sensational exposures (purposely creating body feelings typically felt during emotional experiences) is to help your teen learn to reinterpret body feelings experienced during the emotional experience. Your teen will learn that physical sensations can be experienced without threat or actions taken to lessen their experience. During sensational exposures, your teen will engage in activities that bring about physical sensations (e.g., running in place to intentionally increase heart rate and shortness of breath). When your teen experiences these sensations in an emotional context, it may trigger him or her to engage in emotional behaviors. During the sensational exposure, your teen will learn that these sensations do not need to be avoided and will often naturally decrease. Even when these sensations do stick around for a longer period of time, your teen will learn that they may be uncomfortable, but not harmful, and that one's interpretation of these feelings as threatening is what makes the feelings so distressing.

What Can I Do to Support My Teen with Increasing Awareness of Physical Sensations?

✓ If your teen reports any physical sensations (e.g., headaches, stomachaches, dizziness, tiredness) alongside emotional distress, prompt him or her to use *body scanning* to become more aware of body sensations and help him or her to recognize that these body sensations are uncomfortable but unlikely to cause harm.

✓ Acknowledge that these sensations are uncomfortable, but remind your teen that physical sensations are natural and normal.

✓ Encourage your teen to pay attention to the sensations instead of avoiding or trying to get rid of them.

CHAPTER 5   Core Module 5: Being Flexible in Your Thinking

(Recommended Length: 2 or 3 Sessions)

MATERIALS NEEDED FOR THE MODULE

- Module 5 Workbook Materials:
  1. *Common Thinking Traps* (Worksheet 5.1)
  2. *Evaluating My Thoughts Using Detective Questioning* (Worksheet 5.2)
  3. *Being a Detective—Steps for Detective Thinking* (Worksheet 5.3)
  4. *Detective Thinking* (Form 5.1)
  5. *Getting Unstuck—Steps for Solving a Problem* (Worksheet 5.4)
  6. *Getting Unstuck—Step-by-Step Example of Solving a Problem* (Figure 5.1)
  7. *Tracking the Before, During, and After* (Form 5.2)
- A parent module summary form is provided at the end of this chapter to help support review of module materials with the parent(s) of your adolescent client. You may also use materials from Chapter 9 (Module-P) to help support these discussions.

Assessments to Be Given at *Every* Session:

- Parent and Adolescent Ratings: *Weekly Top Problems Tracking Form* (Appendix 1.3 at the end of Chapter 1 in this Therapist Guide)

This module is designed to help the adolescent be more flexible in the way she is interpreting ambiguous signals or situations in the world, given that youth with emotional disorders often have a first impression or "automatic thought" that such signals or situations are negative or threatening. Learning to do this requires that she is first able to identify these interpretations. During this module, the adolescent will learn to evaluate the interpretations she makes, identifying which of her interpretations seems realistic or likely to be true. She will be presented with a number of tools for making these decisions, including information on "thinking traps" (like cognitive distortions, for those therapists more familiar with that phrase), and she will be introduced to "Detective Thinking" as a means of evaluating her interpretations. Finally, the adolescent will be taught a series of steps for solving a problem; this is also designed to increase cognitive flexibility, particularly as it applies to selecting adaptive behavioral solutions. We practice the latter in both a neutral, fun context and more personally relevant ones, which may include interpersonal conflict scenarios.

- **Goal 1:** Introduce the concept of flexible thinking: automatic and alternative interpretations.
- **Goal 2:** Teach the adolescent the common "thinking traps."
- **Goal 3:** Introduce and ensure understanding of the Detective Thinking skill.
- **Goal 4:** Introduce and ensure understanding of the Problem Solving skill.

Continued use of the *Tracking the Before, During, and After* Form for home learning can be used to help the adolescent record and remember the thoughts, physical sensations, and behaviors she experiences during emotionally evocative situations throughout the week. These experiences can then be applied during the identification of thinking traps and the practice of Detective Thinking.

Therapist Note—Unified Protocol Theory

Core Module 5 presents a number of traditional cognitive-behavioral therapy (CBT) strategies, but their application is unique in the Unified Protocols. While the presentation of cognitive reappraisal in this module is not especially different from other CBT programs for youth anxiety or depression, in the Unified Protocols there is a strong emphasis on using this cognitive technique in the antecedent condition or before the adolescent has a more intense emotional reaction to a situation in which distress is anticipated. The rationale for this is that adolescents may be less likely to use this common CBT technique effectively during a more emotional event, when the cognitive load associated with strong emotions is very high. Therefore, re-evaluating challenging thoughts ahead of time may be more useful in promoting adaptive youth behavior. Problem Solving in the Unified Protocol is a technique that is as much cognitive (in the sense that adolescents are being asked to be more flexible in their thinking about possible solutions to challenging problems identified) as it is behavioral (considering other responses that are at least different, if not fully opposite, actions to their emotional behavior[s]). In this approach, we also emphasize usage of Problem Solving for challenging interpersonal problems, in particular, such as problems with peers, romantic relationships, or parent–child conflict, to allow for a developmentally sensitive application of this technique. It can be particularly helpful to engage an adolescent client in new, less emotional behaviors through what may be highly valued interpersonal interests or goals.

Ways to Divide the Material Across Sessions

You may choose to structure the material in this session several ways. One option is to present the material on identifying one's automatic appraisals and thinking traps in the first session. The second session might then focus on Detective Thinking or reappraisal, such that the adolescent is provided multiple opportunities to practice the use of this skill. The third session would then focus on the Problem Solving steps. If the adolescent picks up Detective Thinking skills quickly, Problem Solving may be included in the second session, making a third unnecessary.

Core Module 5 Content (Divided by Goals)

Goal 1
Introduce the concept of flexible thinking: automatic and alternative interpretations.

How We Make Sense of the World

Every day we have to sort through huge amounts of information. Based on our experiences, we learn to quickly sort through this information, deciding what's important and what's not. Although we may think about what we were experiencing initially to better understand it, with time most people develop automatic ways of interpreting the world without having to think much about it. While these **automatic interpretations** can be useful, they may also get us into patterns (or cycles) that end up causing a problem for us. This may be especially true if the way we're evaluating the world is resulting in emotional behaviors. Therefore, learning to be more flexible in our thinking while we consider the accuracy of these automatic interpretations is an important skill; this will be the focus of this portion of the treatment.

Tell the adolescent that you will be showing her an image and all you'd like her to do is tell you what she "sees" first. Although she may continue to describe any number of interpretations, take special note of what she describes first (e.g., "I see a frog. Wait, I think if I turn it another way, I see a horse"). A number of suggested images/optical illusions are described below in Table 5.1. Images such as these are readily available online, and you should plan to bring at least two to show to the adolescent in session. Feel free to choose additional optical illusions that you find online and that you feel are developmentally appropriate for your adolescent client to further illustrate this "flexible thinking" concept.

Once the adolescent has talked about at least two of the images, ask her what she noticed about the exercise more generally. After allowing her to share her impressions, you will want to discuss the purpose of the exercise more specifically.

Table 5.1 Examples of Optical Illusions and Likely Interpretations

Image	Likely Interpretations
Vase/faces in profile ("Rubin's Vase Illusion")	▪ One vase (white content) ▪ Two faces in profile (black content)
Young lady/old lady	▪ A young lady looking off to the left ▪ An old lady (her nose in the "young lady's neck"; her eye is the "young lady's ear")
Drawing of tree, bridge, lady	▪ A lady in a cape walking near a tree and a bridge ▪ A face is in the background; the bridge forms one eye, the tree branch forms another, the "lady" forms the nose
Elephant Optical Illusion	▪ Pencil-drawn image of an elephant has at least five distinct legs ▪ Elephant has fewer than five legs
Rabbit/Duck Illusion	▪ A duck with its beak facing left ▪ A rabbit facing right, with its ears on the left
Frog/Horse Illusion	▪ A frog looking to the left, sitting on a patch of grass on a pond ▪ Rotating the image to the left, the frog's head is the horse's nose, its hind legs are its ears.

Why We Interpret Things the Way We Do

Discuss with the adolescent that there may be several possible interpretations for (or ways to think about) each of the pictures. There is no single correct answer. Different people, for whatever reason, may tune into different elements of what they are presented with and may see different things as a result. The first interpretation we arrive at usually occurs without much mental effort. Once this first interpretation is arrived at, it may require more effort to identify a second or alternative interpretation. Additionally, focusing on one interpretation may make it more difficult to keep a second possibility clearly in mind. The idea of **flexible thinking** involves simply considering that there may be more than one interpretation of vague or ambiguous stimuli or situations around us.

For many people, when they are experiencing a strong emotion they may make even quicker interpretations about what they see AND they may have more difficulty changing that interpretation. For example, if you are feeling down or upset and look at a picture of someone with a blank look on her face, you might assume that she is thinking about something sad or is upset rather than assuming that she is just bored and watching TV. Alternatively, someone who looked at the picture after having just been in a fight might automatically interpret that she is angry and thinking about getting back at the person she is mad at. This occurs because our emotions influence our interpretations of the world around us. And it makes sense that this would be true. Remember our thoughts are just one part of our emotional experiences and they impact (and are impacted by) our emotional experiences.

It may be harder to be flexible when we feel intense emotions, but, with some effort, it is still possible to become more flexible in our thinking. Learning to evaluate whether our first interpretation is accurate, or whether we're missing out on a more accurate interpretation because our emotions are keeping us focused on just one, is a useful skill and the focus of this part of the treatment.

Try to identify a recent emotionally salient example with the adolescent. (If the adolescent cannot identify one, you may choose to start with the example below.) Help the adolescent understand that the interpretations she makes can influence her emotional experiences:

> *"Imagine you are practicing a presentation for class with your friend. When you're done, your friend says you did an excellent job organizing a lot of information. He also mentions that you should try to speak a little slower because you were talking kind of fast and, with all the information you presented, it was hard to remember everything you were saying."*

Ask the adolescent how she would feel if she received this feedback from her friend. Then, explore how her interpretations might affect the emotions she would experience:

> *"Even in this simple scenario there are several different parts that you might focus on. Focusing on the compliment you received (that you did a good job organizing a lot of information) will probably make you feel pretty good. However, you may also focus on the fact that your friend said you spoke too fast. Focusing on this element, you may believe that he gave you the compliment just to try and soften the criticism he offered and that he didn't really mean the nice stuff he said.*
>
> *Of course, there are any number of ways you could interpret this situation. The emotions you are experiencing and the thoughts you are having Before, During, and After a given situation will impact the way you interpret what happened;*

your interpretations will also impact the emotions you experience During and After that situation."

How We View the World: Identifying Our Interpretations

This component of Goal 1 focuses on identifying more emotionally salient thoughts, with an overarching target of identifying "core beliefs" that maintain intense and distressing emotional states over time. While it's a worthwhile goal, it may also be "over the head" of some adolescents, and the use of the **downward arrow technique** described below may prove challenging as a result. Thus, you may consider skipping this section based on the developmental and cognitive level or awareness level of your client and move on to identifying thinking traps in the next section of this module.

In the previous section of this module, you focused on helping the adolescent identify the automatic interpretations she makes. Now we are going to focus a little more heavily on helping her become aware of her **emotional thoughts**. You may want to use the following example to give the adolescent a better idea of how to identify emotional thoughts:

> *"Let's say that I think spiders are gross. When I see one, I run away, calling for someone to help me. After seeing a spider in my bedroom, I choose not to sleep in there for the next two nights. This is obviously a pretty big reaction, but remember—my automatic interpretation when I think of a spider is just that they are gross. My running away, calling for help, and staying away from the room seems like a pretty big reaction for just thinking something is gross. Do you think that the reaction I had is justified just by thinking spiders are gross? Is it possible that I also had other thoughts about spiders that are causing such an intense reaction? Like what?"*

Explain to the adolescent that a reaction like this might be influenced by other interpretations, too. For instance, you might be thinking that if you are near a spider it will bite you and you will be poisoned and probably die. Fear of this extreme outcome (dying) is a more likely explanation for your intense reaction. So in this case fear of dying would be one "emotional thought" that is going to be really important for the adolescent to identify if she wants to be able to change her emotional behaviors.

As the adolescent begins to understand the idea of "emotional thoughts," you should practice getting to the "emotional thought" associated with one of her intense emotional reactions. An example of how to do this (the downward arrow technique) is provided here.

Try to use an example that the adolescent has described previously or that you think would be particularly impactful to the adolescent for something similar to the following discussion:

> *"You've mentioned before that you're afraid of sitting next to someone you don't know at lunch because you may not have anything to say. Now, you've also told me that because this makes you nervous, you eat your lunch in the library at school every single day even though you'd really like to find someone to sit with. It sounds to me like the interpretation we've identified so far, 'worrying you won't have anything to say to someone,' is relatively small, at least compared to the impact it's having on your life (eating alone in the school library). I'd guess there are some bigger—and scarier—'emotional thoughts' about what would happen if you sat next to someone new. Let's try to find out together.*
>
> *So, you said that if you sat next to someone new you wouldn't have anything to say. What would be so bad about that?"*

The adolescent may say any number of things, such as:

ADOLESCENT: *"We'd just sit there not saying anything . . ."*

THERAPIST: *"I can imagine how uncomfortable that would be, but can you tell me what would be so bad about that?"*

ADOLESCENT: *"I'd feel so uncomfortable. They'd probably just ignore me and act like I'm not even there."*

THERAPIST: *"Wow, I can imagine feeling really uncomfortable in that situation, too. So is your concern that you might feel uncomfortable for the one lunch period?"*

ADOLESCENT: *"No, it's that I'd also see these people around school and every time I saw them they'd remember I was that weird kid who sat next to them and didn't say anything. I'd be uncomfortable around them until I graduated!"*

THERAPIST: *"Now I think I'm starting to see . . . sitting next to someone else at lunch is anxiety-provoking because there is not just the possibility of not having anything to say, but also because you think you'll be uncomfortable for the whole lunch period AND you'll be uncomfortable for the rest of high school because everyone will know you're the kid who sat there one lunch period and had nothing to say. That sounds a lot more like an 'emotional thought' big enough to keep you from wanting to try and sit with others . . . I wonder if that is the only possible way that situation could play out . . ."*

Suggested Home Learning Assignment: Flexible Thinking

If stopping session at this point, assign Form 5.2: *Tracking the Before, During, and After* to encourage review and practice of the material covered in session, with an emphasis on identifying automatic interpretations in the Before and During conditions.

Goal 2

Teach the adolescent the common "thinking traps."

Return to the idea that there are many ways of interpreting, or thinking about, any given situation. However, an individual's emotional thoughts may tend to be similar across situations. In fact, people may come to believe that only a few ways of looking at a situation are likely (e.g., "if I walk into a classroom and people are laughing, they must be laughing at me"). Some people get stuck in the same interpretations again and again and are unable to get out of these patterns on their own. These patterns of thinking will be referred to as **thinking traps** because it is easy to get stuck (or trapped) in them if you're not careful. Thinking traps are not limited to uncomfortable emotions; however, the time-limited nature of this therapy suggests that only those that are problematic should be focused on in the course of this therapy. These are likely to be associated with uncomfortable emotional experiences (e.g., anger, fear, sadness, anxiety). You can introduce thinking traps using this description:

"We all have certain ways of thinking about the world. At times these patterns may be really useful. At other times, they may not be (e.g., thinking all spiders are able to kill with one bite). Evaluating similar situations the same way again and again—despite evidence that they may be different—is called a thinking trap, because it's easy to fall into it again and again.

There are many thinking traps that people can fall into, and once you fall into one, it can be hard to get out. We'll plan to talk about just a few, although you'll find there are many more described in your workbook."

Therapist Note

The adolescent may wonder whether thinking traps are all bad. You may wish to answer in any number of ways. For instance, you may emphasize that a quick response to the environment is often useful (e.g., when there is a real, physical danger) and that these automatic ways of thinking help us respond quickly in such situations. However, many situations, even those *that make us feel afraid, are not actually dangerous. Therefore, if there is no immediate risk, it is important to **BE FLEXIBLE** and allow for other interpretations of the situation. Otherwise, we may continue getting caught in these thinking traps.*

*The adolescent may comment that she feels as though many situations **do** pose a threat, even if it is a more minimal threat. If so, validate the adolescent's concern and gently remind her that, when discussing an immediate threat, we are focusing on an **actual, physical threat** such as a car coming down the road toward you, a person choking, or someone drowning. For situations that feel uncomfortable or scary, but where there is no clear or immediate danger, we can practice evaluating how dangerous the situation may actually be. The goal is generally to expand the number of possible interpretations one allows for while figuring out which one is most accurate.*

The most common thinking traps are presented here. A longer list of thinking traps is included in Worksheet 5.1: *Common Thinking Traps.*

The Most Common Thinking Traps

The first thinking trap is *Jumping to Conclusions.* This is the tendency to overestimate the likelihood that something will happen, be it a panic attack, failure on a test, or an unfriendly person. In a situation where the chances of something bad happening are quite high (e.g., I'll probably get caught if I cheat on that test; staying out past curfew will probably mean I'll be grounded), overestimating the likelihood of a bad outcome may help motivate us to avoid that bad outcome. However, this tendency becomes a "thinking trap" when one is almost always overestimating the chances that an unpleasant event will happen, particularly when the chances are actually quite low. If the adolescent thinks that it is 80 percent likely that she will die as a result of having a panic attack (i.e., she overestimates the likelihood of dying as a result of a panic attack), she might ignore evidence that an alternative interpretation is possible. If the adolescent is accurately evaluating a threatening event, it may be more useful to accept the emotions she is experiencing and to use the Problem Solving skill introduced later in this module to try and improve the situation.

A second thinking trap is *Thinking the Worst.* This thinking trap refers to the tendency to think that the worst possible outcome is going to happen. For example, someone with repetitive thoughts/behaviors might believe that if she doesn't wash her hands a certain way, she will contract a terrible disease. As a result, she feels very anxious after touching anything that potentially has germs on it and has difficulty coping with this uncomfortable emotion. In this scenario, even if the adolescent really doesn't touch anything harmful, she is framing the outcome as catastrophic even though failing to wash one's hands in a ritualized way does not typically produce any disastrous outcomes. Moreover, it is clear that the adolescent could cope with being anxious (and has in the past) if she were unable to wash her hands right away or in her ritualized way. A key element of this thinking trap is the belief that the adolescent could not cope with the event if it did occur. Of note, people often believe they would be unable to cope with the feared outcome, even if they do not identify the outcome as the "worst possible."

Another thinking trap is *Ignoring the Positive*. This thinking trap refers to the tendency to focus on the negative aspects of a situation while ignoring the positive. Recalling the earlier example of the feedback given by a friend about an oral presentation, someone who engages in this thinking trap might focus on the "criticism" and ignore or discount the compliment she received.

Refer to Worksheet 5.1 for a list of common thinking traps, and review with the adolescent those that seem most relevant for her. One way to do this is to have the adolescent review the list and ask her which seem most important or common in her own way of thinking. The adolescent may come to realize that she experiences more than one thinking trap at the same time. In fact, it isn't always necessary to know which thinking trap one is stuck in or to identify the thinking trap accurately every time; rather, just knowing that thinking traps exist can help us figure out whether we need to challenge our automatic interpretations. This latter point is important because these thinking traps overlap and share certain features, sometimes making it challenging to tell them apart. That is okay—this is not a test!

Additionally, be careful to avoid a discussion where you are trying to convince the adolescent that she is engaging in specific thinking traps. Your job at this point is not to convince the adolescent that this is true for her; rather, the goal should be that she understands that these thinking traps exist and that she might benefit by observing her thoughts to figure out if this is true for her. Hopefully walking through the steps outlined in the Detective Thinking section (later in the chapter) will allow the adolescent to see whether her interpretations are truly accurate.

Goal 3

Introduce and ensure understanding of the Detective Thinking skill.

As noted above, everyone has certain patterns of thinking. For some people these patterns include getting stuck in emotion-provoking interpretations of the world around them. Getting stuck this way again and again is referred to as a "thinking trap." Helping the adolescent identify her interpretations and whether these interpretations reflect her falling into thinking traps is a huge step. Once the adolescent is able to do this, she will be ready to learn the skills needed to get herself out of these thinking traps, which will include evaluating the interpretations she makes (in the context of thinking traps) to figure out if they are realistic. This process of cognitive restructuring or reappraisal, which will include looking for evidence and/or clues, will be referred to as **Detective Thinking**.

> **Therapist Note**
> *Why we use Detective Thinking BEFORE: When we are in an emotionally provoking situation, it can be hard to remember that our interpretations or thoughts are not necessarily the only interpretations or thoughts possible. Therefore, it is useful to remind the adolescent that identifying and evaluating her interpretations BEFORE entering a given situation can be extremely helpful. Emotion theory suggests that this is actually the most effective way to reduce our experiences with uncomfortable emotion.*

Detective Questioning

In order to begin teaching the adolescent to think like a detective, introduce the concept of **Detective Questioning**, or specific ways to question one's thoughts or interpretations (looking for "clues" to see if one's thoughts are realistic). Present the following rationale.

With the adolescent, turn to Worksheet 5.2: *Evaluating My Thoughts Using Detective Questioning* in the workbook. This worksheet contains a list of Detective Questions, which are questions that the adolescent can use to help investigate (like a detective) the thoughts she is experiencing. These Detective Questions can help the adolescent figure out how realistic her interpretations truly are. There are many types of evidence available to us, and the adolescent may wish to gather any number of them. Examples of Detective Questions include:

- Am I 100 percent sure that _____ will happen?
- What is the worst thing that could happen?
- If _____ did happen, could I handle it?
- Can I really tell what someone else is thinking?
- How likely is it that _____ will happen?
- How many times has _____ happened in the past?
- Is this really as bad as I think?

Steps for Detective Thinking

The first step in Detective Thinking is to identify the interpretation. With the adolescent, turn to the section in the workbook titled "Using Detective Thinking to Challenge Your Automatic Interpretations," and look at the five Detective Thinking steps. In the example provided in the workbook, the interpretation is that "if I don't get straight A's on my report card, I'll never get into a good college." In this example, the adolescent is falling into the Thinking the Worst thinking trap because she is assuming the chances of something bad happening (not getting into a good college) are greater than they actually are and implying that one could not cope well with such an outcome. Thinking the Worst and Ignoring the Positive might also apply to this situation. After discussing this example, work with the adolescent to identify a situation in which her automatic interpretation may not have been the most realistic or accurate. After identifying the interpretation, see if the adolescent can tell you which of the thinking traps (if any) she thinks she may be falling into with this interpretation. Ask the adolescent to use Worksheet 5.3: *Being a Detective—Steps for Detective Thinking* to write down her automatic interpretation and thinking trap(s).

Now that you've identified the interpretation and which thinking trap the adolescent has fallen into, use the following strategies to evaluate the evidence. First, go through the Detective Questions on Worksheet 5.2: *Evaluating My Thoughts Using Detective Questioning* to evaluate the interpretation. Have the adolescent write at least two Detective Questions she asked (and her corresponding answers) in the appropriate section on Worksheet 5.3: *Being a Detective—Steps for Detective Thinking*. This will help the adolescent evaluate how realistic her interpretation truly is.

Indicate to the adolescent that another part of Detective Thinking may involve identifying her ability to cope with a situation despite an intense emotional reaction. Assist the adolescent in providing evidence that she and others have coped with very difficult things in the past (have the adolescent provide examples—e.g., she was sad but was able to cope when a relative died), if appropriate. After completing the Detective Thinking steps, work with the adolescent to identify a more realistic outcome, as well as how she would cope with the outcome if it were to occur.

Now that you have worked through an example of Detective Thinking to counter the adolescent's interpretation, it may be useful to practice Detective Thinking further by role-playing with the adolescent. An example of this type of role-play, as well as a potential segue to Goal 4 (Problem Solving) is provided here:

ADOLESCENT: *"I got in a fight with my best friend on the way here. I don't even know what it was about, right now. I can't believe it. We'll probably never talk to each other again! And if we stop talking, I won't be able to hang out with the friends we have in common either."*

THERAPIST: *"I'm so sorry; I can imagine how upsetting that must be. I don't know what this means, but I wonder if we could use this example to practice Detective Thinking and see if your (automatic) interpretation is the most realistic? Let's try it. Remember, our job right now will be to gather some evidence, just like a detective might. I'm not asking you to change your mind, just to figure out what the evidence is."*

ADOLESCENT: *"I'll try, but I'm pretty sure this fight will be the end of our friendship. Okay, well, the first step is to identify what I'm thinking, right? I just said it really; I'm thinking that after this fight, I'm going to lose my best friend and all my other friends, too!"*

THERAPIST: *"That's a lot to sort through. Let's try and take it one piece at a time. First, let's try to identify whether you're falling into any thinking traps."*

ADOLESCENT: *"Okay, I guess maybe Thinking the Worst . . . I can't know for certain our friendship is over for good, but it sure feels like it!"*

THERAPIST: *"That's a good start. You recognize that you may be falling into a thinking trap. Now, why don't you look for evidence as to whether or not you're going to lose your best friend because of the fight you just had. How would you start?"*

ADOLESCENT: *"Well, I see on this worksheet that I'm supposed to try and evaluate the evidence . . . I don't have any evidence. We've never had this fight before."*

THERAPIST: *"Hmm, so that is tricky . . . What are some of the questions you can ask yourself to get more evidence?"*

ADOLESCENT: *"Well, let's see . . . Have I been in this situation before? No. Have I been in a similar situation? . . . I did fight with my best friend about something else a few weeks ago. But it wasn't this big a fight . . ."*

THERAPIST: *"Okay, so you fought before, even though it wasn't as big a fight as this one. What happened after that fight?*

ADOLESCENT: *"We didn't talk for a few days and then she called me. I was so relieved she finally called."*

THERAPIST: *"Okay, so last time there was something similar she called you and you were relieved. So even if the fight wasn't as big then, you were able to resolve the fight. That's great information to keep in mind. You don't have to believe the alternative thought, but just having made room for some other interpretation, did your emotional experiences change at all? "*

ADOLESCENT: *"I feel a little hopeful . . ."*

THERAPIST: *"Excellent! And when there's hope there is reason to try and work toward a solution. If there is no hope, why should you even try? I think this is a good time to practice our Problem Solving steps."*

Once again, it should be emphasized that these new interpretations are ways the adolescent can think about a given situation. While they may be useful during and particularly after a situation (especially in cases of social anxiety or depression—where the adolescent may become particularly negative in her thinking after leaving a situation), they will be most useful BEFORE entering a given situation. You should also emphasize that this process is about REALISTIC THINKING rather than just thinking positively. The whole activity of Detective Thinking should be summarized as follows:

- Learn to evaluate what is really likely to happen in a situation.
- Reconsider thoughts that might be thinking traps.
- See how this process impacts our emotional behavior in those situations.

Goal 4

Introduce and ensure understanding of the Problem Solving skill.

This section should be introduced as a series of steps the adolescent can use to get out of situations where she may feel "stuck," or unable to come to a good solution. It may be useful to remind the adolescent that situations such as these are often associated with strong, uncomfortable emotions.

Steps in Problem Solving

The first Problem Solving step is to *define the problem*. How you define the problem will influence the solutions you come up with. Try to define the problem in the simplest and most straightforward terms possible. The next step is to *identify some solutions*. Encourage the adolescent to think of as many solutions as possible. At this point, the solutions are not to be evaluated or judged. Though most of the time we have a sense of solutions that are "good" and those that are "bad," when strong emotions are involved we may choose to dismiss a solution because we'd feel uncomfortable in the short term even though that solution might help us meet our larger goals. Therefore, judging our options too soon might result in missing out on some decent solutions.

Therapist Note

Generally, you should allow the adolescent to generate the solutions; however, some adolescents may have difficulty generating solutions or may frequently miss some possibilities. At these times, you may wish to help the adolescent, noting that during periods of high emotion it can be difficult

> *to pick any solution except the one that you think you need to do to reduce your uncomfortable emotional experiences.*

After generating a list of possible solutions, the next step is to *list the good and bad things about each solution*. Try to think of at least one good thing and one bad thing that may be associated with each solution. Based on your review of the good and bad things about each solution, the next step is to *pick one to try*. Be specific; instead of saying "I will try that solution sometime in the next week," say "I will try that solution Friday after school." Afterwards, *evaluate how the solution worked*. If it did, great! If it didn't, you can either try a second one or go back to step one and try again. It may help to change the way you defined the problem or to think of other solutions.

Next, you and the adolescent will go through the Problem Solving steps using an example or two. As you go through an example, have the adolescent follow along using Worksheet 5.4: *Getting Unstuck—Steps for Solving a Problem*.

Below are two scripts for practicing Problem Solving. The first is an emotionally neutral problem that may be useful to start with for some adolescents. The second is an example of how to go through the Problem Solving steps for a problem that evokes strong emotions for the adolescent. This text is not meant to represent the only way the material can be presented, but rather to provide an example of how this discussion may proceed. Following the scripts, there are other examples of problems you can use to practice the Problem Solving skills with the adolescent.

Problem to Solve—Example 1 (Emotionally Neutral)

THERAPIST: *"Let's practice using these steps. I'd like you to figure out how to move this binder from the desk to the other side of the room. However, for this challenge you will not be able to use your hands. Using the steps we just discussed, how would you go about solving this problem?"*

ADOLESCENT: *"Well, I guess I have to move the binder across the room, right? But I can't use my hands."*

THERAPIST: *"That's the perfect definition of the problem! Now what might some solutions be?"*

ADOLESCENT: *"I guess I could use my elbows, or my feet, or my nose, or my head."*

THERAPIST: *"Excellent! Those are all options. And you did a wonderful job not evaluating those options yet. You just threw them out there and didn't get stuck trying to find the 'right one'."*

ADOLESCENT: *"Well, I guess that using my nose might hurt, and it wouldn't be easy to move the binder. I could probably push the binder with my elbow pretty easily, though."*

THERAPIST: *"Alright, so which option do you think you'd like to try?"*

ADOLESCENT: *"I'm going to try to use my elbows! And I'm going to try it right now. I'll see how it goes and then figure out where to go next."*

THERAPIST: *"Great, let's see how it goes then!"*

Problem to Solve—Example 2 (Strong Emotion)

THERAPIST: *"Let's practice using the Problem Solving steps. I'd like you to think about something that results in your experiencing a strong emotion, perhaps a situation where you haven't been able to find a solution you were pleased with . . . Anything come to mind?"*

ADOLESCENT: *"Well, I've been feeling really angry that my best friend didn't call me last Friday night, even though she got together with a bunch of our friends."*

THERAPIST: *"That's a great problem to try and solve! How might you define that problem?"*

ADOLESCENT: *"Hmm, that I'm angry at my best friend for not calling me to hang out with friends."*

THERAPIST: *"Excellent! Now what might some solutions be?"*

ADOLESCENT: *"Well, I haven't said anything to her about it yet."*

THERAPIST: *"Sounds like that's one option, not to say anything. What might others be?"*

ADOLESCENT: *"I guess I could tell her that it bothered me. I could also talk to another friend about how much she hurt me . . . Or, next time I know they're out I can just join them without being called."*

THERAPIST: *"Those all sound like options you could try. And you did a wonderful job not evaluating those options yet. You just threw them out there and didn't get stuck trying to find the 'right one.' What are the good and bad things about each option?"*

ADOLESCENT: *"Well, if I talked to another friend about it, she might make me feel better or invite me next time, but it might get back to my best friend and she'd be angry at me for that. If I told her how much she hurt me, it might mean she won't do it again but I'd feel really uncomfortable and anxious when I was talking to her. If I don't say anything, nothing will change, but I won't feel uncomfortable either. If I just go join them, I wouldn't be missing out, but it wouldn't really solve the problem of my friend not calling."*

THERAPIST: *"Alright, so which option do you think you'd like to try?"*

ADOLESCENT: *"I'm going to not say anything for now."*

THERAPIST: *"That's a valid choice. Why don't we plan to check in next week and see if that solution has worked for you?"*

Additional Examples to Use for Practicing Problem Solving Skills

1. The adolescent forgot her password to her email account.
2. The adolescent cannot find her cell phone.
3. The adolescent received the wrong order at a fast-food restaurant.
4. The adolescent is scared of spiders and sees a small spider in her bedroom.
5. The adolescent keeps letting her friend borrow her videogames, but the friend never returns them.
6. The adolescent forgot to complete her homework for English class today.
7. The adolescent did not understand the math lesson in school today.
8. The adolescent's friend won't reply to her text messages, and she is now worried that her friend is upset with her.
9. The adolescent's parents won't let her go to the big party this weekend.
10. One of the adolescent's friends keeps posting negative comments on social media about her.

You may also wish to use Figure 5.1: *Getting Unstuck—Step-by-Step Example of Solving a Problem* to help the adolescent see yet another example of using the Problem Solving steps.

Before ending the discussion of Problem Solving, you should be sure to go through the steps using an example from the adolescent's own life. Ideally, this example will be a problem that the adolescent is either experiencing now or anticipates she will experience in the future, and it should also be one that brings up some strong emotions for the adolescent.

Therapist Note

Some therapists find that Problem Solving is an excellent strategy to help solve interpersonal conflicts that the adolescent client is experiencing with peers, in romantic relationships, and with parents and/or others. For example, it may be useful to have the parent and adolescent use the Problem Solving steps together at the end of this session to further illustrate the concept with regard to a recent conflict or disagreement. Be careful not to let this exercise descend into high levels of interpersonal negativity in the therapy room. Identify and validate any strong emotions raised and reinforce that this is a good strategy for approaching conflicts in a productive and adaptive manner at home.

Suggested Home Learning Assignment: Problem Solving

Assign the following handouts to encourage review and practice of the material covered in session:

- Form 5.2: *Tracking the Before, During, and After*
- Worksheet 5.4: *Getting Unstuck—Steps for Solving a Problem.* Have the adolescent practice the Problem Solving steps at home using this worksheet. If the adolescent does not experience a problem she believes she needs to use the skill for, instruct her to complete the worksheet with a hypothetical situation.

Parent Summary Form for Core Module 5: Being Flexible in Your Thinking

Core Module 5 is designed to help your teen learn to identify the ways he or she interprets the world and to evaluate whether these interpretations are the most realistic. The human brain naturally focuses on certain aspects of a situation and interprets events without thinking about it. These are called *automatic thoughts* or *interpretations*. Our automatic interpretations can influence our emotional experiences and vice versa. There are usually a number of different ways to think about a given situation. For example, a friend not saying "hi" when walking by could be interpreted as him just not seeing you or him ignoring you on purpose. The way we interpret a situation then affects the entire emotional experience. Becoming more aware of automatic interpretations can help your teen identify *thinking traps* (i.e., inaccurate/unrealistic/unhelpful automatic interpretations) he or she may fall into and identify more realistic interpretations.

Detective Thinking

What Is a Thinking Trap?

When people tend to think about situations in an unrealistic or unhelpful way, they can get stuck in a pattern of making these interpretations again and again, and they may be unable to get out of these patterns on their own. Your teen will learn when he or she is getting stuck in these thinking traps and how to get unstuck! Your teen will also receive a list of common thinking traps.

Detective Thinking is a skill that directs your teen to think about his or her interpretations more objectively, the way detectives might—looking for clues to tell them what may or may not be really happening in a situation. What is your teen's automatic interpretation? Is your teen falling into a thinking trap? Is there evidence to support your teen's interpretation? Your teen will learn to use *Detective Questioning* of his or her interpretations. Detective Thinking is helpful to use before entering difficult situations.

Examples of Detective Questions

- Am I 100 percent sure that _____ will happen?
- What is the worst thing that could happen?
- If _____ did happen, could I handle it?
- Can I really tell what someone else is thinking?
- How likely is it that _____ will happen?
- How many times has _____ happened in the past?
- Is this really as bad as I think?

Problem Solving

Problem Solving is another skill that can help your teen get unstuck in difficult situations, and it is especially useful for conflicts or academic/time management problems, among others. Problem Solving steps are helpful to identify an effective solution when you are feeling stuck. Try it yourself next time you are not sure how to solve a problem in your life!

Problem Solving Steps

1. What is the problem you are trying to solve?
2. What are all the possible things you could do in this situation?
3. What are the good things about each solution?
4. What are the bad things about each solution?
5. Identify the solution you think is the best one and try it out!
6. If the solution you choose doesn't work, go through the process again.

What Can I Do to Support My Teen with Being More Flexible in Thinking?

✓ Share alternative interpretations of situations and events with your teen. Identify multiple ways you can interpret one situation.

✓ Prior to situations that are emotionally intense for your teen, prompt him or her to use Detective Thinking skills.

✓ Help your teen identify potential solutions to problems, but give your teen the independence to test out solutions he or she chooses.

CHAPTER 6

Core Module 6: Awareness of Emotional Experiences

(Recommended Length: 1 or 2 Sessions)

MATERIALS NEEDED FOR THE MODULE

- Module 6 Workbook Materials:
  1. *Notice it, Say Something About it, Experience it* (Worksheet 6.1)
  2. *Awareness Practice Monitoring* (Form 6.1)
  3. *Emotion Story* (Worksheet 6.2)
  4. Media device for practicing nonjudgmental awareness exercises
  5. *Tracking the Before, During, and After Form* (Form 6.2)
- A parent module summary form is provided at the end of this chapter to help support review of module materials with the parent(s) of your adolescent client. You may also use materials from Chapter 9 (Module-P) to help support these discussions.

Assessments to Be Given at *Every* Session:

- Parent and Adolescent Ratings: *Weekly Top Problems Tracking Form* (Appendix 1.3 at the end of Chapter 1 in this Therapist Guide)

In this module, you will first work with the adolescent to increase awareness of his experiences more broadly. Then, you will work with the adolescent to put such strategies into action to increase his awareness during emotionally evocative situations. Awareness training is an important step in the treatment process. This module will assist the adolescent in adopting a practice of present-moment and nonjudgmental awareness in different situations and across varying triggers of increasing intensity, which may in turn eventually reduce attempts to avoid uncomfortable emotional experiences. Even if present-moment or nonjudgmental awareness is not fully understood or achieved during this module, you may return to these concepts and techniques and practice them again during situational emotion exposures in Core Module 7.

- **Goal 1:** Introduce the rationale for present-moment awareness and practice present-moment awareness activities in session.
- **Goal 2:** Introduce the rationale for nonjudgmental awareness and practice nonjudgmental awareness activities in session.
- **Goal 3:** Introduce generalized emotion exposures and practice nonjudgmental and present-moment awareness in context, identifying and processing any subtle avoidance behaviors observed with the client.

Therapist Note—Unified Protocol Theory

In many different ways up to this point in the UP-A, you have been encouraging present-moment awareness of intense emotional experiences with your adolescent client. Starting in Core Module 2, you introduced the idea of being more aware of and observing the reactions he had to emotional triggers using the Before, During, and After form. In Core Module 4, you reinforced practice of greater body awareness using the body scanning technique. In Core Module 5, you encouraged the adolescent to develop awareness of potential thinking traps. Here in Core Module 6, we are extending this practice through effortful attention to our emotional experiences during any given "present moment." You can think of these strategies as an opposite action to the distraction, rumination, and suppression that often occur when we perceive thoughts or situations within or around us that are difficult to experience or process in the moment. By purposely moving in this module from less intense practice experiences to more intense emotional situations, you are also shaping this awareness behavior in increasingly naturalistic situations and settings.

Goal 1

Introduce the rationale for present-moment awareness and practice present-moment awareness activities in session.

Therapist Note

- *Don't forget to start each session re-rating top problems with the adolescent and parent.*
- *Don't forget to give the parent the Core Module 6 summary form to aid in understanding this module's important material. Spend some time in one session during this module to review this form with the parent.*

Introducing Present-Moment Awareness

As indicated in the Unified Protocol Theory discussion above, you can start this module by discussing how you have encouraged the adolescent in prior modules to work on greater and greater awareness of the different parts of his emotional experience. In this module, you will be introducing another way to be more aware of his entire response to a trigger, as well as the situation your adolescent client is in while having this response. This new type of awareness is called *present-moment awareness*. Whereas the cognitive techniques discussed in Core Module 5 are most effective when utilized *before* entering a potential emotionally provoking situation, present-moment awareness can be practiced *before, during, or after* an emotionally provoking situation in order to increase engagement with the facts of the current situation. When practicing present-moment awareness, it is important to allow oneself to fully participate in the "here and now," not in the future (which hasn't happened yet) or in the past (which we can't change). Not focusing on the present moment is sometimes referred to as being on *autopilot*. When we are on autopilot, we are likely unfocused and not being fully aware of our present thoughts, emotions, or experiences because we are distracted by our own judgments or thoughts about the future or past. Being on autopilot can keep us stuck in our emotion twisters:

> *"Present-moment awareness means we are fully engaged in the 'here and now.' We are not thinking about the past or the future, but only about what is happening in the moment. We are focusing on one thing at a time and letting go of distractions.*

I'd like to suggest that it is okay to just notice and say something to yourself about what you are experiencing and leave it at that, so you can participate in the present moment. In the end, this may help slow down the emotion twisters you experience, which will help you better manage your emotions in the future."

Explaining Why Present-Moment Awareness Is Important

- When explaining **present-moment awareness** to your adolescent client, it can be helpful to start off by describing some sort of situation that might allow the practice of present-moment awareness to make more sense (i.e., a situation that causes strong emotions for your client).
- The particular situation will differ by client, and it is important to relate the concept to the client's individual experience.
- You should explain that when we feel strong emotions, it is natural to think about our problems (or what might be causing our strong emotions).
- Then, introduce the issue that your adolescent client may have experienced before—indicating that strong emotions may cause him to think about too many things at once or to think over and over about negative things in life, causing him to feel overwhelmed.
- Explain that present-moment awareness can help him slow down these thoughts and focus on one thing at a time. Note that, when we are able to do that, we are then in a more helpful frame of mind to approach the problem at hand and manage strong emotions.

Introducing "Noticing It, Saying Something About It, and Experiencing It" as Parts of Present-Moment Awareness

You will recall that in Core Module 4 we discussed using the framework of noticing, saying something about, and experiencing when we were teaching the adolescent to use body scanning to increase his awareness of how physical sensations change over time. In this module, we are returning to that framework, but this time to remind the adolescent how he might be more "present-moment aware" of the emotional and less emotional triggers in his environment. You can help the adolescent to recall the meaning of these terms as they relate to present-moment awareness by discussing the following terms along with examples:

1. *Notice it* (wordlessly notice your environment and emotional experiences): When at the beach, noticing that I smell the ocean, I see the people, I hear the birds chirping, I feel the sand between my toes

2. *Say something about it* (label the details of your experience): When at the beach, telling myself that the ocean smells salty, the people are wearing bright colors, the birds are chirping loudly, the sand feels soft and fine beneath my toes

3. *Experience it* (use all of your senses to fully experience the moment without distractions): Repeatedly bringing myself back to these sensations that represent my beach experience

Engaging in Present-Moment Awareness Exercises

Use Worksheet 6.1: *Notice It, Say Something About It, Experience It* to practice present-moment awareness exercises in session. In-session present-moment awareness exercises should focus on helping the adolescent notice, say something about, and experience the here and now using a variety of non-emotional stimuli to begin with. Using all of the adolescent's senses to build awareness should be emphasized. Examples of present-moment awareness exercises are provided here. It is important to choose exercises that will be interesting to your client. Be creative. Present-moment awareness can be practiced during any activity. Although no one exercise is better than the others, it is important to try and gauge which one might be the best fit for the particular adolescent. Use at least one exercise to practice this skill in session and encourage further practice of present-moment awareness at home. Remind the adolescent that present-moment awareness can be practiced anywhere and at any time. While learning to use this skill, it is important that the adolescent set up times to practice. Once he understands the use of the skill, he may not need to practice at predetermined times and may use the skill in his daily life instead. The following are some suggested present-moment awareness practice exercises.

General Breathing Awareness

Instruct the adolescent to do the following:

1. *Assume a comfortable posture lying on your back or sitting. If you are sitting, keep the spine straight and let your shoulders drop.*
2. *Close your eyes if it feels comfortable.*
3. *Bring your attention to your belly, feeling it rise or expand gently on the in-breath and fall or recede on the out-breath.*
4. *Keep your focus on your breathing, "being with" each in-breath for its full duration and with each out-breath for its full duration, as if you were riding the waves of your own breathing.*

5. *Every time you notice that your mind has wandered off the breath, notice what it was that took you away and then gently bring your attention back to your belly and the feeling of the breath coming in and out.*

6. *If your mind wanders away from the breath a thousand times, then your "job" is simply to bring it back to the breath every time, no matter what it becomes preoccupied with.*

7. *Practice this exercise for 5 to 15 minutes at a convenient time every day, whether you feel like it or not, for one week and see how it feels to incorporate present-moment practice into your life. Be aware of how it feels to spend time each day just being with your breath without having to do anything.*

Awareness of Physical Sensations—Exploring a Candy Exercise

Instruct the adolescent to do the following:[1]

1. *Take one small (unwrapped) candy (e.g., a Starburst), and hold it in your hand. Focus on this one piece of candy and imagine that you just dropped in from Mars and have never seen candy like this before in your life.*

2. *Take this candy and hold it in the palm of your hand, or between your finger and thumb. Pay attention to seeing it. Look at it carefully, as if you had never seen a candy before.*

3. *Turn it over between your fingers, examining the highlights where the light shines and where it is darker.*

4. *While you are doing this, notice any thoughts that come to mind, such as "what a weird thing we are doing" or "what is the point of this?" or "I don't like these." Just note them as thoughts and bring your awareness back to the details of the candy.*

5. *And now smell the piece of candy, take it and hold it beneath your nose, and with each breath in carefully notice the smell of it.*

6. *Slowly put the candy on your tongue, maybe noticing how your hand and arm know exactly where to put it, or noticing your mouth watering as it comes up. Notice it without biting it, just exploring the sensations of having it your mouth.*

7. *And when you are ready, very consciously take a bite into it and notice the taste it releases.*

8. *Slowly chew it. Notice the saliva in your mouth and the change in the consistency of the object as you chew it.*

---

[1] This exercise was adapted from Williams et al., 2007.

9. *Then, when you feel ready to swallow, see if you can first notice your mouth deciding to swallow, so that even this is experienced consciously before you actually swallow it.*

10. *Finally, see if you can follow the feelings of swallowing, sensing the candy moving down to your stomach.*

Mindful Walking

Go for a walk to practice present-moment awareness. Instruct the adolescent to do the following:

"Begin by feeling the connection of your body to the ground or the floor and then become aware of the surroundings, spending a few moments taking in any sights, smells, tastes, sounds, thoughts, emotions, or other sensations. Then mindfully begin to focus solely upon walking as your weight shifts from left leg to right leg, and you begin to lift your right foot up, then left foot up, and then back down on the ground to move each foot forward one at a time. Start off by walking slowly and paying attention to sensations on the soles of the feet, heels, and toes as they touch the ground. Then notice how your body moves as you walk with your arms either swinging back and forth or placed behind, beside, or in front of you. Continue your walk with this awareness, one step at a time."

Play-Doh Exercise

To use present-moment awareness skills with Play-Doh, have the adolescent hold and look at a ball of Play-Doh without squeezing it. Have the adolescent notice his urge to squeeze the Play-Doh. Then have him describe what he notices about the Play-Doh using his senses: the temperature, scent, texture, shape, color, and so forth. Then have the adolescent participate by making something out of the Play-Doh.

Guessing the Flavor

Using jellybeans or other multi-flavored food, have the adolescent close his eyes and slowly eat one piece at a time. Have him use his present-moment awareness skills to guess the flavor of the piece he is eating.

Guessing the Scent

Using spices, candles, food, lotion, and so forth, have the adolescent close his eyes and use his sense of smell to identify different items based on their scent.

Pebble Identification

Collect multiple stones or pebbles with different shapes, sizes, and textures. Have the adolescent close his eyes and pick one of the pebbles. While his eyes are closed, have him use his other senses to become familiar with the pebble he picked. After a few minutes, have him place the stone back in the pile with the other pebbles. With his eyes open and using his other senses, have him identify which pebble was his.

Goal 2

Introduce the rationale for nonjudgmental awareness and practice nonjudgmental awareness activities in session.

Defining Nonjudgmental Awareness

Nonjudgmental awareness is a compassionate, kind, and accepting form of present-moment awareness of what is going on inside and around us. We can also think of it as an opposite action to worry or other efforts to suppress, control, or distract from uncomfortable thoughts the adolescent may be having. We do not want the adolescent to evaluate his experiences as right, wrong, good, or bad. Instead, we want him to approach his emotional experience with empathy and understanding, much like we would toward a friend. Sometimes when we are paying close attention to what we're thinking and feeling, we can become critical and judgmental of our thoughts and feelings, and may try to change them or distract ourselves because this judgment-filled awareness is uncomfortable. For example, when the adolescent is talking to someone, he might notice that his voice shakes, and he may think, "I am such an idiot! What's wrong with me? This person will never like me if I can't calm down." These critical or judgmental thoughts may actually make us feel worse and potentially even avoid things like hanging out with friends. Being nonjudgmentally aware means paying attention to what is happening around us and inside of us, letting go of the judgment, and just acknowledging and accepting our experiences for what they are. We are not necessarily accepting that a given situation is dangerous or threatening. Instead we are focusing on acceptance of our emotional reaction to it, before possibly acting in a different way.

The same general present-moment awareness skills reviewed earlier in this module should be applied when practicing nonjudgmental awareness more specifically. For example, if the adolescent had been practicing nonjudgmental awareness during that conversation when his voice shook, he might say to himself, "This is how it is right now (notice it), there go my thoughts again (say something about it)," and would then gently bring his attention back to the person and the conversation (experience it). This may sound different, unrealistic, or hard to do. It can be hard to do at first, but it's not impossible; it just takes practice. Importantly, it is not something that the adolescent has to do perfectly in order to have it be helpful. The more we practice, the more natural it becomes. The following may be one way to personalize the concept of nonjudgmental awareness to your client:

> "Nonjudgmental awareness means that while becoming more aware of our emotions we are also being sure not to react to or judge the emotions that we are experiencing, but rather notice and accept our emotions for what they are. Having an emotion is not a bad thing! One way to rethink your reactions to your emotional experiences is to consider how you would respond to a friend who came to you with the same concerns. Would you say that your friend was 'stupid' or 'wrong' for feeling a certain emotion? Or would you have some empathy for your friend's experience and tell her that it is okay to feel that way? This is the same nonjudgmental perspective to practice with your own feelings. This new way of looking at your emotions will allow you to be able to let go of them more easily, because it's easier to move past things that are less scary and threatening. The more you tell yourself that your feelings are 'bad' or that you are 'bad' for feeling that way, the more you will get caught up in them."

Engaging in Nonjudgmental Awareness Exercises

You can reinforce the concept of nonjudgmental awareness with the adolescent at this point. You can do this in a non-emotional context by bringing in a few everyday objects and having the adolescent notice and talk about these objects without judgment. To further reinforce the non-judgmental component of this present-moment awareness practice, you can also conduct a role-play. You can play the "friend" who is experiencing an emotional situation (perhaps one similar to the adolescent's own experiences) and allow the adolescent to assist you with nonjudgmental awareness and offer you empathic statements toward "your" feelings in the situation. Additional examples of nonjudgmental awareness exercises are provided below. After at least one exercise to practice this skill in session, encourage further practice of nonjudgmental awareness at home. Remind the adolescent that nonjudgmental awareness can be practiced anywhere and at any time and is most helpful when used during a strong emotional experience.

During this practice, introduce nonjudgmental awareness activities so the adolescent can bring nonjudgmental awareness to his entire emotional experience (i.e., thoughts, bodily sensations, and behaviors). You can also use the activities described in the *Engaging in Present-Moment Awareness Exercises* section of this module by adding an emphasis on the adolescent's nonjudgmental awareness of his entire emotional experience during these same activities. Nonjudgmental awareness can also be practiced by applying these skills to examples of past experiences during which an adolescent experienced a strong emotion. Alternatively, these skills can be practiced during the generalized emotion exposures that your client will be introduced to in the next section of this module. Again, for adolescents who particularly benefit from this practice, an additional session focusing on alternate nonjudgmental awareness and mindfulness activities may be added. The following activities can be used to practice nonjudgmental awareness in session with your client:

Awareness of Thoughts

"This is an exercise to practice observing your thoughts and allowing them to flow in and out of your mind without judging or acting upon them. Close your eyes and imagine that you are sitting by a quiet river watching the water flow downstream. Notice how the water quietly continues to flow. It doesn't stop or get stuck, it gently keeps moving downstream. Take a few moments to watch the water as it flows. Now begin to notice your thoughts. What are you currently thinking? Gently place that thought onto the river and watch as your thought flows away with the water. Do not interfere or interrupt the thought, simply watch as your thought moves away with the water. If you have another thought, again place it on the river and watch it flow downstream without interrupting it. Just notice. If at some point the water has stopped flowing or you become distracted by a thought, that's okay, just notice that and return to your thoughts and place them on the river. Continue this exercise for a few minutes and then gently open your eyes."

Awareness of Emotions Exercise

Use this for a salient emotional event from the week:

"First, begin to get centered by focusing on your breathing . . . Then, begin to notice the room around you. Notice things you can see in the room, the sounds you can hear, any smells . . . Next, spend a few moments focusing your attention on

sensations in your body. For example, notice the feeling of your body in the chair or on the floor, and any other sensation as they come and go . . . Now, gently shift your attention to the thoughts as they run through your mind, and the emotions that you are having. Just notice the experience, without attempting to alter or judge it. When you notice that you are trying to change your experience, or you notice that you are labeling or judging your experience, just notice that and then shift your focus back to the thought and emotions. Notice the efforts to push away or hold onto certain feelings. Notice how the emotions you are having change, or how they remain constant."

Suggested Home Learning Assignment: Present-Moment and/or Nonjudgmental Awareness Practice

If ending a session before practicing generalized emotion exposures, you may wish to assign the following home learning to encourage review and practice of the material covered in session:

- Ask the adolescent to monitor a non-emotional or minimally intense emotional experience while practicing present-moment and/ or nonjudgmental awareness using Form 6.1: *Awareness Practice Monitoring*. Brainstorm when/where the adolescent can practice over the next week.
- Conversely, these new behaviors can be tracked on Form 6.2: *Tracking the Before, During, and After*, if assigning multiple home learning forms is problematic for your adolescent client.

Goal 3

Introduce generalized emotion exposures and practice nonjudgmental and present-moment awareness in context, identifying and processing any subtle avoidance behaviors observed with the client.

Generalized Emotion Exposure

In order to guide the adolescent to become more aware of his emotional experiences and allow them to exist rather than try to suppress them or avoid them, you should encourage him to participate in a number of exercises that may induce emotional experiences. These exercises may include listening to or watching a piece of media, reading or writing a narrative (using Worksheet 6.2: *Emotion Story*), or engaging in some other activity. These types of exercises will be referred to as *generalized emotion exposures*. Regardless of what exercise you choose, the goals are (1) to help the adolescent practice using present-moment and nonjudgmental awareness regarding his internal and external experiences during such exercises, and (2) to notice that the thoughts, feelings, and behaviors that he wants to engage in during these experiences may change in intensity over time.

> **Therapist Note**
> *For time-saving purposes, you may elect to incorporate generalized emotion exposure practice into Core Module 7, but we generally encourage some level of emotion-focused practice of present-moment/nonjudgmental awareness before moving forward.*

Generalized emotion exposures are designed not only to help the adolescent become more emotionally aware, but also to provoke emotions that the adolescent may not be comfortable experiencing or that he may be coping with in maladaptive ways. Therefore, generalized emotion exposures are designed to allow the adolescent to experience relevant emotions while encouraging him to use emotion regulation skills presented in this manual, which will help him solidify his use of these new skills.

As with any emotion exposure, the goal is to have the adolescent experience an emotion he has been responding to in a maladaptive way, while choosing to respond to that emotion in an alternative manner, whether these are "positive emotions" or more "negative" ones. However, it is often helpful—for both rapport purposes and for the purposes of introducing generalized emotion exposures—to use a balance of positive emotion cues (those that evoke joy, happiness, and so forth) and more distressing ones, starting with the former and moving to the latter. Often starting with an exposure that is more positive (e.g., a song or video that makes the adolescent laugh or want to sing and dance), then continuing with one that contains a blend of positive and negative emotional triggers (e.g., watching a video of family reunions at the airport), and concluding with one that is more overtly sad or difficult to watch or listen to (e.g., watching part of a movie where someone is sick or someone's relative passes away) may be a good progression. In the end, the goal is to help the adolescent learn that he does not need to avoid experiencing uncomfortable emotions and can use his awareness skills effectively while observing his responses to such.

Before assigning media exposures, you may wish to speak to the adolescent's parents to ensure you understand family rules/expectations around the adolescent's media viewing (e.g., the adolescent is not allowed to watch R-rated films). If there is reason to believe these rules should be altered for the purposes of generalized emotion exposure, talk to the parent about that possibility (e.g., perhaps the adolescent isn't allowed to watch horror films, but that's in part because of how fearful he becomes when watching films such as these). The following dialogue may be used with the adolescent to introduce the practice of generalized emotion exposures:

> *"Up until now, we've been working to understand your emotional experiences. Now we're going to practice monitoring your emotional experiences as they're happening. To do this we'll practice some things that are meant to help you experience your emotions. I know some of your emotions feel really uncomfortable and you may not want to experience them anymore. But practicing being present and aware of your experiences and doing so without judging them will help you change your responses to strong emotions.*
>
> *Now we are going to practice what is called an emotion exposure exercise. We are going to do this by looking at these pictures/watching these video clips/listening to these songs/writing/recording some past experiences you have had/playing this game/doing this task. Your job is just to pay attention to both the emotions you experience by 'noticing it,' then 'saying something about it' (even if to yourself), and making sure you are fully 'experiencing it.' If you notice yourself thinking that any part of your emotional experience is bad or wrong, or if you notice yourself trying to get rid of any part of your emotional experience, practice using the nonjudgmental awareness exercises we used. We are going to try to bring up a few different types of emotions."*

Subtle or Overt Avoidance Behaviors

During generalized emotion exposures, it is important that the adolescent remain aware of his emotional experience. Monitor his efforts to distance himself from this experience. For instance, during a media-based exposure, ensure the adolescent does not turn away from the screen to try to avoid experiencing the emotion. You may counter this by having the adolescent "sportscast" his thoughts and reactions while watching an emotionally evocative video clip or take breaks during the playing of a song to elicit such responses as they occur.

For adolescents who are highly avoidant of uncomfortable emotions or who are significantly depressed, you may wish to stick to activities meant to induce pleasant emotions, which might include a physical activity (e.g., a quick game of trash-can basketball), and practice awareness of emotional responses to such. Regardless of the chosen activity, ask the adolescent to record the Before, During, and After associated with this task using Form 6.2: *Tracking the Before, During, and After.*

Suggested Home Learning Assignment: Generalized Emotion Exposures

Assign the following home learning to encourage review and practice of the material covered in session:

- Assign generalized emotion exposures that the adolescent can do during the upcoming week and have him track his use of present-moment/nonjudgmental awareness using Form 6.1: *Awareness Practice Monitoring.*
- You can also assign continued tracking of the Before, During, and After of additional emotional experiences (using Form 6.2.: *Tracking the Before, During, and After*). However, if doing both home learning forms feels like a lot more work than your client can complete in one week, prioritize practice of awareness exercises.

Parent Summary Form for Core Module 6: Awareness of Emotional Experiences

Not focusing on the present is sometimes referred to as being on automatic pilot or *autopilot*. When your teen is on autopilot, he or she may not be focusing accurately on the details of what's going on around him or her. This may sound a bit strange, as you might feel that your teen is always stuck in the details of his or her emotional experiences. But, in reality, he or she may just be very aware of unhelpful ideas he or she is having about the past or future during these times—not the present moment!

Present-moment awareness and *nonjudgmental awareness* are skills that your teen can use to help focus his or her attention when having a strong emotion in a way that might lead to a calmer idea of what to do during these difficult moments. During this module, we will eventually introduce these skills in more emotionally challenging situations to encourage "real world" practice of awareness skills.

Present-Moment Awareness

Present-moment awareness means fully participating in the "here and now," not the future (which hasn't happened yet) or the past (which we can't change). *Noticing it, saying something about it,* and *experiencing it* will be the terms we use with your teen to help him or her practice being more aware of the present moment.

Nonjudgmental Awareness

Nonjudgmental awareness is a *compassionate, kind, and accepting* form of present-moment awareness. Sometimes when your teen is paying close attention to what he or she is thinking and feeling, your teen might become critical and judgmental of his or her own thoughts and feelings, and may try to change them or distract himself or herself because they feel so uncomfortable.

Being nonjudgmentally aware means paying attention to what is happening around you and inside of you, and treating these observations similar to how you would treat a friend's observations—meaning in a kinder way than maybe your teen has done in the past.

CHAPTER 7

Core Module 7: Situational Emotion Exposure

(Recommended Length: at least 2 sessions[1])

MATERIALS NEEDED FOR THE MODULE

- Module 7 Workbook Materials:
  1. *Emotional Behavior Form* (Form 7.1)
  2. *Sample Completed Emotional Behavior Form* (Figure 7.1)
  3. *Tracking the Before, During, and After* (Form 7.2)
  4. *Emotion Curve: Avoidance/Escape* (Figure 7.2)
  5. *Emotion Curve: Habituation* (Figure 7.3)
  6. *Emotion Curve: Habituation with Practice* (Figure 7.4)
  7. *My Emotion Ladder* (Form 7.3)
- A parent module summary form is provided at the end of this chapter to help support review of module materials with the parent(s) of your adolescent client. You may also use materials from Chapter 9 (Module-P) to help support these discussions.

Assessments to Be Given at *Every* Session:

- Parent and Adolescent Ratings: *Weekly Top Problems Tracking Form* (Appendix 1.3 at the end of Chapter 1 in this Therapist Guide)

---

[1] No formal maximum number of sessions. This module may be used as much as needed (up to the total number of allowable treatment sessions).

At the outset of Core Module 7, you will review previously discussed skills with the adolescent. Within this module you will be working with the adolescent to identify situations in which she is continuing to use maladaptive emotional behaviors, including behavioral avoidance, cognitive avoidance, aggression, and others to cope with strong emotions. You will work with the adolescent to help her approach and/or use more adaptive behaviors in these situations. Encourage the adolescent to use previously learned skills as a means of remaining in these situations while observing the way her emotions change. Information about additional skills applicable to those with obsessive-compulsive symptoms or needs for social skills development in concert with situational emotion exposure is provided as well.

- **Goal 1:** Review previously learned skills and create the adolescent's *Emotional Behavior Form* (Form 7.1).
- **Goal 2:** Practice entering situations in which the adolescent has previously used maladaptive emotional behaviors, encouraging the adolescent to monitor her emotional reactions to these situations.
- **Goal 3:** (Optional) Adapt situational emotion exposures to special cases—dealing with distress, introducing social skills, and adding response prevention goals.

Therapist Note—Unified Protocol Theory

*In many ways, the heart of any cognitive-behavioral approach to emotional disorders involves practice engaging in opposite action or different, more helpful action when at the height of intense, dysregulated emotions. In Core Module 3, we introduced this concept to your adolescent client and practiced engaging in opposite actions related to sadness. Here in Core Module 7, you will help your adolescent client first take stock of all she has accomplished thus far in treatment and what emotional behaviors remain problematic for her. Following this, you will introduce and practice engagement in an array of opposite actions regarding avoidance and similar behaviors. This technique, referred to as **exposure**, could be considered a therapy unto itself and can last for an unspecified amount of time as you and your client work to achieve remaining emotional behavior reduction goals. It is best practiced directly with your adolescent client to start and in a manner that truly engages her in experiencing her strong emotions, while preventing problematic avoidance and escape behaviors. As you practice exposure, you* *will find yourself using techniques from throughout this manual to encourage awareness of emotional experiences and flexible thinking (in the Before condition), and maybe some occasional problem solving too, in order to maximize the benefits of exposure for your client.*

Core Module 7 Content (Divided into Goals)

Goal 1

Review previously learned skills and create the adolescent's Emotional Behavior Form *(Form 7.1).*

> **Therapist Note**
> - *Don't forget to start* each session *re-rating top problems with the adolescent and parent.*
> - *Don't forget to give parent the Core Module 7 summary form to aid in understanding this module's important material. Spend some time in one session during this module to review this form with the parent.*

Skill Review

This should be a relatively brief review of skills learned up to this point. Begin with an open-ended discussion allowing the adolescent to describe the skills she has learned and identify which ones she has found to be most helpful. The goal is not to enter into a lengthy discussion of the use of each skill or to quiz the adolescent, but to ensure that the skill is available to the adolescent should she need it later. The *Reviewing Your Skills* section in Chapter 7 of the workbook can be used to structure this discussion and remind the adolescent of concepts she has learned thus far.

Create the Adolescent's *Emotional Behavior Form*

As both a review of progress to date and in preparation for conducting situational emotion exposures with the adolescent, you should create an *Emotional Behavior Form* (Form 7.1) with your client *before discussing the rationale for exposure*. Work with the adolescent to identify a number of situations in which she is currently using maladaptive emotional behaviors, as well as the emotional behaviors she is using. Examples of emotional behaviors may include behavioral avoidance, cognitive avoidance (e.g., distraction, rumination), reassurance-seeking or other controlling behaviors, use of safety behaviors, withdrawal behaviors, and even maladaptive approach-oriented behaviors such as physical or verbal aggression.

Once you have worked with the adolescent to identify approximately 5 to 10 such situations and behaviors, you may begin to enter them on the *Emotional Behavior Form* (Form 7.1). It is helpful to refer to the *Sample Completed Emotional Behavior Form* (Figure 7.1) during this activity both for sample item ideas and to help the adolescent understand how to generate ideas for her own *Emotional Behavior Form*. As exemplified within the *Sample Completed Emotional Behavior Form*, for each item, the adolescent should indicate the relevant problematic situation or thing triggering an emotional response, the type of emotional behavior being used in response to the situation/thing, and the intensity of the emotion the situation/thing elicits. Typically items are entered on the *Emotional Behavior Form* in order, with items eliciting the lowest degree of emotion on the bottom and those eliciting the strongest emotions near the top. If you are working with an adolescent who struggles with more than one type of strong emotion, it may also be helpful to write down the emotion the adolescent experiences in the "Emotion" column. As the adolescent begins to engage in the exposures over time, she may indicate when she has completed an exposure by marking a "Y" or "N" in the corresponding "Did You Work on This?" column.

As the therapist, you should think very carefully about being as specific and pragmatic as possible in your choice of items, with an eye toward their realization as situational exposures in this module. When creating the *Emotional Behavior Form* with the adolescent, reviewing Form 7.2: *Tracking the Before, During, and After* and other home learning worksheets may be helpful for identifying the situations and behaviors that are still causing difficulty for the adolescent. You may also wish to consult the adolescent's and parent's *Top Problems* form to identify remaining problem areas that may be addressed through exposure. *For some adolescents, it may be helpful to focus first on identifying situations/triggers and thereafter on identifying emotional behaviors.* This approach may work particularly well for adolescents with fear-based disorders or social anxiety, as the situations resulting in emotional behaviors may be especially obvious. *For other adolescents, however, it may be most helpful to begin by discussing the adolescent's engagement in problematic emotional behaviors.* This approach may work best for some adolescents with OCD as well as for adolescents who struggle with anger and frustration. For these adolescents, the emotional behaviors may be especially obvious or easy to identify (e.g., checking, cleaning rituals, angry outbursts, aggression), but situations that trigger these emotional behaviors may initially be less obvious. The following is a list of emotional behaviors that are useful targets for exposure. You may find it helpful to think about whether your adolescent client is using any of the following unhelpful emotional behaviors when developing the *Emotional Behavior Form*:

- Avoidance
- Escape
- Withdrawal/isolation
- Bringing along other people (e.g., only going to parties with a friend)
- Distraction
- Emotion suppression
- Worry
- Rituals (e.g., checking, cleaning, using special words or phrases, evening)
- Anger outbursts
- Physical aggression

Some adolescents are able to identify very general situational/object-related triggers for their emotional behaviors, but it can be helpful here to work with them to determine the core belief or core fear about the situation that triggers the emotional behavior. For example, going to school in the morning may result in significant avoidance and other emotional behaviors. However, it is difficult to design an effective exposure without obtaining more information from the adolescent about which aspects of school elicit strong emotions and result in emotional behaviors. If you know avoidance is due to worries about being judged negatively by peers while walking through the hallways, it is much easier to design an effective exposure specifically targeting the adolescent's core fears.

Suggested Home Learning Assignment: Tracking Opposite Action Using the Before, During, and After Form

Have the adolescent continue to track her emotional experiences using Form 7.2: *Tracking the Before, During, and After*. In preparation for exposures, instruct the adolescent to begin to practice acting opposite to some of her emotional behaviors and to note how acting opposite affects her emotional experience and its consequences. In this case, the Before would refer to the trigger (e.g., invited to a party and did not want to go), the During would refer to the emotional response while engaging in the opposite action (e.g., thought no one would like her outfit, had butterflies in her stomach, but went anyway), and the After would refer to the consequence of completing the exercise (e.g., sat with distress, was able to have fun with friends).

Goal 2

Practice entering situations in which the adolescent has previously used maladaptive emotional behaviors, encouraging the adolescent to monitor her emotional reactions to these situations.

Situational Emotion Exposure as an "Emotion-Focused Behavioral Experiment"

Situational emotion exposure is defined by engagement with a situation where the adolescent experiences an uncomfortable emotion, including fear, anxiety, sadness, and anger. Frequently, the adolescent has been avoiding or enduring such situations with the aid of other emotional behaviors (e.g., distraction, bringing along an object or person, physical or verbal aggression). By entering and enduring increasingly difficult situations associated with these intense emotions, the adolescent can learn that she does not need to engage in avoidance or other emotional behaviors as a way to manage uncomfortable or intense emotional states. Rather, through exposure, the adolescent can observe that nothing truly dangerous or terrible is happening and adjust her cognitions and behaviors to allow for continued engagement in such situations.

It may be useful to describe situational emotion exposures to the adolescent as another type of emotion-focused behavioral experiment, similar to those in which the adolescent participated in Module 3. For each exposure, the adolescent could define the experimental task (or the exposure task), identify her initial guesses or interpretations (or hypotheses) about what will happen in that experiment, evaluate these guesses to determine if they are realistic (using Detective Questioning and Detective Thinking), and then monitor the progress and outcomes of the experiment through use of good awareness skills throughout the exposure. In the end, the results of the experiment should be compared to her initial guesses. The use of this metaphor is not required, but it has proven useful to many therapists administering this treatment. Emphasize that the goal is to learn that we can experience whatever emotions come up while in any given situation, without doing anything to get rid of them, and that we will still be okay.

Why Does Exposure Work?

The adolescent may fear entering any of the situations she has been avoiding or enduring by using maladaptive emotional behaviors. She may feel these situations are genuinely dangerous or that she may not be able to cope with them. Suggest that if she faces situations that elicit strong emotions, without avoiding them or engaging in any emotional behaviors to lessen her experience of them, her strong emotions will start to feel less intense over time. This happens, in part, because of something called **habituation**.

Habituation involves purposely allowing an intense emotional response to occur when presented with a feared or upsetting situation, without trying to get out of a situation, resulting in the response becoming less intense over time. Looking at Figure 7.2: *Emotion Curve: Avoidance/Escape*, explain that the descent after the peak of the curve has probably been happening as a result of avoidance or use of other emotional behaviors that may quickly reduce the intensity of an emotion. However, explain that avoidance and other emotional behaviors prevent the adolescent from learning that reduction in emotion will eventually occur as a result of staying in the situation and that negative consequences will generally not result from this (other than simply feeling uncomfortable). Use Figure 7.3: *Emotion Curve: Habituation* to illustrate this point.

It may be helpful to emphasize that when we begin to approach uncomfortable situations that we have previously avoided or in which we have used problematic emotional behaviors, our discomfort in those situations may not reduce all the way. In fact, we may still feel some distress or intense emotions the entire time we are in the situation. Emphasize to the adolescent that this is a *completely normal response*. Even if her anxiety does not fully reduce, the next time she approaches the situation or one like it, it will likely not be quite as uncomfortable or anxiety-provoking. This phenomenon is sometimes referred to as **between-session habituation**. You may wish to use Figure 7.4: *The Emotion Curve: Habituation with Practice* to illustrate this point.

Another reason why exposure works so well is that, when a person repeatedly faces situations that cause strong or uncomfortable emotions, she may realize that her initial worst-case automatic interpretation (i.e., thinking trap) of what might happen is not true, or, if it is true, the outcome is not as terrible as she anticipated. This phenomenon is sometimes referred to a **belief disconfirmation**. Similar to what occurs during Detective Thinking, adolescents who repeatedly face situations that cause feelings of anger, sadness, anxiety, or other uncomfortable emotions gradually gather evidence that helps them cope more effectively in similar situations in the future. For example, the adolescent may gather evidence that she is able to survive such an uncomfortable situation, that the worst possible outcome did not occur or was not actually that bad, or that strong emotions become more tolerable as one gets used to experiencing them. As a result, she will become more confident in her ability to cope with difficult situations.

Therapist Note

Habituation during an exposure is not necessary for an exposure to be effective and for strong emotions to reduce over time. However, if habituation does not occur, you may wish to process this with the adolescent's parent(s) following the exposure activity. Parents may view the lack of habituation during exposure as an indication that the child cannot handle exposure work, and they may request that you discontinue or needlessly "dial down" exposures as a result. Some psychoeducation about why lack of habituation may be an acceptable outcome, as well as how to handle any youth distress to follow, would be wise to utilize in this case.

Dealing with Subtle Avoidance and/or Safety Behaviors

During situational emotion exposures it is important that the adolescent remain aware of her emotional experience. Efforts to distance herself from this experience should be monitored. For instance, during the sensational exposures in Core Module 4, you encouraged the adolescent to keep doing those activities, even when physical sensations increased, as opposed to discontinuing the task too soon because of distress, which might be considered an **avoidance behavior**. Avoidance behaviors may be contrasted with frank attempts to leave emotionally evocative situational exposures, which are often referred to as **escape behaviors**. If avoidance or escape behaviors are noted during exposure tasks, the adolescent may need to pause her actions and start over in the task, with overt effort to attend to the things about the situation and her response to it that made her want to avoid or escape. Giving the adolescent a sense of control over which exposures she engages in, and when, can also help minimize avoidance and escape responses.

Additionally, you should keep an eye out for attempts to engage in **safety behaviors** during exposures. Safety behaviors are unneeded actions the adolescent may take in order to make herself believe that a given experience is, in fact, safe. For instance, if the adolescent believes she would only feel safe taking a car ride if her parent were with her, riding in the car only when her parent is present would be a safety behavior. Eventually, the goal should be for the adolescent to understand that she can ride in a car with a whole variety of people and that she is in no more danger on those occasions than she would be at any other time. Cell phones, water bottles, and other objects can also serve as similar **safety objects**, and exposures may need to be initiated or re-initiated without such safety objects to maximize the intensity and effects of the exposure.

Exposure Practice—*My Emotion Ladder*

You can use Form 7.3: *My Emotion Ladder* to break down broader triggers from Form 7.1: *Emotional Behavior Form* into smaller, more approachable steps for exposure. Ask the adolescent to identify a potential exposure to be completed in session (or help derive one for her) using Form 7.1. Then use Form 7.3 to break down any individual item on Form 7.1 into its component steps to approach and eventually achieve the exposure goal. You are not required to use both forms for exposure planning, but it may be useful to map out the smaller steps toward achieving a maximally intense exposure at least one time on the *My Emotion Ladder* form so that the adolescent (and parent[s]) understand how to break down a larger exposure goal into its component, graduated steps.

For example, for an adolescent who has "speaking in front of the class" as an item on her *Emotional Behavior Form*, you might begin by working with the adolescent to simply say hello to an unfamiliar person in session as one step on her *My Emotion Ladder* form, and then fill in the remainder of this plan with at-home and in-session exposure opportunities (e.g., saying hello to two people, reading in front of a friend for 2 minutes, reading in front of two friends for 2 minutes, reading in front of a small group of people who work in the clinic office in session for 2 minutes; then expanding time goals for public speaking). Use as many graduated steps as needed for the adolescent to feel confident about achieving her goal, but be aware that some adolescents may select steps that are too small or break exposure tasks down into too many steps as a means of avoidance. Therefore, you should take care to ensure that the adolescent is working toward achieving more challenging steps at an appropriate pace. You will not always do every step on the *My Emotion Ladder* for each item on the *Emotional Behavior Form*, as this may be practically impossible, but rather communicate clearly to the adolescent that you will progress through less difficult steps before proceeding to more challenging ones.

Therapist Note

Consider the adolescent's motivation level and degree of treatment engagement as she sets forth on difficult in-session exposures. There may also be times where an adolescent struggles to identify situational emotion exposure opportunities, and you may need to be creative in trying out a variety of anticipated triggers, including use of confederates or engaging in exposure opportunities that are similar to the trigger stimuli or situation in order to simply "get the ball rolling." While it will be useful to eventually have the adolescent engage in situational emotion exposures that are directly related to her presenting concerns, it may be necessary to help the adolescent engage in situational emotion exposures that may not appear to be as directly related (e.g., exposures eliciting the same emotions, but in less overtly feared or avoided situations). Frequently, once you attempt to do a few in-session exposures, opportunities for future ones or ideas about pacing of exposures will become more apparent.

Once You Have the First *My Emotion Ladder* Form Ready

Ask the adolescent to identify how she expects to feel when completing this exposure. Pull for as much detail as possible. Get her to describe the emotions she expects to experience, the physical sensations she believes she will have, and the thoughts she expects to be present. Ask her to rate the amount of emotion she expects to have in that situation using a Subjective Units of Distress (SUDS) scale (e.g., from 0 to 8).

Therapist Note

This discussion may increase arousal prior to even a relatively lower-level exposure. However, for the purposes of exposure success, this is not a problem and in fact may be useful to illustrate how habituation might operate. In general, though, lengthy pre-exposure discussions could promote avoidance behavior and should be minimized when not completely needed.

Monitoring can be done simply (before, during, and after the exposure) or in a more detailed fashion (before, at several points during, and after the exposure). You can use SUDS ratings to track the adolescent's response in real time or, if she is poor at self-rating numerically, you can use temperature words (hot, warm, cool, cold) to observe changes in her emotional state during exposure.

It is important to debrief after the exposure. Issues to cover are as follows:

- Was there anything that surprised her?
- Were her guesses supported/did what she expected to happen occur?
- Did she learn anything new about the situation or about her behaviors during the exposure?
- Did her ability to observe the strong emotion she was experiencing improve over time?
- Was her emotion level highest before the exposure began? Did it continue to drop during the exposure? What about after the exposure was over?

You may also want to spend some time discussing the following after each exposure:

- Point out any noticeable patterns in changes in the adolescent's self-ratings over the course of the exposure.
- If the adolescent experiences habituation during the exposure, return to the emotion curves showing that in the past her emotion likely went down at the point she decided to avoid a feared thing/situation and how this response has changed over time through exposure.
- If habituation does not occur during the exposure, encourage the adolescent to verbalize anything new she learned about the situation or about her ability to deal with strong emotions. Emphasize that some situations require repeated practice before the intensity of the emotional response will change.

Therapist Note

Home-based practice of exposures should be focused on expanding the type and breadth of exposure experiences and creating exposures in the actual environments that trigger distress. For the first home learning exposure, it is often helpful for the adolescent to repeat an exposure similar to the one she has already completed in the clinic in a different environment. Repeating an exposure that has already been completed increases the likelihood that the adolescent will be successful, and it facilitates generalization of learning to a new environment. Often, exposures conducted at home or for home learning are those that may be practically difficult to arrange in session. Extensive in-session practice with exposures will help to prepare the adolescent for such at-home activity, and it is often useful to make a specific plan with the adolescent as to when and how she will complete the exposure. You may also wish to work with parents to help monitor safety behaviors and avoidance behaviors at home in order to facilitate the most naturalistic exposures possible.

Suggested Home Learning Assignment: Situational Exposure

Have the adolescent complete approximately **two** situational emotion exposure activities each week between the remaining sessions. Ask the adolescent to monitor her emotional reactions during these exposure tasks using Form 7.2: *Tracking the Before, During, and After.* In this case, the Before would refer to the planned exposure (e.g., planned speech in front of two friends), the During would refer to the emotional response during the exposure (e.g., thought I would make a mistake and everyone would laugh, had butterflies in my stomach, but finished my speech), and the After would refer to the consequence of completing the exercise (e.g., sat with distress, felt better when it was over).

Goal 3

(Optional) Adapt situational emotion exposures to special cases—dealing with distress, introducing social skills, and adding response prevention goals.

Dealing with Distress

The most common thing new therapists working with this module may fear is that their adolescent client will become distressed during these situational exposures. This is a reasonable concern, as exposures are designed to provoke distress! Your best mode of operation with exposures is to be bold and try exposures that are as naturalistic and even "over the top" at times in order to achieve exposure goals, scaling back only if needed to meet the demands of the adolescent's concerns. However, there are times when the adolescent may be reluctant to engage in the bold exposure you have planned. Any step toward an exposure or similar opposite action goal should be encouraged, and sufficient time should be allowed for the adolescent to make the active decision to try these scenarios. While compromises about exposure are sometimes needed to end session on a positive or approach-oriented note, it is okay for the adolescent's distress to not reduce in the planned exposure as discussed above.

Incorporating Social Skill Goals

Some adolescents require more information about *how* to approach a new situation than others. Particularly, adolescents with social anxiety concerns may need more prompting about entering and exiting situations smoothly, maintaining conversations, and selecting appropriate peers or peer groups for exposure opportunities. A good plan of action in these cases is to introduce the social skill goal that will be targeted in the planned exposure (e.g., how to keep a conversation going past simply initiating it), role-play the social skill with a confederate or the therapist, and then practice the new skill in a novel situation or with a novel person.

Incorporating Response Prevention

In the context of obsessive-compulsive symptoms, situational emotion exposures sometimes involve approaching feared situations in a similar manner to that described above, but it is important to understand that these also include what are referred to as *response prevention* techniques as well. Response prevention is when you are literally preventing a youth from engaging in a compulsive or repetitive behavior. This is often an "all or nothing" type of exposure. It can be difficult to only partially prevent a compulsion—although some forms of response prevention may involve simply trying out a different response from the one the adolescent feels she should do or "messing with" the desired compulsive response. Nonetheless, you can delay, reduce, or fully eliminate a compulsive behavior using such techniques within this module.

Parent Summary Form for Core Module 7: Situational Emotion Exposure

Core Module 7 is designed to help your teen enter situations that he or she currently avoids and/or associates with uncomfortable emotions. This will allow your teen to practice skills he or she has learned throughout treatment instead of acting on emotional behaviors. With practice, your teen will learn that he or she *can* experience whatever emotions come up in any given situation without doing anything to get rid of the emotions. The more your teen practices this, the less often problematic emotional experiences may happen, so it's a pretty important skill!

Why Does Exposure Work?

There are several explanations for why exposure is effective. No matter how intense your teen's uncomfortable emotions may be, with practice, he or she will learn to tolerate those emotions without doing anything to get rid of them. Allowing physical sensations, thoughts, and emotions to exist, without trying to escape a situation, will actually decrease the intensity of these sensations and emotions over time. By continuing to approach (rather than avoid) the things that trigger your teen's uncomfortable emotions, your teen will also learn that some of the negative, upsetting, or frightening things he or she expects to happen are unlikely or less likely than other outcomes. Eventually, your teen will experience less difficulty approaching these situations on his or her own or will no longer need to use problematic emotional behaviors to get through the situation.

The *Emotional Behaviors Form* and *My Emotion Ladder*

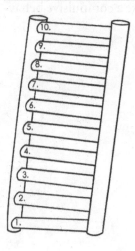

You, your teen, and his or her therapist will create an *Emotional Behaviors Form* and use it as a guide for selecting situations for exposures. Your teen's therapist will start working with your teen on tolerating the situations that are less intense and then gradually work toward completing more emotionally intense or difficult exposures. Your teen and therapist will also work together to identify specific steps that need to be completed at home and in session to work toward approaching difficult situations. This is known as the *My Emotion Ladder* form.

Thinking About Exposures as Experiments

Situational exposures can also be described as experiments, much like those your teen completed during Core Module 3 of this treatment. Like a scientific experiment, your teen has guesses or hypotheses about what will happen in an emotional situation. Your teen will be evaluating how realistic those guesses are (using Detective Thinking) before the exposure occurs. Then, your teen will try out these guesses in an experiment where he or she exposes himself or herself to a situation that brings up strong emotions without engaging in emotional behaviors like avoidance, distraction, or aggression. Finally, your teen will evaluate the results to see if his or her hypotheses about what would happen in the situation turned out to be true. As more experiments are conducted, your adolescent will begin to see that his or her initial guesses may not have been the most realistic ones and that he or she can get through the situation without acting on emotions.

What Can I Do to Support My Teen with Situational Emotion Exposures?

✓ Reward your teen's *effort*! Even if he or she seemed to struggle during the exposure, praise or reward your teen just for trying.

✓ If your teen appears to be struggling during exposures, remind him or her of the skills learned in therapy. It may also be helpful to remind your teen of the long-term benefits of feeling uncomfortable in the short term.

✓ Be creative! Think of creative ideas to help your teen enter situations he or she previously avoided.

✓ Encourage your teen to practice exposures every day. Just like learning an instrument or playing a sport, overcoming anxiety, depression, and other emotional disorders takes practice and effort!

✓ Live the "exposure lifestyle." If you notice any situation during which your teen appears to be having a hard time, think of how to turn that situation into an exposure or behavioral experiment.

✓ Remember that your teen will likely feel discomfort at the beginning of exposures. This is sometimes difficult for parents to see, but remember that this is normal and it is important for your teen to learn that he or she can overcome these strong emotions *independently*.

✓ Avoid accommodating or allowing your teen to engage in avoidance behaviors. Sometimes an exposure may prove to be more difficult than expected and your teen refuses to do it as planned. It is always better to make the exposure a bit easier (we call this "dialing it down") rather than allow your teen to quit the task altogether, which can reinforce avoidance.

CHAPTER 8

Core Module 8: Reviewing Accomplishments and Looking Ahead

(Recommended Length: 1 Session)

MATERIALS NEEDED FOR THE MODULE

- Module 8 Workbook Materials:
  1. *Skills I Know and How to Use Them* (Worksheet 8.1)
  2. *Taking Stock of All I've Accomplished* (Worksheet 8.2)
  3. *Becoming My Own Therapist!* (Worksheet 8.3)
  4. Copy of *Emotional Behavior Form* already filled out by adolescent (Form 7.1)
- A parent module summary form is provided at the end of this chapter to help support review of module materials with the parent(s) of your adolescent client. You may also use materials from Chapter 9 (Module-P) to help support these discussions.

Assessments to Be Given at *Every* Session:

- Parent and Adolescent Ratings: *Weekly Top Problems Tracking Form* (Appendix 1.3 at the end of Chapter 1 in this Therapist Guide)

Overall Core Module 8 Goals

By the end of treatment, you have worked closely with the adolescent to learn what skills are most effective for him to manage his intense or uncomfortable emotions, and your client has done what he can to make progress toward adjusting problematic emotional behaviors. For this final session, it will be important to review all the skills covered as well as the progress that your adolescent client has made in order to emphasize his ability to effectively address strong or intense emotions that he may experience in the future. It will also be helpful for you as a therapist to get feedback about what he found helpful in treatment and what he did not find to be useful, as this will impact which skills you should emphasize in planning for future challenges. As the adolescent has gained a support system by coming to therapy each week, it may be unsettling for therapy to end. Helping your client plan for future stressors and decide what skills to put in place will help prevent a relapse to pretreatment levels of distress. In this module, you will find a number of worksheets, activities, and optional exercises that can facilitate review of skills and treatment progress. If you are covering this module in a single session (the typical module length), you are unlikely to be able to cover all of the materials presented and should select those that you feel will be most helpful and appealing to your adolescent client.

- **Goal 1:** Review skills that have been most useful to the adolescent.
- **Goal 2:** Review progress by discussing changes in the adolescent's (and parents') Top Problems ratings and Form 7.1: *Emotional Behavior Form* ratings.
- **Goal 3:** Make a post-treatment plan in order to prevent relapse.

Therapist Note—Unified Protocol Theory

Core Module 8 provides an opportunity to revisit how your adolescent client has benefited from the Unified Protocol approach. There are a multitude of potential topics you may be covering from past modules as you approach termination with your client, with a key emphasis on ascertaining which aspects of this approach have been most useful to him in effectively managing intense emotions and problematic emotional behaviors. You will want your client to leave therapy on a positive and empowering note. Frequently, adolescents who reach this point in treatment have overcome significant or problematic roadblocks and have achieved a healthier, more adaptive manner of approaching (rather than avoiding) intense or challenging emotions in their lives. This is a time to relish such success and plan for an outstanding future of healthy coping.

Goal 1

Review skills that have been most useful to the adolescent and progress made in treatment.

Therapist Note

▪ *Don't forget to start each session re-rating top problems with the adolescent and parent.*

▪ *Don't forget to give the parent the Core Module 8 summary form to aid in understanding this module's important material. Spend some time reviewing this form with the parent.*

Skills and Progress Review

While in the waiting room or with you at the start of this module, have the adolescent client complete Worksheet 8.1: *Skills I Know and How to Use Them*, as this will be useful in guiding discussion in session.

Once in session, spend time reviewing the skills mentioned on the worksheet, making sure to assess the adolescent's familiarity with each skill, and provide clarification about skills as needed. You should not spend time here extensively reviewing skills, but you can direct the adolescent back to relevant sections of the workbook to read on his own after treatment. Focus on encouraging the adolescent to personalize skills learned in treatment by having him articulate and note what he found most helpful about each skill.

You should also engage the adolescent in a discussion of how he will continue to use his skills in the future to manage situations or triggers that elicit strong emotions. Some skills, such as present-moment awareness, may be helpful to practice every day, and you may wish to help the adolescent make a plan for how and when to do so. Others, such as situational emotion exposures and problem solving, may be more situation-dependent. Now that you know the adolescent quite well, you will likely be able to anticipate and suggest situations in which the adolescent would benefit from continuing to practice specific skills.

Goal 2

Review progress by discussing changes in the adolescent's (and parents') Top Problems ratings and Emotional Behavior Form ratings.

Reviewing Changes in Top Problems

You have been asking the adolescent and his parent(s) to rate top problems every week throughout treatment, and these ratings are likely to have decreased substantially by the final session. Reviewing changes in top problems with the adolescent can help build his self-confidence, promote his sense of self-efficacy, and develop motivation for him to continue using skills to face his uncomfortable emotions after treatment. When reviewing changes in top problems, it is important to both celebrate the adolescent's successes and identify areas that he should continue to work on after treatment. Later in this session, you will be helping the adolescent to develop a plan for continuing to make progress in these areas.

To facilitate the discussion of changes in top problems, it is often helpful to create a graph or other tool *before session* that visually illustrates changes in top problems over time. This is easily accomplished using Microsoft Excel or other computer programs, but you can also create such graphs by hand. Regardless of how you choose to represent changes in the adolescent's top problems, it is often helpful to discuss the following points:

- **When did the adolescent's top problems begin to decrease?** Did it occur during or right after the presentation of particular skills? If so, you may wish to help the adolescent identify how a particular skill may have contributed to the decrease.
- **Did any top problem ratings fluctuate, going up and down frequently over time?** If so, normalize this pattern for the adolescent. Emphasize that some problems do not decrease steadily over time, and draw the adolescent's attention to the overall downward trend (if there was one). You may also wish to address external factors that may have contributed to frequent fluctuations (e.g., for an adolescent with test anxiety, ratings might increase during standardized testing and finals and decrease over the summer).
- **Did any top problem ratings remain high until the onset of situational emotion exposures in Core Module 7?** If so, discuss how some problems really begin to improve when individuals start

to approach situations that elicit strong emotions without engaging in avoidance or other emotional behaviors.

- **Did any top problem ratings decrease minimally or not at all?** If so, you may wish to help the adolescent discuss which skills he has used in an attempt to address the problem area, as well as why he feels those skills have not been very successful. Later in this session, you will help the adolescent make a plan for continuing to address these remaining problem areas. Normalize this pattern by discussing that some problems may take longer to improve than others. In fact, it is very common to see further decreases in some problem areas occur months or more later, once the adolescent has had more time to practice using his skills in a range of situations. It is also important to note that even if the adolescent's rating has not changed, he may have experienced changes in the type or extent of emotional behaviors he uses in response to the problem or in his ability to deal with discomfort in his body during intense emotions. Explore these possibilities with the adolescent and highlight such changes where applicable.

You may also wish to engage the adolescent's parent(s) in a discussion of how their top problems ratings have changed over treatment. You can provide parents with a graph of changes in their own ratings of the adolescent's top problems at the beginning of session and ask them to review the graph in the waiting room. Near the end of the session, parents may then be brought into the therapy room to discuss changes in their own ratings and to discuss the adolescent's plan for making continued gains.

Re-rating the Emotional Behavior Form

If you have not done so recently, also have your client re-rate his *Emotional Behavior Form* (Form 7.1). Review differences in both emotional behaviors used and reported intensity of emotion for each situation. You may wish to have the adolescent cross out situations that are no longer problematic and use a blank copy of the *Emotional Behavior Form* to plan exposures or other behavioral experiments he would like to continue to practice on his own after treatment.

Often, discussing changes in top problems and *Emotional Behavior Form* ratings can serve as an opportunity to celebrate the adolescent's successes and progress during treatment. It is, of course, possible that your client has not made significant gains during treatment, but that the decision has been made for treatment to end anyway. Even under these circumstances, it is important to keep the final session positive and hopeful, despite minimal progress or when some of the adolescent's goals have not yet been achieved. Be open and honest with the family about your thoughts on why treatment gains were or were not made so that future therapy might be more effective and/or current gains may be capitalized upon.

Taking Stock of Accomplishments

By discussing changes in the adolescent's top problem and *Emotional Behavior Form* ratings, you have provided him with data-driven evidence of progress he has made during treatment. Sometimes it can also be helpful to encourage your adolescent client to verbalize and/or record more global changes in his responses to strong emotions. You may wish to structure such a discussion by using Worksheet 8.2: *Taking Stock of All I've Accomplished*. You can use this worksheet to encourage the adolescent to consider difficult situations he has learned to manage, changes in the way he reacts to strong emotions, and changes in his overall functioning.

Goal 3
Make a post-treatment plan in order to prevent relapse.

Making a Plan for the Future

It will be important to let the adolescent know that he is likely to experience at least some anxiety, sadness, anger, or other intense emotions in the future. These are, after all, normal emotional responses to situations in our lives. It is more likely the adolescent will experience these emotions more intensely during times of stress. Inform the adolescent that a recurrence of some symptoms is natural and normal, and this does not mean his emotional disorder has returned. Rather, this would be an ideal time to take out his workbook and to review the knowledge, skills, and strategies he has attained during this treatment, all of which he can now use to address any symptoms that he may be experiencing. Therefore, it is important to remember to utilize the skills learned in treatment during periods of stress.

It may be helpful to define the terms *lapse* and *relapse* to clarify for the adolescent (and his parents) what the difference is between a temporary return of symptoms during a brief, stressful time (lapse) and a more significant and impairing return of symptoms (relapse). In the clinical research literature, a two-week timeframe is often cited as the minimum amount of time needed to count symptom return as a relapse, but the adolescent and parent should also consider the frequency (how often the problem is happening), duration (how long the problem has persisted), and relative impairment (how impactful the problem is in the adolescent's day-to-day life) of these symptoms, as well as how they compare with those at the start of this treatment, before deciding to return for additional intervention.

As the skills learned in treatment can be used at any time, emphasize that the adolescent can continue to make significant gains even though he is no longer meeting with you; however, this will require that he does not avoid situations that might bring on uncomfortable emotions. Emphasize that he will see the greatest gains if he continues to practice the skills he has learned in treatment on a regular basis so that the cycles that kept him from facing intense emotions previously don't recur.

Also emphasize that it will be important to be proactive when faced with stressors by implementing a plan of action based on Worksheet 8.3: *Becoming My Own Therapist!* You may use this worksheet to encourage the adolescent to identify remaining challenges and devise a plan for approaching these challenges using the skills he has learned in treatment. When completing this worksheet with the adolescent, you may find it helpful to use the *Weekly Top Problems Tracking Form* (in Appendix 1.3) and Form 7.1: *Emotional Behavior Form* to identify remaining challenges to focus on within the next four weeks. Be as specific as possible about behavioral goals to be accomplished in the upcoming month and the timeframe for accomplishing these goals.

Optional Activities for this Module

A number of potential activities for use in this module have been detailed below. Feel free to select an activity based on what you believe the adolescent will benefit most from in order to make his experience of using the Unified Protocol more meaningful or memorable as you complete treatment.

- If your client enjoys writing, he might enjoy writing a poem or brief narrative about his treatment gains.
- To facilitate a review of skills learned in treatment, you may wish to present the adolescent with a series of hypothetical situations he might plausibly encounter after treatment and ask him to describe which skills he would use in each situation.

- Sometimes it is helpful to have your client do a situational emotion exposure that he found quite difficult in the beginning but can do without struggle now. This is a concrete way of emphasizing the progress he has made, especially if he is not verbalizing that he is proud of his successes.

- Have your client discuss hopes and dreams about the future and empower him with the idea that the skills and behaviors he has learned will help him reach his goals.

- We often use the term "exposure lifestyle" in the UP-A to emphasize that once adolescents have achieved their goal of approaching previously avoided situations, they may feel empowered to continue doing so as they face new challenges. You may wish to use this term with your successful client as well. Ask the adolescent for concrete examples of how he might embody the "exposure lifestyle" in his life after treatment.

Parent Summary Form for Core Module 8: Reviewing Accomplishments and Looking Ahead

Core Module 8 is designed to review the skills covered and progress made in treatment. This module is also designed to plan for future stressors and decide on what skills to put in place.

Reviewing Skills and Progress

> **What Can I Do to Support My Teen With Reviewing Accomplishments and Looking Ahead?**
>
> ✓ Emphasize the gains, even if they are less than you would like, that your teen has made in treatment!
> ✓ Identify times that are likely to be stressful for your teen in the future and help him or her identify specific skills that can help your teen confront his or her emotions.
> ✓ Encourage your teen to continue to practice the skills and conduct emotion-focused behavioral experiments or exposures even though he or she is no longer in treatment.
> ✓ Know the signs that may indicate additional treatment is needed.

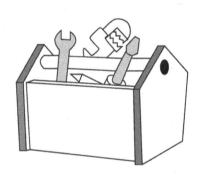

By this point in treatment you and your teen have learned a lot! It is important to recognize the changes your teen has made in dealing with strong emotions on a day-to-day basis and to provide him or her with positive feedback on progress. Your teen's therapist may review changes in your ratings of your teen's top problems over the course of therapy in order to point out areas in which he or she has made progress as well as problems your teen may wish to continue working on in the future. Identifying the skills your teen has found useful for dealing with uncomfortable emotions will assist him or her in dealing with such experiences helpfully and appropriately in the future.

Planning for the Future

Your teen is likely to experience at least some anxiety, sadness, or other strong emotions in the future. Strong emotions can be, after all, normal responses to events in our lives and do not necessarily mean his or her emotional disorder has returned. It is likely that your teen will experience these emotions more intensely during times of stress. Therefore, it will be important to help him or her remember to use the skills learned in treatment during periods of stress. Your teen should see continued gains if he or she continues to practice awareness, exposures, and other skills learned in therapy so that behaviors that previously kept him or her from facing and dealing with emotions more helpfully don't recur.

CHAPTER 9

Module-P: Parenting the Emotional Adolescent

(Recommended Length: as needed; typically 1–3 sessions)

MATERIALS NEEDED FOR THE MODULE

- *Sample Double Before, During, and After* (Figure 9.1 near the end of this chapter)
- *Double Before, During, and After* (Figure 9.2 near the end of this chapter)
- A parent module summary form is provided at the end of this chapter to help support review of module materials with the parent(s) of your adolescent client.

Assessments to Be Given at *Every* Session:

- Parent and Adolescent Ratings: *Weekly Top Problems Tracking Form* (Appendix 1.3 at the end of Chapter 1 in this Therapist Guide)

Overall Module-P Goals

The overall goal of Module-P is to introduce parents to the idea that the parenting behaviors they use in response to their adolescent's strong emotions may maintain or even amplify their adolescent's emotional responses. In this module, parents are encouraged to identify their own emotional responses to their adolescent's strong emotions, as well as the parenting behaviors they use to manage both their own and their adolescent's distress. Parents are then introduced to four parenting behaviors or "pitfalls" common to families of children and adolescents with emotional disorders, as well as "opposite parenting behaviors" that may be more effective in helping their adolescent to manage strong emotions. Each of these parenting behaviors may then be reviewed in more depth, depending upon the needs of the parents.

It is important to note that a brief review of current adolescent functioning and session topics may be accomplished *at the end of individual adolescent sessions* by using the Parent Module summary forms at the end of each UP-A chapter in this book; some of the topics reviewed in Module-P may also be incorporated in such discussions.

Additional parent-directed sessions (as covered in this module) are meant to review the topics below in greater depth than a brief meeting at the end of a given session would allow. Suggestions for when to provide more in-depth, parent-directed time in sessions are given in this module; however, this material may also be incorporated at any time, at your discretion. If the adolescent and family require more parent-directed time than this to negotiate major issues outside of those specified below or if a parent with his or her own psychopathology requires individual therapy for himself or herself, this is outside of the specifications for this module and referrals should be discussed. With this in mind, the specific goals of this module are as follows:

- **Goal 1:** Introduce parents to Figure 9.1: *Double Before, During, and After* (Double BDA) to increase parents' awareness of their own emotional responses to adolescent distress.
- **Goal 2:** Introduce parents to four emotional parenting behaviors that are generally thought to be ineffective or less effective ways of responding to adolescent distress.
- **Goal 3:** As applicable, discuss each emotional parenting behavior and its opposite parenting behavior in further detail.

Therapist Note—Unified Protocol Theory

Module-P is meant to support and reinforce all adolescent-directed therapy goals specified in the Unified Protocol. The materials provided in this module can likely benefit all parents. We provide these materials here as a whole section, rather than divided up throughout the core modules, to give you the flexibility to decide when and to what extent to use them. Some parents will only need a general introduction to the idea that their parenting behavior

---

impacts their adolescent's distress and emotional behaviors. For such par-
ents, potentially with fewer needs for clinical attention, you may wish to
use these materials more informally in the last 5 to 10 minutes of each
session, along with providing the Core Module Summary forms for each
session. Other parents might need focused attention on specific emotional
behaviors in the context of their adolescent's distress, particularly as you ask
the adolescent to change her emotional behaviors. For these latter parents,
we recommend using the material provided below for a partial or entire
session as you introduce emotion-focused behavioral experiments in Core
Module 3 and/or as you plan for situational emotion exposures in Core
Module 7. Additional suggestions for when to incorporate these materials
can be found in Therapist Notes throughout this module.

Module-P Content (Divided by Goals)

Goal 1

Introduce parents to Figure 9.1: Double Before, During, and After *to increase parents' awareness of their own emotional responses to adolescent distress.*

Parenting an emotional adolescent can be exhausting and confusing. Sometimes parents have their own mental health issues or environmental stressors that make parenting these adolescents even more challenging. However, even in families without such difficulties, the distress and requests for assistance and reassurance that some emotional adolescents present pose a unique parenting challenge. During these times, an adolescent's strong emotions and behaviors may be the trigger for an emotional response in the parents, and the parents may act on their own frustration, anxiety, or anger in a way that maintains or even amplifies their adolescent's emotions in the short and/or long term. If you notice this cycle occurring with an adolescent and parents, you may wish to schedule a parent session to begin to build parent awareness of how their own parenting behaviors may be reinforcing their adolescent's cycle of avoidance or cycle of other emotional behaviors. Use Figure 9.1: *Sample Double Before, During, and After* to guide discussion of this topic and Figure 9.2: *Double Before, During, and After* to walk the parents through an example of how this might apply to their specific situation.

> **Therapist Note**
>
> *As a default and as noted above, just before or during Core Modules 3 and 7 are helpful times to schedule a parent-only session dedicated to a discussion of emotional parenting behaviors. It is important to build parents' awareness of how their own distress may impact the adolescent's practice of emotion-focused behavioral experiments or exposure activities introduced in these modules. However, you may also wish to introduce the concept of emotional parenting behaviors earlier in treatment if it becomes clear that a parent is frequently utilizing any of the emotional parenting behaviors discussed in this module. If you wait until Module 7 to introduce these topics, parents who struggle significantly with overcontrol or inconsistency, for example, may not have enough opportunity to work on monitoring and changing these behaviors to be effective coaches for their adolescent during emotion exposures.*

If you determine that parents involved in treatment struggle with any of the emotional parenting behaviors discussed in this module, it is best to present these topics by first aligning with the family members over their struggle to parent their adolescent as best as they can. You should normalize the struggles parents face when parenting an adolescent with an emotional disorder, and you should be sure to praise parents for attempting to support their adolescent and manage their adolescent's behavior as best they can. Also, it is relevant to note that most of the difficulties demonstrated by parents of emotional adolescents may result from a normal, appropriate desire to *lessen* their adolescent's distress rather than encourage it. The problem is that such strategies typically operate to unintentionally limit the adolescent's interaction with upsetting situations or stimuli, thereby accidentally reinforcing the adolescent's emotional disorder symptoms over time.

Begin to introduce the idea of emotional parenting behaviors by asking the parents to take a look at Figure 9.1: *Sample Double Before, During, and After*. Be sure to emphasize the relationship between the example adolescent behaviors and the parent's emotional experience on the figure. Also review short- and long-term consequences and discuss how these parent and adolescent interaction patterns lead to future emotional experiences for both the parent and the adolescent. Once you have read through the example with the parents, have the parents think of a recent occasion when their adolescent experienced a strong emotion. The example should be one where the parents were at least present but ideally where they responded in some way to their adolescent's experience—verbally, behaviorally, or both. Using Figure 9.2: *Double Before, During, and After*, ask the parent to identify the Before (i.e., trigger), the During, and the After for their *adolescent's* emotional experience first. Note that parents may be unable to provide information about certain aspects of their adolescent's emotional experience, particularly their adolescent's thoughts or body clues. This is okay—encourage the parents to identify as many aspects of the experience as they can or at least describe what they perceived occurring in the given situation. When completing the Before, During, and After for their adolescent, parents should be instructed to focus on the short- and long-term consequences of the emotional and behavioral responses exhibited by the adolescent rather than those exhibited by the parent.

Next, explain to the parents that observing their adolescent having a strong emotional response or engaging in emotionally driven behaviors can often trigger an emotional reaction in a parent. Thus, in the "Parent" portion of the figure, parents should note in the "Before" section the portion of the adolescent's emotional experience that they observed and that triggered their own emotional reaction. Assist the parents in identifying the emotion they were experiencing, all the while normalizing any feelings of anxiety, frustration, anger, or sadness that may have occurred for the parents. Encourage the parents to identify the three parts of their own emotional response, including their thoughts, body sensations, and behaviors. When exploring short- and long-term consequences with the parents in the "After" section of Figure 9.2: *Double Before, During, and After*, encourage the parents to identify how their own emotional parenting behaviors may have had short- and long-term consequences both for themselves and for their adolescent. Refer back to Figure 9.1: *Sample Double Before, During, and After* to help illustrate this concept.

You should have the parents complete at least one or two examples at home over the course of treatment so that you have ample opportunities to point out the relationship between emotional parenting behaviors and the adolescent's future emotional responding. If you suspect that the parents may struggle with any of the common emotional parenting behaviors listed below, it may be helpful to complete a *Double Before, During, and After* for that parenting behavior.

Goal 2

Introduce parents to four emotional parenting behaviors that are generally thought to be ineffective or less effective ways of responding to adolescent distress.

In addition to introducing parents to the general concept that parenting behaviors may have an important impact upon an adolescent's current or future emotional behaviors, you may want to spend time focusing on some specific parenting behaviors that appear to be problematic for the particular parent(s) you are working with. Table 9.1 illustrates the types of emotional parenting behaviors that are common in parents of adolescents with emotional disorders, examples of each type of parenting behavior, potential consequences of the behavior, and the interventions that will be introduced in this module as opposite actions to each type of emotional parenting behavior. Depending upon the parents, you may find it useful to introduce all four of these emotional parenting behaviors or to focus on just one or two that seem most relevant to the concern you observe. If you have not observed such reactions, nor have they been identified by the adolescent or parents previously, it may not be worth spending excess time discussing such pitfalls in session, as parents may react defensively to this presentation.

Regardless of how many emotional parenting behaviors you choose to discuss, be sure to emphasize that:

1. These behaviors are extremely common in parents of adolescents with emotional disorders;
2. These behaviors feel very natural at times or may be utilized commonly with youth without emotional disorders (without a problem), and thus it is easy to find oneself using them repeatedly; and
3. Changing emotional parenting behaviors is not easy and may take time and patience on the part of the parent.

Model a nonjudgmental stance when reviewing the four emotional parenting behaviors listed in Table 9.1, and encourage parents to approach their previous attempts to manage their adolescent's difficult emotions in a nonjudgmental way.

Introduce parents to the idea that in this treatment, just as parents will be an emotional "coach" for their adolescent, you will serve as a "coach" for the parents to help them learn to identify their own emotional parenting behaviors and replace them with alternative parenting behaviors:

"Let's think of you as a 'coach' who is going to cheer on your teen as she works to succeed, supporting her appropriately and reinforcing healthy behaviors when she is feeling overwhelmed by strong emotions. In these parenting sessions, I can also be your coach as you learn how to reinforce appropriate behavior and how to deal with difficult emotions that may arise when your adolescent is overcoming these obstacles."

Table 9.1 Common Emotional Parenting Behaviors and Their Opposite Parenting Behaviors

Emotional Parenting Behavior	Examples of Emotional Parenting Behavior	Potential Long-Term Consequences for Adolescent	Opposite Parenting Behavior Taught in This Module
Overcontrol/ Overprotection	▪ Speaking for the adolescent in social situations ▪ Arranging social activities for the adolescent ▪ Not allowing the adolescent to engage in age-appropriate activities for fear something might happen to him or her ▪ Making excuses to others for the adolescent's withdrawal or avoidance behaviors	Low adolescent self-efficacy; increased avoidance; poor social skills	Healthy independence-granting
Criticism	▪ Excessively attending to the adolescent's mistakes or misbehaviors ▪ Focusing on the negative aspects of the adolescent's behavior and ignoring the positive aspects ▪ Subtle behaviors such as eye rolling, head shaking, or sighing ▪ Telling the adolescent that he/she shouldn't feel a certain way or should stop feeling a certain way	Low adolescent self-efficacy; down mood; giving up easily; excessive people-pleasing behaviors; behavior problems	Expressing empathy, using positive reinforcement, active ignoring
Inconsistency	▪ Not following through with rewards when promised ▪ Punishing naughty behavior sometimes but allowing the adolescent to get away with it at other times ▪ Frequently changing household rules ▪ Encouraging approach behaviors at certain times and avoidance behaviors at other times	Increased behavior problems; increased avoidance; increased anxiety	Using consistent discipline/praise
Excessive Modeling of Intense Emotions and Avoidance	▪ Extreme reactions to and avoidance of objectively non-threatening situations ▪ Expressing adult worries in front of the adolescent ▪ Suppression of emotion and refusal to talk about sad events that impact the family ▪ Using aggressive behaviors or swearing excessively when angry ▪ Isolating from the family when angry or upset	Increased emotional reactivity and avoidance	Healthy emotional modeling

Goal 3

Discuss each emotional parenting behavior and its opposite parenting behavior in further detail.

Overcontrol and Overprotection Versus Healthy Independence-Granting

Emotional Parenting Behavior: Overcontrol/Overprotection

Adolescents with emotional disorders often have a reduced sense of self-efficacy, which can serve to maintain or worsen their feelings of anxiety, depression, and other strong emotions. Often, parents will do things for their adolescent (e.g., speak for their adolescent in a social situation) or allow their adolescent to continue with avoidant behaviors in order to help reduce their adolescent's emotional distress. The urge to do this is quite natural, as it arises from a healthy protective urge to reduce adolescent distress. Overcontrolling and overprotective parenting practices often help both adolescents and parents to feel better in the short term: adolescents are able to avoid something they do not want to do, while parents feel like they are helping to reduce the adolescent's distress. However, by using these overprotective parenting responses repeatedly in the context of the adolescent's distress, parents inadvertently reinforce the adolescent's emotional behaviors and decrease the adolescent's confidence in her ability to function independently. The adolescent may feel even more helpless to solve her own problems, which generally ends up contributing to increased avoidance and symptoms of anxiety and depression. By encouraging independence in their adolescent, parents can help increase her confidence and self-efficacy, thereby reducing feelings of helplessness, the use of avoidance behaviors, and overall anxiety and depression.

> **Therapist Note**
> *If you have noticed a parent making statements such as, "She cannot do that on her own," or "I am afraid he will lose control if he has to do that alone," there is a good chance that the parent is employing the emotional parenting behaviors of overcontrol/overprotection and would benefit from learning specific strategies to reduce these behaviors. If a parent appears to be helping an adolescent avoid feared situations, making excuses for the adolescent, or helping the adolescent with tasks she can do on her own (e.g., therapy home learning), these may be additional indications that a discussion of overcontrol/overprotection is needed.*

Opposite Parenting Behavior: Healthy Independence-Granting

No parent is comfortable when his or her adolescent is in distress, and it can be difficult to break overcontrolling or overprotective tendencies. However, for many parents, simple identification of overprotective and overcontrolling behaviors, illustration of their ineffectiveness, and suggestions of more productive methods for helping their adolescent deal more appropriately and independently with his or her emotional disorder symptoms sufficiently reduces counterproductive parental behaviors.

Other than promoting awareness via the *Double Before, During, and After,* parents can use the following techniques for increasing independence and decreasing overprotective or overcontrolling parental behaviors:

1. *Labeled praise* **of good coping techniques.** Praise of a desired behavior effectively increases the likelihood that the behavior will occur again in the future. By praising positive and independent coping behaviors, parents increase the likelihood that their adolescent will behave this way in the future (e.g., "I like how you started your homework today without me asking you to do it").

2. *Planned ignoring* **of minor inappropriate behaviors or distress signals while the adolescent is upset.** As mentioned, any attention to a behavior increases the likelihood that this behavior will occur in the future. By selectively ignoring the adolescent's minor inappropriate behaviors such as whining, crying, and excessive reassurance-seeking, the adolescent is more likely to figure out how to deal with an emotional situation independently. Conversely, when parents run to their adolescent's aid in such situations, the adolescent learns that these inappropriate behaviors or distress signals lead to parental attention and the parent helping to solve the problem. Unfortunately, this results in decreased self-efficacy and a greater chance that the adolescent will continue to use these behaviors when upset in the future. Thus, gently prompting the adolescent to use a therapeutic skill and then ignoring these behaviors is extremely important (e.g., ignoring whining and reassurance-seeking from the adolescent).

3. *Differential reinforcement of other behaviors* **that are more adaptive when distressed.** Even when an adolescent is behaving in an inappropriate fashion in an emotional situation (e.g., throwing a fit over choosing an outfit in the morning), parents can still praise or reward the components of the adolescent's behavior that are desirable in order to increase those components and, at the same time, ignore and help

reduce the frequency of less desirable components (e.g., "I like how you picked out your own shirt even though it was hard for you").

Use of these techniques with one scenario is illustrated below (although these strategies may be applicable across several other examples and types of emotional distress as well):

PARENT: *Sometimes I feel like Magda doesn't even care about having friends anymore. She would just rather sit at home and play on the computer.*

THERAPIST: *It sounds like you are really frustrated with how Magda is handling her emotions around peers right now. You are concerned that she is no longer interested in making friends.*

PARENT: *I am not sure if that's exactly what I mean. I know on some level that she still wants to make friends. She just doesn't seem to try anymore. I just know what can happen if she gives up on making friends . . . She'll just be alone and will start to feel really down again. I don't want that for her.*

THERAPIST: *I can hear how concerned you are about Magda and that you want to help her build friendships. Is she doing anything right now to build new friendships or maintain old ones, in your opinion?*

PARENT: *Well, she definitely still texts a lot and I see her on social media from time to time. I just feel like she isn't making that same effort in person AT ALL and I don't want her to become totally isolated.*

THERAPIST: *So, you do see some forms of interaction still happening with friends, but not as much in person. Do you think that's very different from how her current friends interact? Sometimes teens with higher social anxiety prefer online interactions to in-person ones and may need to be cautious about not becoming too isolated from their friends.*

PARENT: *I guess it's hard to tell how different it is. Her friends definitely communicate more by text than in person as well. But I can sense how things are shifting with her and she just seems less interested in communicating overall. So, yes—I'm definitely concerned that this is her social anxiety at work and maybe some sadness about her friendships too.*

THERAPIST: *That helps me understand better. Thank you. So, how do you think you could encourage that face-to-face interaction more?*

PARENT: *I guess I could praise her for trying, like you mentioned earlier, or offer her opportunities to go hang out with friends more. I think maybe I stopped offering to take her to the mall and whatnot as often because it feels like she always says no.*

THERAPIST: *Focusing on the positives and trying to build new or restore old approach behaviors with friends are really good ideas. I get what you are saying that Magda might shoot down your suggestions for how to help here. Let's maybe use some problem-solving steps to figure out what else we could do to get her motivated around this issue.*

Notice how in this interaction the therapist acknowledges the validity of the concerns raised by Magda's parent, but does not indulge in negative talk about the adolescent's behavior. Rather, the therapist reinforces insights and attempts to encourage prosocial and interactive behaviors. Then, the therapist prompts the parent to continue brainstorming ways to encourage Magda to increase approach-oriented behaviors.

In addition to the behavioral parenting strategies noted above, parents who limit their adolescent's autonomy or independence can be encouraged to utilize *shaping* principles to encourage successive approximations of increasingly independent, appropriate activities. This procedure is not unlike the exposure strategies used with their adolescent for engaging with specific emotionally related situations she is avoiding and can be explained as similar to such. Similar to exposure, shaping involves encouraging or rewarding successive approximations toward a desirable behavior. For example, if an adolescent is unable to successfully plan an outing with a friend, a parent might first praise or reward any text to a friend, then later reward a text to a friend about what the friend is doing this weekend, then an attempt at setting up a short and simple outing, and finally attending a socially oriented outing.

Some parents become extremely distressed during behavioral experiments or exposure and may require additional coaching to support their adolescent's independence-building goals. They may find it very hard to observe their adolescent in distress, even though you have explained this is only a short-term outcome and they can look to the long-term goal of reduced adolescent emotional difficulty as a benefit of tolerating these tough moments. You may need to help these parents institute distress tolerance plans (e.g., using appropriate parental self-care during adolescent distress, gaining social support, swapping out parents if one is better at tolerating the adolescent's distress) for managing their own strong emotions.

Other families may be dealing with an adolescent who needs more rudimentary help with independence-building beyond simple avoidance. For example, some adolescents may lack basic self-advocacy skills or self-care skills that will allow them to engage in new tasks or situations with greater confidence. You may find that building step-by-step plans with parents for addressing these underlying deficits may be reinforcing to both parent and adolescents.

Emotional Parenting Behavior: Criticism

Many adolescents with emotional problems feel that they "can't do any-thing right." This perception may in part reflect the distorted thinking that many emotional adolescents engage in, but it is also true that many adolescents with emotional problems get the message from teachers, friends, coaches, and even parents that they aren't doing what they are supposed to be doing, don't measure up, aren't trying hard enough, or are letting others down. Adolescents with emotional disorders may be espe-cially sensitive to criticism, so they may be more likely than other adoles-cents to pick up on such messages even when they are communicated very subtly or ambiguously.

Introduce parents to the impact of criticism on their adolescent by asking them to consider a time when a boss, coworker, or family member criti-cized them in some way. Ask the parents how this criticism impacted both their emotions and their future behavior. Then, ask the parents to think of another time when they were praised for something they did. Which was more motivating—the criticism or the praise? Which resulted in more long-lasting changes in behavior? Once parents consider the impact of criticism on their own emotions and behavior, they are often able to understand how critical comments or gestures might impact their adoles-cent. To reinforce this point, it may be helpful to explicitly mention and discuss some of the potential consequences of criticism, including low self-esteem, withdrawal, loss of motivation, heightened negative emotion, and others mentioned in Table 9.1 If you have observed the adolescent's parents making critical comments, or if the parents disclosed making them, this may be a good time to gently point such comments out to the parents and ask them to reflect upon how such comments might influ-ence their adolescent's emotions or behavior.

Avoiding criticism does not mean that parents cannot correct their ado-lescent's mistakes or misbehaviors. If parents appear confused about the distinction between criticism and correction, you can reassure them that teaching their adolescent right from wrong is an important job of par-enting. One difference between criticism and correction is that criticism often occurs in response to minor mistakes or concerns that could just as well be overlooked, while correction is a response to a significant mis-behavior or concern and serves as a "teaching moment." Criticism often involves the use of global "always" or "never" statements, while correction sticks to the issue at hand. Finally, criticism often denies or invalidates the adolescent's emotional experience, while correction validates the adolescent's emotions, despite the fact that the adolescent may have made the wrong decision.

If you have noticed parents making comments that deny, minimize, or judge their adolescent's emotions or experiences more generally, this may be a good opportunity to point out that such comments are a form of criticism, as they suggest that the adolescent is "wrong" for feeling the way she does. These types of comments can sometimes arise from good intentions. When parents notice that their adolescent's emotional reaction appears extreme and out of proportion to a particular trigger, it is natural for them to want to point this out to their adolescent. However, parents must be careful to do so in a way that acknowledges without judging their adolescent's emotional experience, a topic that will be discussed below.

Therapist Note

Many parents are quite sensitive and even defensive when it comes to the topic of criticism. If you do not observe or hear from the adolescent about any of the forms of criticism mentioned above, it may not be beneficial to discuss this emotional parenting behavior. However, even non-critical parents may have difficulty expressing empathy at times. Therefore, you may still wish to briefly cover the following section on empathy at some point during treatment, even if you did not discuss criticism.

Opposite Parenting Behavior: Empathy

You have already been building the parents' empathy for their adolescent's struggles during this treatment, and it may be helpful to take a moment to point this out to the parents. Through use of module summary forms and brief meetings with the family weekly, you have been sharing with the parents what types of skills you are teaching their adolescent and how they can help reinforce these through home-based practice. You should continue to do this, but you can also ask the parents themselves to engage in treatment activities (e.g., behavioral experiments, exposure examples) to increase their empathy and respect for how difficult it is to engage in new behaviors during distress.

Empathizing with an adolescent who is experiencing intense emotional distress may seem like a relatively straightforward skill to reinforce, especially to therapists, for whom empathizing comes quite naturally.

However, for many overly critical parents, expressing empathy may be difficult, and it can be helpful for them to learn some specific, concrete steps for expressing empathy for their adolescent's emotions and experiences. The following steps can be introduced to parents:

1. *Label the emotion you perceive the adolescent to be experiencing* (e.g., "It looks like you are feeling sad right now").
   a. Note that if the adolescent rejects the parent's label and endorses a different emotion, it is important to express acceptance, even if the parent may disagree.
2. *Convey that you understand why the adolescent might feel this way, given the trigger or situation* (e.g., "It makes sense that getting a C on a test you studied really hard for would make you feel sad").
   a. Note to the parents that they may be having difficulty understanding their adolescent's emotional response, and they may feel the response is out of proportion to the trigger. It is of course okay for the parent to feel this way, but one essential component of empathy is acknowledging that the adolescent's emotional response makes sense *from the adolescent's perspective.*
3. *Encourage the adolescent to use one of her skills and support her in doing so as needed.*
   a. An adolescent who is experiencing a strong emotion may have difficulty thinking flexibly about which skills to use or recalling how to use therapeutic skills in the moment. If the adolescent appears receptive, parents may help suggest and guide their adolescent in using skills.

You may wish to conduct a role-play with the parent by pretending to be a distressed adolescent and encouraging the parent to practice expressing empathy.

An additional opposite parenting behavior to criticism is combining positive reinforcement, such as praise, with active ignoring of minor emotional reactions or misbehaviors.

Inconsistency Versus Consistent Use of Discipline and Praise

Emotional Parenting Behavior: Inconsistency

Adolescents with emotional disorders often display high levels of irritability, anger, and general negative affect, especially when facing situations that trigger difficult emotional experiences. For example, a socially anxious adolescent may become irritable, dysregulated, or noncompliant in the moments or even days prior to having to give a speech in front of her class. Parents of adolescents with emotional disorders may not be sure how to handle such behaviors, and they may respond to their adolescent in ways that increase the behaviors. Some parents provide decreased or inconsistent discipline in response to their adolescent's inappropriate emotional behaviors, which can inadvertently increase these behaviors. Parents may also provide inconsistent reinforcement or praise of brave or coping behaviors, which can decrease these desired behaviors.

Parents who use inconsistent discipline with their emotional adolescent are often responding this way due to frustration, a reluctance to punish their adolescent for acting out when they feel the adolescent's actions are the result of an emotional disorder (e.g., parents who do not punish their adolescent for not doing her homework if the parent suspects that anxiety is playing a role in the behavior), and/or a lack of knowledge about how best to intervene. While not punishing an adolescent for engaging in emotionally driven behaviors, even when such behaviors are disruptive, is empathetic in nature, it may become problematic in some families if the adolescent is allowed to engage in rule-breaking behavior repeatedly. By inconsistently disciplining disruptive behaviors, parents teach their adolescent that she can sometimes get away with certain disruptive behaviors. Some parents also become emotionally dysregulated themselves in the face of their adolescent's misbehavior. Parent dysregulation is often the source of harsh parenting techniques and also provides increased attention to the misbehavior, which in turn may increase emotional dysregulation and misbehavior in adolescents.

Some parents of youth with emotional disorders may also provide insufficient praise when their adolescent engages in emotionally triggering situations that might not appear to be difficult to the average person but require a lot of effort for the specific adolescent. For example, parents might not praise a depressed or anxious adolescent for going to the movies with her friends, even when this is extremely difficult for the adolescent, because this type of activity is expected to be fun. The lack of response to an adolescent's effortful and prosocial coping behavior from her parent may reduce the chance that the adolescent will continue to use coping behaviors in the face of similarly difficult emotional experiences. However, consistent use of praise and other reinforcers can increase the adolescent's willingness and ability to face her difficult emotions.

Generally speaking, the UP-A protocol does not address more severe conduct or oppositional defiant problems more directly. If the problems that the parents are indicating are of that level of severity and/or have become the primary focus of treatment as time has progressed, you may wish to consider referring or adapting your treatment plan to include a greater focus on behavioral parent training skills.

Opposite Parenting Behavior: Consistent Use of Discipline and Praise

Rewards and Reinforcements: Increasing parental use of consistent rewards, especially as adolescents begin to approach and cope with intense emotional experiences in more prosocial ways throughout treatment, can greatly increase treatment-related gains. Often, implementation of consistent praise and reward for brave and compliant behaviors is best achieved via working with parents (with input from their adolescent) to create a reinforcement system. Reinforcement systems are structured ways to ensure that praise and rewards are being provided consistently when adolescents behave in desirable ways (e.g., approaching difficult emotional situations, coping with difficult emotions). When praise and rewards are consistent, adolescents learn that they will experience a desirable outcome when they do things that are difficult. This association makes it more likely that adolescents will continue to engage in previously avoided situations and to cope with their emotions prosocially.

When creating a reward or reinforcement system, review the importance of rewarding an adolescent for non-avoidant and appropriate behaviors as soon as possible after behaviors occur to increase learning and the likelihood that she will act this way again and to help her see that her parent recognizes how hard she is trying to approach difficult situations. When rewards are not feasible, *specific, labeled praise* (mentioned above) and *enthusiasm* about the adolescent's behavior should be used in the moment to acknowledge achievements (e.g., parents should be a "cheerleader" for their adolescent).

If covering this section of Module-P, it may be useful to spend some time generating a reward list with both the adolescent and parents. Let the adolescent and parent know that rewards *should not* be costly. Make sure you come up with a range of ideas—some smaller rewards (like getting a small sum of money or screen time) and some bigger ones (like going to a movie or concert). Rewards can be split up into categories (smaller rewards for doing things that are less challenging and increasingly desired rewards for doing more challenging things). For ideas on creating a reward list, refer to the example rewards on the Parent Summary for Module-P, at the end of this chapter. Some adolescents can still appreciate a token system (e.g., a jar that can be filled with marbles or other objects that can be cashed in for a larger reward) or a reward chart. Others may find such token economy systems to be too young or silly and need to be reinforced through more direct praise or reward opportunities.

Therapist Note

Some parents find the prospect of rewarding their adolescent for behaviors that might seem to be already rewarding, if not for their emotional disorder symptoms (e.g., spending time with friends or going to school), to be off-putting and frustrating. If parents indicate this, acknowledge their concerns and explain the rationale for rewarding such behaviors. You may explain to the parent that currently the adolescent is engaging in very little or none of the approach behaviors targeted for reward and that reward may provide motivation to "push through" difficult exposure opportunities. You can also discuss fading of reward once a new behavior is established. In fact, learning theory tells us that once a new behavior is established, it is actually preferable to reward it more intermittently to maintain that new behavior over time, rather than at each instance of its occurrence.

Behavior Management: The UP-A does not currently target youth behavior problems as primary presenting problems, as noted. However, youth with emotional disorders often become behaviorally dysregulated or engage in anger-related behaviors in the face of their emotional challenges. When this occurs, it is important to implement appropriate behavior management strategies in a consistent manner. Only when behavior management techniques are implemented fairly, calmly, and consistently do adolescents respond well to such techniques.

Below is information about several behavior management strategies you may wish to address with parents during Module-P sessions. Other strategies, such as planned ignoring (see above) and giving choices to increase the adolescent's sense of control over a situation, may also be employed. It should be reiterated that poor consistency in the use of behavior management skills may actually worsen problem behaviors over time, and thus parents must be able to fully commit to consistent usage.

1. *Creating Appropriate House Rules:* For parents with few or no overt rules regarding aggression or defiance, you may wish to begin by

establishing just one clear, behaviorally grounded house rule (e.g., no hitting) and discussing how they might enforce this rule if it were broken. Role-play of verbal responses and consequences to rule-breaking should be practiced between caregivers or with you to promote confidence. Once an initial rule is established and maintained, others can be added gradually over time.

2. *Using Effective Commands:* Coach the parents on effective command strategies. An effective command should include the following steps:

   a) Gain the adolescent's attention (e.g., "Emily, please look at me").

   b) Once attention is gained, use a firm (but not angry) voice requesting that the adolescent do something.

   c) Issue only one command at a time and provide a brief interval for compliance to occur (e.g., "Emily, turn off the computer").

   d) After a brief wait, if compliance does not occur, re-issue the command. If compliance does occur, reward should be given.

   e) If an additional prompt does not result in compliance, a consequence warning may be given (e.g., "If you don't turn off the computer, you will lose screen time for the night.).

   The parent should be prepared to praise and/or reward any compliance behavior and provide the stated consequence if compliance does not occur.

3. *Response Cost Procedures:* As noted under the effective commands section above, one strategy for delivering consequences involves the removal of a preferred activity or item for a specified period of time. Typically, this timeframe should be brief (i.e., no more than one day), and the parent should make sure to clearly state a command **and** a warning before removing privileges.

Excessive Modeling of Intense Emotions and Avoidance Versus Healthy Emotional Modeling

Emotional Parenting Behavior: Excessive Modeling of Intense Emotions and Avoidance

It is often the case that parents of some adolescents with emotional disorders are, in fact, experiencing (or have experienced in the past) some level of difficulty with emotional disorders themselves. Even if the parent does not have a clinical disorder per se, he or she may be exhibiting high levels of avoidance behaviors, safety behaviors, or other emotional behaviors that can be easily perceived as "the norm" in the household.

In the scope of this protocol, it is certainly relevant to gently point out instances of such modeling of emotional disorder symptoms and, more pertinently, avoidance-oriented behaviors to parents. Many parents are unaware of their own engagement in emotional behaviors and, if they are aware, may tend to normalize or minimize them. For such parents, it is helpful to point out that one way children and adolescents learn is by observing how the important people in their lives (particularly their parents) think and act. Therefore, by excessively expressing strong emotions, voicing distorted thinking, and engaging in emotional behaviors in front of their adolescents, parents may be inadvertently teaching their adolescent to respond to emotions in the way they themselves do.

Opposite Parenting Behavior: Healthy Emotional Modeling

When addressing modeling as an emotional behavior, it is important to remind parents that they are certainly allowed, expected, and even encouraged to have their own emotional experiences! Remind them that the purpose of this treatment is not to get rid of emotions but to learn when we are reacting to our emotions in a way that is not helpful and to change the emotional behaviors we are using. Emotions are of course normal, natural, and not harmful for parents as well as for adolescents.

Encourage parents to reflect on emotional behaviors they might have used over the past several weeks, and ask them to consider what their adolescent might have learned about the situation by observing the parents' emotional responses. For many parents, just pointing out how these behaviors may be reinforcing avoidance as a norm in their household is enough to motivate changes in parent behavior. However, some parents may require more assistance to adjust such behaviors using techniques outlined for adolescents in this protocol, as they are similar in many ways to those available in the Unified Protocol for adults.

It may also be helpful to more explicitly teach parents to model their emotions in a healthy manner. Parents may accomplish this by using the following steps when they are experiencing a strong emotion:

1. *Model appropriate labeling of their emotion and the trigger* (e.g., Mom is feeling anxious right now, because we are late for therapy).
2. *Verbally adopt a nonjudgmental stance to the emotion* (e.g., It is okay to feel anxious—lots of people get nervous when they're running late to something important).

3. *Identify and use an appropriate skill or coping strategy for managing the emotion* (e.g., I am going to use my present-moment awareness skills to help me pay attention to driving and experience our conversation, rather than continuing to worry about how late we'll be).

It may be helpful to role-play these steps for healthy emotional modeling in session, using recent examples from the parents' experiences.

Following the introduction of parenting skills, it might be helpful to provide parents with a copy of *Ways to Support My Adolescent* (Parent Summary for Module-P), which provides a shorthand review of some tips for providing empathy and rewards for adolescents coping with difficult and strong emotional experiences.

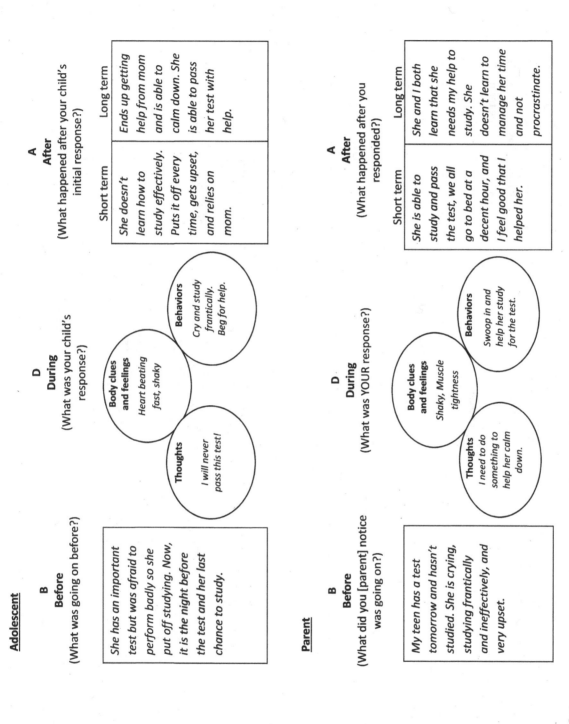

Adolescent

B
Before
(What was going on before?)

She has an important test but was afraid to perform badly so she put off studying. Now, it is the night before the test and her last chance to study.

D
During
(What was your child's response?)

Body clues and feelings
Heart beating fast, shaky

Behaviors
Cry and study frantically. Beg for help.

Thoughts
I will never pass this test!

A
After
(What happened after your child's initial response?)

Short term

She doesn't learn how to study effectively. Puts it off every time, gets upset, and relies on mom.

Long term

Ends up getting help from mom and is able to calm down. She is able to pass her test with help.

Parent

B
Before
(What did you [parent] notice was going on?)

My teen has a test tomorrow and hasn't studied. She is crying, studying frantically and ineffectively, and very upset.

D
During
(What was YOUR response?)

Body clues and feelings
Shaky, Muscle tightness

Behaviors
Swoop in and help her study for the test.

Thoughts
I need to do something to help her calm down.

A
After
(What happened after you responded?)

Short term

She is able to study and pass the test, we all go to bed at a decent hour, and I feel good that I helped her.

Long term

She and I both learn that she needs my help to study. She doesn't learn to manage her time and not procrastinate.

Figure 9.1

Sample Double Before, During, and After

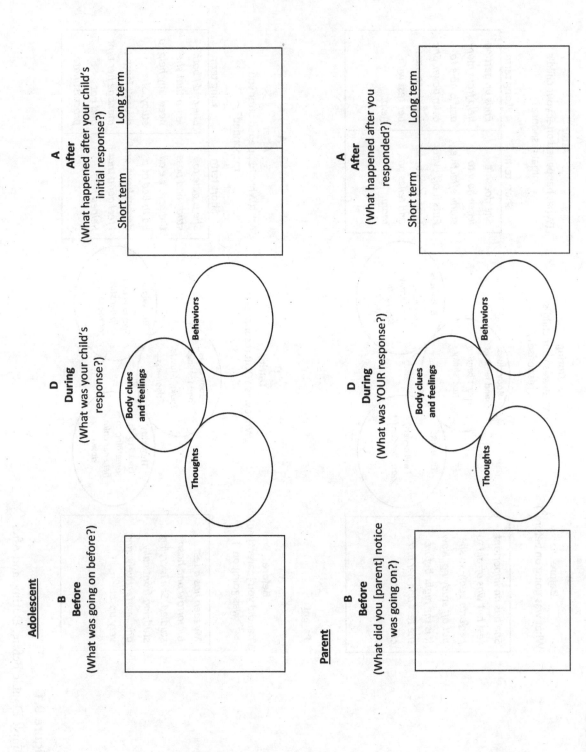

Adolescent

B
Before
(What was going on before?)

D
During
(What was your child's response?)

Body clues and feelings

Thoughts

Behaviors

A
After
(What happened after your child's initial response?)

Short term | Long term

Parent

B
Before
(What did you [parent] notice was going on?)

D
During
(What was YOUR response?)

Body clues and feelings

Thoughts

Behaviors

A
After
(What happened after you responded?)

Short term | Long term

Figure 9.2

Double Before, During, and After

Parent Summary Form for Module-P:
Parenting the Emotional Adolescent

Ways to Support My Teen

✓ Provide your teen with specific, *labeled praise* when your teen does something you would like him or her to keep doing.

<u>For example:</u>

"I like it when you clean your room."

"Nice job getting to school today even though it was hard for you."

"Good job calling your friend on your own."

Labeled praise includes supportive, positive statements that reinforce your teen for dealing appropriately with strong emotions.

✓ Label your teen's emotions to show that you understand and empathize with what your teen is feeling. Let your teen know that it makes sense to be feeling that way, given the situation or what has happened in the past.

<u>For example:</u>

"You are feeling scared right now."

"I know this is tough for you because you are sad."

"It makes sense that you are feeling frustrated right now. I know this situation isn't going the way you wanted it to go."

✓ If your teen is struggling with a difficult emotion, try not to step in and help right away. Express empathy for how your teen is feeling and encourage him or her to try out a skill from treatment. Remember: the goal is to help your teen learn to solve problems and cope with emotions independently.

✓ Reward your teen for non-avoidant behaviors or effective coping as soon as possible after behaviors occur. This increases the likelihood that your teen will act this way again and helps your teen see that you recognize how hard he or she is trying to overcome intense emotional experiences.

<u>For example:</u>

A small amount of cash or small gift card towards a desired gift

Special activity with friends or family

Family hike

Candy (in moderation)

Choosing restaurant or meal/dessert at home

Screen time (using device/game/show of choice)

Getting to stay up late one time

PART TWO

Children (UP-C)

CHAPTER 10

Introduction to the *Unified Protocol for Transdiagnostic Treatment of Emotional Disorders in Children* (UP-C)

Structural and Pragmatic Considerations in Using the UP-C

General Overview

Whether you have fully reviewed the UP-A chapters in this Therapist Guide before starting this chapter or whether this is the very first page you are turning to, welcome! This section will introduce you to important structural and pragmatic considerations for delivering the *Unified Protocol for Transdiagnostic Treatment of Emotional Disorders in Children* (UP-C). As you will see, we also refer to the UP-C as the "Emotion Detectives" program in many places, including across both the Therapist Guide and the accompanying child- and parent-directed workbook. This alternative naming scheme reflects the guiding treatment metaphor used in this version of the Unified Protocol—teaching children to "solve the mystery of their emotions," as detectives might—as well as the developmentally sensitive nature of this adaptation.

Please review the introduction to this entire Therapist Guide (the very first chapter in this book), where you will find a detailed theoretical rationale for the UP-C and history of the evidence base supporting this approach. If you have already reviewed that introduction, the unique purpose of this separate introduction will be clearer: to introduce you to the structure and usage of the UP-C specifically.

Intended Audience for the UP-C

The UP-C is intended for children between the ages of 7 and 13, although children slightly above or below this age group may benefit from this format for the presentation of Unified Protocol skills. We generally suggest that adolescents above the age of 13 use the UP-A materials presented in the first half of this Therapist Guide and the companion adolescent workbook, as the UP-C materials and the central "Emotion Detectives" metaphor may seem too juvenile to adolescents and may consequently hinder their treatment engagement and motivation. However, adolescents with more limited cognitive abilities or particularly limited emotion knowledge may benefit from utilizing some UP-C (versus UP-A) materials on an as-needed basis according to the therapist's judgment. Additionally, we have successfully used this treatment format with children younger than 7, though the ability of younger children to benefit from this program may depend on their reading level and the degree of parental involvement and child cognitive development.

Just like the UP-A, the UP-C is intended to reduce the intensity and frequency of symptoms common to youth with *emotional disorders*. The UP-C accomplishes this by using core evidence-based treatment strategies in a broad manner that applies to a wide range of aversive emotional experiences characteristic of youth emotional disorders (i.e., anxiety, depression, other internalizing disorders). Many anxiety, depression, adjustment, traumatic stress-related, or obsessive-compulsive or related disorders would be appropriate targets for this intervention, although other problems in which the main goal of treatment is to reduce distress in response to strong emotions could be treated within this intervention. This is not necessarily a treatment that targets primary behavioral problems in children, such as oppositional or noncompliant behaviors. However, behavioral dysregulation co-occurring with emotional disorders, along with other co-occurring problems such as attention-deficit/hyperactivity disorder (ADHD), may be targeted in part through this treatment's focus on anger and on "opposite parenting behaviors" that are helpful for managing emotion dysregulation more generally. However, the therapist and caregivers should clearly understand that the main goals of the UP-C are to target emotional problems primarily through extinction of distress and anxiety in response to strong and aversive emotion states.

UP-C Is Presented as a Group Therapy

The structure and delivery of the UP-C are distinct from those of the UP-A in several important ways. First, you will notice that the forthcoming chapters introduce the UP-C as a *group therapy* approach. You will also notice that we suggest conducting the child and parent groups of the UP-C on the same session day. These decisions were predicated on the fact that the UP-C has been tested only as a group therapy and in the delivery manner specified within this guide in a previous randomized controlled trial. This decision is also based on our belief that this intervention is particularly well accepted by child clients and parents in this type of concurrent group setting. Children find the support of their peers to be a huge benefit, especially while practicing emotion-evoking experiments and exercises. Further, parents have often remarked that the cohesive parent group approach yields an extraordinarily supportive environment in which to practice new, opposite parenting behaviors. The combination of these child-alone and parent-alone aspects of each session, along with conjoint child and parent time at the beginning and end of each session, facilitates smooth and easy collaboration between all relevant parties in the delivery of each UP-C skill.

Chapter 23 of this Therapist Guide directly addresses changes to the intervention that therapists should consider if implementing UP-C as an *individual therapy*. Anecdotally, our experience suggests that the use of the UP-C as an individual therapy involves relatively simple adaptations, which we explain in further detail in Chapter 23. In our research trials, we have delivered this treatment with two therapists dedicated to the child group component and two therapists dedicated to the parent group component. However, we understand that the implementation of this intervention in varying clinical settings, as well as limitations on therapist availability, may require that this treatment be conducted differently from its structure in our research setting. One option may be to hold parent and child group components simultaneously but reduce the number of therapists assigned to each group. We believe that it is likely feasible to conduct this group with two therapists assigned to the child component and one to the parent component, but may be challenging with fewer unless the group is quite small. We have also conducted the UP-C parent group following the child group (both parent and child sessions back to back in the same day) with little disruption to the quality of the service, but therapists should know that the time involved will be slightly greater (since the parent group time is added cumulatively to the child group time) and may require two full hours dedicated to each session. It would also certainly be possible to conduct the parent component of the UP-C at a different time or on a different day, without the children present, as long as the parent is present during the child sessions as well (to take part in together time at the end of each session).

UP-C Content

The UP-C includes 15 consecutive sessions, typically delivered over approximately 15 weeks. Table 10.1 provides a session-by-session overview of the UP-C and a brief outline of the child- and parent-directed content covered during the 15 sessions of treatment. Those familiar with the UP-A will immediately notice in Table 10.1 that the treatment skills in the UP-C mirror content from the UP-A in terms of the order in which skills are delivered and the general focus of treatment sessions. However, a major difference between the UP-C and UP-A is that the UP-C skills are presented and organized around the acronym "CLUES" and that the young "Emotion Detectives" participating in this intervention are being actively encouraged to learn these Emotion Detective skills (also referred to as the CLUES skills in discussions with child clients) in order to "solve the mystery of their emotions." The acronym CLUES stands for:

C—Consider How I Feel
L—Look at My Thoughts
U—Use Detective Thinking and Problem Solving
E—Experience My Emotions
S—Stay Healthy and Happy.

The parent group component of this treatment has three primary functions:

1. To introduce parents to the Emotion Detective skills their children are learning in the child component of this treatment
2. To introduce parents to some less helpful "emotional parenting behaviors" they may be using in response to their child's strong emotions, as well as some more helpful "opposite parenting behaviors" to consider
3. To foster support and camaraderie among the parents.

The last of these goals occurs throughout all 15 parent sessions, in part as a natural consequence of parents sharing their experiences and concerns with other parents in similar situations. Therapists also foster support and camaraderie among the parents by leading them in skills practice as a

Table 10.1 Session by Session Overview of the UP-C

CLUES (Emotion Detective) skills	Session	Child group goals	Parent group goals
C Skill (Consider How I Feel)	**UP-C Session 1:** Introduction to the *Unified Protocol for Transdiagnostic Treatment of Emotional Disorders in Children* [Chapter 11 in this Therapist Guide]	1. Introduce children to treatment model and structure 2. Identify top problems and treatment goals 3. Develop rapport among group members and between therapists and group members 4. Introduce children to the purpose of emotions and begin to build emotional awareness	1. Introduce parents to treatment structure and CLUES skills 2. Introduce parents to the three-component model of emotions 3. Discuss the cycle of emotional behaviors
	UP-C Session 2: Getting to Know Your Emotions [Chapter 12 in this Therapist Guide]	1. Learn to identify and rate intensity of different emotions 2. Continue to normalize emotional experiences 3. Introduce the three parts of the emotional experience 4. Introduce the cycle of avoidance 5. Identify rewards for new behaviors	1. Introduce parents to the *Double Before, During and After* (BDA) tracking process 2. Introduce parents to the "emotional parenting behaviors" and their "opposite parenting behaviors" 3. Discuss positive reinforcement as the opposite behavior for criticism
	UP-C Session 3: Using Science Experiments to Change Our Emotions and Behavior [Chapter 13 in this Therapist Guide]	1. Learn about the concept of "acting opposite" 2. Practice using science experiments to help with acting opposite/emotional behaviors 3. Learn the connection between activity and emotion 4. Introduce emotion and activity tracking as an experiment	1. Introduce parents to the idea of science experiments 2. Discuss how parents can support their children in completing science experiments 3. Discuss ways to reinforce children
	UP-C Session 4: Our Body Clues [Chapter 14 in this Therapist Guide]	1. Describe the concept of body clues and their relation to strong emotions 2. Learn to identify body clues for different emotions 3. Teach the skill of body scanning to develop awareness of body clues 4. Help children practice experiencing body clues without using avoidance/distraction	1. Introduce the concept of somatization 2. Teach parents the skill of body scanning 3. Introduce sensational exposures and practice them as a group 4. Teach parents how to express empathy

(continued)

Table 10.1 Continued

CLUES (Emotion Detective) skills	Session	Child group goals	Parent group goals
L Skill (Look at My Thoughts)	UP-C Session 5: Look at My Thoughts [Chapter 15 in this Therapist Guide]	1. Introduce the concept of flexible thinking 2. Teach children to recognize common "thinking traps"	1. Introduce cognitive flexibility 2. Introduce four common "thinking traps" 3. Discuss the emotional parenting behavior of inconsistency and its opposite parenting behavior of consistent reinforcement and discipline
U Skill (Use Detective Thinking and Problem Solving)	UP-C Session 6: Use Detective Thinking [Chapter 16 in this Therapist Guide]	1. Introduce Detective Thinking 2. Apply Detective Thinking	1. Introduce Detective Thinking 2. Practice Detective Thinking 3. Introduce emotional parenting behavior of overcontrol/overprotection and its opposite parenting behavior, healthy independence-granting
	UP-C Session 7: Problem Solving and Conflict Management [Chapter 17 in this Therapist Guide]	1. Introduce Problem Solving 2. Apply Problem Solving	1. Introduce Problem Solving 2. Discuss Problem Solving for interpersonal conflicts 3. Discuss reassurance-seeking and accommodation
E Skill (Experience My Emotions)	UP-C Session 8: Awareness of Emotional Experiences [Chapter 18 in this Therapist Guide]	1. Learn about the E skill 2. Teach children about present-moment awareness 3. Introduce nonjudgmental awareness	1. Discuss the importance of learning to experience emotions rather than avoiding them 2. Introduce and practice present-moment awareness 3. Introduce and practice nonjudgmental awareness 4. Begin completing the *Emotional Behavior Form*
	UP-C Session 9: Introduction to Emotion Exposure [Chapter 19 in this Therapist Guide]	1. Review Emotion Detective skills learned to date in the UP-C 2. Review the concepts of emotional behaviors and "acting opposite" in preparation for a new type of science experiment called "exposure" 3. Complete a demonstration of an exposure using a toy or other object 4. Work together with children and parents to finalize *Emotional Behavior Forms*	1. Introduce parents to the concept of situational emotion exposure, a different type of science experiment 2. Explain the parent's role in practicing exposures at home 3. Introduce parents to the emotional parenting behavior of excessive modeling of intense emotions and avoidance and its opposite parenting behavior, healthy emotional modeling 4. Continue to develop the *Emotional Behavior Form* in preparation for upcoming exposures

Table 10.1 Continued

CLUES (Emotion Detective) skills	Session	Child group goals	Parent group goals
	UP-C Session 10: Facing Our Emotions—Part 1 [Chapter 20 in this Therapist Guide]	1. Review the concept of using science experiments to face strong emotions 2. Introduce the idea of safety behaviors and subtle avoidance behaviors (e.g., distraction) 3. Practice a science experiment to face strong emotions as a group (sample situational emotion exposure) 4. Make plans for future science experiments for facing strong emotions (individualized situational emotion exposures)	1. Review the concept of a situational emotion exposure and discuss applications of exposure to different symptom presentations 2. Introduce and discuss the concept of safety behaviors 3. Explain how parents can use all of their "opposite parenting behaviors" to support their child's exposures 4. Introduce the *Emotion Ladder* for exposures and assist parents in finalizing *Emotional Behavior Form*
	UP-C Sessions 11–14: Facing Our Emotions—Part 2 [Chapter 21 in this Therapist Guide]	1. Plan and execute initial situational emotion exposure in Session 11 2. Plan and execute additional situational emotion exposure activities in Sessions 12–14	N/A
S Skill (Stay Healthy and Happy)	**UP-C Session 15:** Wrap-up and Relapse Prevention [Chapter 22 in this Therapist Guide]	1. Review Emotion Detective skills learned in the UP-C program 2. Plan for facing strong emotions in the future 3. Celebrate progress made in treatment program	1. Review Emotion Detective skills and "opposite parenting behaviors" 2. Discuss and celebrate each child's progress 3. Create a plan for sustaining and furthering progress after treatment 4. Distinguish lapses from relapses and help parents recognize warning signs of relapse

group and encouraging them to share their successes and struggles with one another. That being said, therapists should prioritize skills acquisition and practice in the parent sessions, rather than dedicating significant session time to promoting its "support group" function. Throughout treatment, therapists leading parent group sessions are referred to as "group leaders" in order to prevent parents from feeling like they are receiving therapy, when the identified client within this treatment is their child.

In general, therapists are encouraged to present these skills and sessions in the order suggested. However, some variations are highlighted in the forthcoming chapters where appropriate.

Use of Parent Materials

Another unique feature of the UP-C versus the UP-A is the extensive parent involvement in the UP-C. As noted, there is an entire parent group curriculum presented in the UP-C, along with parent-directed workbook materials in the latter half of the UP-C workbook. We highly encourage you to implement and foster this high level of parent involvement in the treatment, as we believe parents are key to the longer-term management of behavioral experiments and emotion-focused exposure components believed to be vital to the efficacy of this approach.

Accordingly, you will notice that each parent session typically contains several home learning assignment options for parents to complete between sessions. In general, parent home learning assignments fall into one of several categories: (1) assignments for developing parents' ability to monitor their child's emotional experiences and their own parent reactions; (2) assignments for helping parents master the Emotion Detective skills that their children are learning in the child sessions; and (3) assignments for helping parents notice their "emotional parenting behaviors" and practice "opposite parenting behaviors" instead. We have included these different types of materials to provide therapists with different options for home learning assignments, and because we think that parents can benefit from all of them! However, it may not be feasible for parents to complete all of the home learning assignments or in-session worksheets included in the workbook, and you should use your clinical judgment when choosing the number and type of home learning assignments to assign to parents. Some parents have the time and motivation to learn and practice as much as they can, and these parents should be encouraged to complete all parent materials if they would like to do so. For other parents, you may need to consider the types of home learning assignments they would most benefit from at different points in treatment. You may also wish to allow parents to choose which of several possible home learning assignments they complete, depending upon what type of assignment seems most beneficial in a given week.

This focus on parental involvement in the UP-C does not imply that we believe parent involvement is unimportant in the UP-A, but rather that it may be more difficult to routinely involve the parents of adolescents in a weekly intervention. Hence, we include the more flexible approach to parent involvement in the UP-A. Therapists using the UP-A who wish to engage parents even more in the intervention should feel free to include the parent-directed materials for the UP-C as part of their weekly UP-A intervention approach, as these materials are largely appropriate for a broader age range than specified for the UP-C alone.

The Increased Importance of Rewards in UP-C

An additional, unique feature of the UP-C is the more frequent use of positive reinforcement for participating in therapy-related activities, both delivered by therapists in session and delivered at home by parents. Using consistent and frequent reinforcement is particularly important in this age group, as behavioral experiments and exposure activities may be new and challenging for some children and families to initiate and maintain. Therapists use tokens (e.g., poker chips) throughout each session and CLUES badges at the end of each treatment section to encourage and reinforce appropriate child engagement and productive behavior. Other reinforcements (e.g., puzzle pieces) uniquely target completion of home learning assignments and help the group as a whole achieve a group-level reward at the end of treatment. For example, we have often selected a 50- or 60-piece puzzle depicting a celebration with treats or prizes, distributed these puzzle pieces during treatment for home learning completion, and allowed children to put the puzzle together in the final session to reveal the end-of-treatment celebratory reward. Parents are also encouraged and supported in the delivery of praise and tangible reinforcements to encourage new, brave child behaviors. Attention is paid both to concerns that parents may have about the delivery of such reinforcements and problem solving if rewards are not effective.

General Materials and Preparation Guidelines for the UP-C

In each chapter of the UP-C Therapist Guide, you will find a description of materials and preparation required for each session. Most of the materials required for this treatment are cheap and easy to obtain and are commonly found in many clinical settings. In addition to materials required for individual sessions, certain materials are required for several or even all sessions of this treatment. As noted in the previous section, we have used tokens such as poker chips and puzzle pieces as reinforcements for brave, on-task, and prosocial behaviors in our research and clinical practice of the UP-C. You should bring these materials (or any alternative reinforcements you choose to use) to each session. Children collect and store these tokens in a "CLUES kit," a Tupperware or cardboard box (which you should have available for each new child client prior to beginning Session 1 of treatment) that the children decorate in the first session. Rather than allowing the children to take their CLUES kits home with them, we have generally found that it works best for therapists to collect these kits at the end of each session and bring them to the following session. You may wish to allow the children to exchange their tokens for a small prize from a prize box every third session or so. We have followed this practice in our clinic and often include prizes such as small toys, bouncy balls, paper airplanes, nail polish, bean bag animals, or hair clips from which the children may choose. We also find it helpful to bring pens, pencils, crayons/markers, and art supplies to sessions.

Finally, be aware that children are awarded a CLUES badge at the end of each corresponding session of treatment. For example, children receive a C badge at the end of Session 4, the L badge at the end of Session 5, and so on. We have typically used either small, foam sticky letters that children may affix to their CLUES kits or laminated cardboard cutout letters that children can place inside their CLUES kits. It is important to be aware of when each section of treatment ends so that you can be sure to bring the appropriate CLUES letter to the appropriate session.

A Final Word about the UP-C

Overall, we hope that you, as the therapist, find the UP-C to be a fun, useful, and effective intervention for the children and families that you serve. By targeting strong or tough emotions in this skills-based manner, we believe that you will be helping to foster healthy adaptation and reduce impairment in the lives of children with emotional disorders.

CHAPTER 11

UP-C Session 1: Introduction to the *Unified Protocol for the Transdiagnostic Treatment of Emotional Disorders in Children*

C Skill: Consider How I Feel

MATERIALS NEEDED FOR GROUP

- For Each Child Group Session:
  1. Detective CLUES kits (small plastic container or shoebox for each child)
  2. Poker chips (or other tokens to collect and redeem for individual rewards)
  3. Puzzle (with approximately 60 pieces depicting a reward, such as a party or treats)
  4. Prize box filled with small prizes (<$1 each, such as erasers, stickers, small figurines)
  5. Large piece of paper or whiteboard to record children's answers for any group activities
- For Session 1 Only:
  6. Nametags
  7. Art supplies (e.g., stickers, markers, puff paint)
  8. UP-C Workbook Chapter 1
     a. *What Do Detectives Do?* (Worksheet 1.1)
     b. *My Goals for Emotion Detectives* (Worksheet 1.2)
     c. *CLUES Skills* (Figure 1.1)
     d. *How to Deal with Strong Emotions* (Worksheet 1.3)
     e. *Normal, Natural, and Harmless* (Figure 1.2)
- For Home Learning:
  9. *My Emotions at Home* (Worksheet 1.4)

- Assessments to Be Given at Every Session:
  10. *Weekly Top Problems Tracking Form* (Appendix 11.1 at the end of this chapter)
- For Parent Group Session:
  11. UP-C Workbook Chapter 13
      a. *Treatment Schedule* (Figure 13.1)
      b. *CLUES Skills for Parents* (Figure 13.2)
- For Parent Home Learning:
  12. *C for Parents* (Worksheet 13.1)

Therapist Preparation

In preparation for this session, purchase medium-size plastic or other inexpensive containers so that each child can have one for his or her "detective CLUES kit." It may also be helpful to have other arts and crafts materials available to give children the opportunity to decorate their detective CLUES kits. Poker chips, or other small tokens, will be introduced in this chapter as reinforcers for in-session brave and adaptive behaviors (such as following the rules, paying good attention, and trying difficult activities), so you will need those as well. Typically, these tokens are redeemable for prizes from a prize box (make sure to have these on hand) or another larger reward throughout treatment, at your discretion. Puzzle pieces will be introduced as a group reward that can be earned by completing home learning assignments or for other designated behaviors of interest each week. Puzzle pieces may be redeemed at the end of treatment for a small prize depicted on the puzzle (such as a party or treats).

Therapist's Note

Parent and child portions of this group can occur simultaneously, sequentially, or even independently. Content is presented as if groups are occurring simultaneously, with separate therapists leading child and parent groups and with groups meeting all together at the beginning and end of each session. If child groups are run separately or independently from parent groups, together time before and after each session should be completed for each child group session. Even in the absence of a separate parent group occurring simultaneously to the child group, together time portions of the treatment are necessary as some parent involvement is required for this treatment.

The main goal of this session is to introduce the model of treatment to the children and their families, and to begin fostering a relationship among the children, between the children and therapists, and between family members and therapists. To that end, it is most important for you to focus on rapport building and **motivational enhancement** throughout the first session. If motivation for treatment appears to be a concern, you may wish to supplement this session with some of the motivational enhancement materials from Module 1 of the UP-A (Chapter 1 in this Therapist Guide).

- **Goal 1:** Introduce children and caregivers to the treatment model and structure.
- **Goal 2:** Identify top problems (Weisz et al., 2011) and treatment goals.
- **Goal 3:** Develop rapport among group members and between therapists and group members.
- **Goal 4:** Introduce children to the purpose of emotions and begin to build emotional awareness.

Therapist Note

Some children may be very worried, upset, or afraid when attending the first session. It may be helpful to warn parents ahead of time that the first session could be difficult for their child, and to offer them some strategies for encouraging participation. The UP-C is meant to be very engaging and enjoyable in the first session, particularly, and parents can be advised that many children leave feeling as though they had fun and even potentially met children who are experiencing similar issues to themselves. Let parents know that it is always most difficult for children to attend the first session, but there is a high probability that they will enjoy treatment and want to come back. It may also be helpful for parents to tell their child that some of the other kids may also seem upset at the first session, but that everyone will work together to make this experience a good one for all.

Session 1 Content (Divided by Goals)

Session 1, Goal 1
Introduce children and caregivers to the treatment model and structure.

Getting to Know One Another and Welcome to Emotion Detectives

As families enter the office for this first session, ask both the child and parent to fill out or decorate name tags for themselves as they await the arrival of any additional group members. Once all child clients and family members have arrived, the therapists introduce themselves, one by one, and they state a magical power they wish they had (or another similar statement, such as an animal they wish they were). Next, the parents and children go around the room and do the same. Following these introductions, each child is given the UP-C workbook.

Therapist Note

The UP-C workbook contains all child-directed materials for each of the CLUES skills sessions in the first half of the workbook and all the parent-directed materials for these same sessions in the latter portions of the workbook. It also introduces the overarching "Emotion Detective" theme of UP-C, as further described below.

Instruct the children and their families to open their workbooks to *Welcome to the UP-C and Emotion Detectives* (p. 1 in workbook), and work with the children and their families to go over the purpose of treatment using workbook content as a guide. This may be done in the following way:

> *"Emotion Detectives is a special program that helps kids and their families learn about feelings like being happy, sad, joyful, angry, worried, and scared. Emotion Detectives also helps kids and their families learn how to deal with some of the tough emotions that kids need to handle sometimes. Everyone has emotions, even tough ones, and emotions are important. Sometimes, strong or tough emotions can lead us to do things that can be less helpful and can also cause us to be really upset, make us want to miss out on time with people we love, give us trouble sleeping or eating, lead us to feel like we don't want to do fun things we used to like doing, or even cause us to have big arguments or fights with our friends or family. In this program, which we call the Unified Protocol for Children (UP-C), we will work with you to learn new, more helpful ways to deal with some of these tough emotions that you might be having."*

Provide families with time to go over *UP-C Session 1* (p. 3 in workbook), which summarizes the goals for Session 1 of treatment.

Then, instruct the children and their parents to turn to Worksheet 1.1: *What Do Detectives Do?* and introduce the detective theme inherent in the UP-C treatment. You may choose to introduce this idea in the following way, using workbook material as a guide:

"In this group, you will be learning to be an Emotion Detective! Does anyone know what a detective does?"

Provide the children and their parents with time to brainstorm ideas about what detectives do. (For younger children, who may be less likely to understand the concept of a detective, parents can help think of ideas of what detectives do.) Solicit answers from the group. An answer could be: Someone who looks for clues and tries to solve a mystery. Children may also state that a detective helps people figure things out.

"Sometimes our emotions feel like mysteries, similar to a mystery that a detective might be working to solve. In this group, we are going to become Emotion Detectives to better notice and deal with our strong emotions when they occur."

Then describe the concept of Emotion Detectives more specifically. This may be done in the following way:

"In our case, instead of solving mysteries like those you might see on TV or read about in books, Jack and Nina are going to help us solve the mystery of our emotions or the feelings we all have that you might call sadness, fear, worry, and anger! To help you do this, you each get your own detective workbook. This is a place where you will have all of the worksheets, home learning forms, and other helpful information we will use each week as we become Emotion Detectives. There is also information at the back of your workbook for your parent(s) to use as they help you learn to become an Emotion Detective. You and your family can take the workbook home with you, but remember to bring it back each week!"

Confidentiality

Next, discuss the importance of **confidentiality** and the limits of confidentiality. This can be accomplished by introducing the principles of confidentiality as a "detective code," in accordance with the unifying theme of this manual.

First talk about how you will maintain client confidentiality (e.g., notes, home learning, and forms will be kept private) and then state the limits of confidentiality relevant to the clinic or institution where the session is being held. Then explain that the clients also have a responsibility to follow the detective code for the rest of the group members.

It may be especially helpful to present this information in a Socratic way and ask the children for examples of people they can talk to about group in general and about people they can talk to about the other group members (that is, no one). For example, it is okay to talk to family members about their own emotions and things that they have learned in group, but it is not acceptable to discuss content related to any other group member, even with their own family, or with people that group member may know. You may also provide scenarios and ask participants whether this is a breach of the detective code or not. (For example, you know one of the group members prior to group and see his friends outside of group. Can you talk about the group member and group with his friend, or does that go against the detective code?)

Treatment Structure and Model

In this first session, the **structure of treatment sessions** should be reviewed with child clients and their parents (understanding that the structure of treatment may differ depending on whether the parent group is being conducted simultaneously, sequentially, or separately from the child group). It is suggested that each group therapist be assigned to work primarily with some subset of the group members (depending on the ratio of families to therapists) in order to provide families with a person to contact about missing group sessions as well as someone to check in with during home learning review and other individualized portions of the group.

You then describe the **model of treatment** to the children and parents together, which might sound something like this:

> *"During group, we'll meet and work together each week to address some of the feelings and concerns each child and family may be having. Everyone here may be feeling sad, scared, or angry about things at times (along with happy and joyful too, of course!). At the same time, everyone is different! Each of you may be different in terms of what you feel afraid of, what you worry about, and what you do about that. We're going to learn skills to help us deal with our feelings and problems a little differently."*

Session 1, Goal 2
Identify top problems and treatment goals.

My Goals for Emotion Detectives

Next, instruct the children and parents to turn to Worksheet 1.2: *My Goals for Emotion Detectives* and tell the children to work with their parents to write down three problem areas that the child would like to address during treatment. Problems should be specific and relevant to the UP-C treatment model. If needed, you can find more specific guidance on generating appropriate top problems in Chapter 1 of this Therapist Guide. Work with your assigned family/families to help them generate these problem lists. You should also share that this problem list will be private for now, but that the group will be talking about some goals at the end. Instruct the children to leave the "goals" portion of their worksheets blank for now.

> **Therapist Note**
>
> *As noted in Chapter 1 of this Therapist Guide, some youth may be reluctant to discuss their concerns as "problems" or feel irritated by this framework. In that case, you may reformat this exercise as one in which they identify their "top three goals" for treatment.*

Work individually with each family to have the child and parent generate severity ratings for each top problem area. These ratings should then be entered on the *Weekly Top Problems Tracking Form* (found in Appendix 11.1 at the end of this chapter). Bring the *Weekly Top Problems Tracking Form* for each child to all future sessions and obtain weekly severity ratings from both the parent and child at the beginning of each session.

Following this activity, if parent and child groups are occurring simultaneously, the parents will leave and go to the parent group (discussed starting on p. 197 below), while the children and therapists stay together for the child group. If child and parent groups are occurring sequentially, parents still leave the room for the following child-only portion of group.

> **Therapist Note**
>
> *Separation from the parent can trigger anxiety or other strong emotions for some of the children. Be on the lookout for these signs and address them proactively in session. For some children who need more time to warm up to a new group of people, you might consider asking specific families to arrive 10 to 15 minutes early to the first group session to allow such children adequate time to acclimate to the new environment before being asked to interact with unfamiliar people. It is important that you reinforce the potentially enjoyable nature of the UP-C and model approach-oriented behavior and not avoidance behavior at this stage of treatment.*

Session 1, Goal 3

Develop rapport among group members and between therapist and group members.

Child Group Alone

Normalization of Emotions

The child-alone portion of this session begins by reviewing the concept of an "Emotion Detective" as a person working to figure out how to notice, understand, and deal with strong emotions. You might begin by saying:

> *"As we discussed earlier, in this group we will all be **Emotion Detectives**. Let's talk about what this means some more. First, who knows what an 'emotion' is? How do you know if you are having an emotion?"*

Solicit answers from the group and remind them that emotions are things we feel in our bodies that can feel very strong sometimes. This may be a good opportunity to begin briefly talking about the idea that an emotion has three parts: what you think, what you feel in your body, and what you do. It may also be helpful to ask the children to name some different emotions. Although this manual distinguishes the idea of body feelings or "body clues" from emotions, it is not necessary to discuss this distinction in detail just yet.

> *"Okay, now who can tell me what we said detectives are and what they do? You can look back at your workbook for some ideas!"*

This is an excellent opportunity to brainstorm lists of famous detectives and their helpers, such as Sherlock Holmes and Dr. Watson; Dora the Explorer; Harry Potter, Ron, and Hermione; Nancy Drew; Harriet the

Spy; and Scooby Doo and the Scooby Gang or other currently relevant examples. Ask the group of children:

"Do you think detectives are more successful when they work alone, or with other people like Jack and Nina?"

Reinforce the idea that working together as a team might help children solve the mystery of their emotions faster and more effectively. Note that the therapists present, and the children's parents, siblings, and friends, along with other group members, may be helpful members of the team working on the mystery of our emotions.

Team-Building Activities

Next, you can initiate team-building activities to help generate cohesion and greater rapport between group members. This session of the UP-C is meant to be as fun as possible, so you are encouraged to be a bit silly and certainly enthusiastic throughout the session and in these team-building exercises. The first team-building exercise, generating the group name, can be particularly silly and fun, while the second—establishing group rules—may feel a little more serious or focused in its presentation by comparison.

1. *Group Name:* To strengthen team identity, each group should select its own name. Encourage a name choice that reflects either the detective theme (e.g., "Mystery Solvers") or a type of animal, object, or activity that is brave or deals with stress well (e.g., "The Tigers"). Make sure to elicit both "serious" name options and more "silly" ones, similar to how we encourage children to generate any possible solution later in treatment during problem-solving activities. Write potential names on the board and then vote (quickly) or come to a consensus.

Next, introduce the detective rules as the first activity you will do as a new group:

2. *Detective Rules:* To keep the group a safe space, rules are needed. To introduce this topic, you might say:

"We need to have some group rules to make sure everyone feels safe and gets the most out of this group."

The group now brainstorms rules to be listed on a whiteboard or chalk-board. Encourage the following rules in addition to those generated by the group:

- Listen
- Keep hands to yourself
- Take turns speaking
- Try everything
- Work together
- Have fun

Introduce the CLUES Skills

Direct the group to turn to Figure 1.1: *CLUES Skills*. In this figure, the word "CLUES" is presented as an acronym, meaning that the letters C-L-U-E and S each stand for something. In this case, they stand for **CONSIDER** How I Feel, **LOOK** at My Thoughts, **USE** Detective Thinking and Problem Solving, **EXPERIENCE** My Emotions, and **S**TAY Healthy and Happy. As you introduce the **CLUES skills**, emphasize that a mystery is something that is difficult to understand, and it helps if we have *clues* to solve it. Here is an effective way to begin:

> *"Sometimes, when there is a mystery, even a silly one like 'who stole the cookie from the cookie jar' or 'how many doors are there in this building,' you may think you know the answer, but as detectives we will use CLUES to help find 'evidence' or information to help solve the mystery."*

You may continue:

> *"Just like the mysteries we have discussed so far, we ALSO need to use CLUES to solve the mystery of our emotions. So throughout the course of this group, Jack and Nina will be helping us learn the CLUES skills, which are special skills meant to help us become expert Emotion Detectives like them! These skills will help us learn about and deal with our strong emotions—like fear, anxiety, sadness, or anger."*

Next, have children volunteer to read out what the letters stand for:

- **C**onsider How I Feel
- **L**ook at My Thoughts
- **U**se Detective Thinking and Problem Solving
- **E**xperience My Emotions
- **S**tay Healthy and Happy

Indicate that by using the CLUES skills, we will be learning even more helpful ways to deal with our strong emotions over the next several weeks, while reducing our use of less helpful ways of dealing with them at the same time.

Ask the group to turn to Worksheet 1.3: *How to Deal with Strong Emotions*. First, ask for volunteers to read the example (of a behavioral response to sadness) provided and then instruct children to brainstorm what are *helpful* versus *less helpful* ways to deal with different strong emotions like fear, sadness, or anger. Allow time for children to share their answers with the group. Using a large board or paper, write down examples shared by each child.

Make Detective CLUES Kits

At this point in the session, it is time to have the children create their own personal **CLUES kit**. Pass out small boxes (such as clear plastic containers or shoeboxes), along with stickers, markers, crayons, colored pencils, glitter glue, and any other available art supplies. Explain to the children that, in addition to the workbooks they've received, these containers are a place for them to keep their materials from group (such as reward tokens, which will be explained later). For now, instruct the children to decorate their containers however they please, using the materials provided. Encourage them to either put their name on the container or make sure that they will be able to identify their own container later. You may wish to keep these containers in your office for the duration of group to ensure their safe-keeping and utility in subsequent group sessions, allowing children to take them home after the last group session.

While the children are busy decorating, introduce the importance of the CLUES kits. Each time children learn and master a CLUES skill, each group member is given a letter to keep in/on his or her CLUES kit. These letters will help the group members remember their CLUES skills down the road and reinforce the idea that they are moving toward achieving the goal of becoming an Emotion Detective! You should explain to group members that whenever they are having a tough time in the future with their emotions, they can come back to this kit and remember the skills learned in this program.

Describing the Importance of Home Learning Assignments Between Sessions

This program works best when the children practice their CLUES skills between sessions. Although attendance and practice in session are helpful, completing home learning tasks between sessions will allow children to build upon their skills and generalize them to other, more natural, situations. Explain the importance of practicing these skills between sessions using examples the children can relate to, and suggest that such practice will allow them to feel more prepared to deal with their strong emotions skillfully (e.g., learning to ride a bike, practicing skills in soccer, or rehearsing for a play). Also indicate that children can earn a puzzle piece to go in their CLUES kits for each home learning assignment they complete. At the end of group, these puzzle pieces will be shared and put together to reveal a prize that everyone has earned.

One other way to describe the purpose of home learning is:

> *"You already have a lot of homework and schoolwork. Why do you do homework or schoolwork? The home learning assignments we do for group help us practice the skills we learn here, too. The more we practice these skills, the better detectives we can be. But if we don't practice them, we might forget these skills when we need to use them. So, the more we practice, the easier it will be to remember during a hard time."*

Rewards for Following Rules

Introduce the concept of poker chips or other similar tokens that can be used as reinforcement for *following the rules, participation, and any other positive behaviors that need to be reinforced*. In general, children in the group environment should be rewarded consistently for the same types of behaviors. However, some youth with more challenging in-session behaviors may need additional goals and rewards to maintain attention and participation. The chips can be redeemed for a trip to the "prize box" or similar reward store at the end of every session or every other session. Inexpensive prizes (e.g., stickers, small games, inexpensive miniature figures or stuffed animals) can be purchased from the internet or local stores to create this prize box. Group leaders should determine the schedule for visiting the prize box and should adhere to that schedule consistently throughout treatment. For example, you may offer a trip to the prize box in exchange for three tokens every session or five tokens every other session. Make the threshold for going to the prize box high enough that it motivates the children to follow group rules and so forth, but not so high as to limit opportunities to gain such rewards.

If there is any time left over in the child session, the children can continue to decorate their CLUES kits while the group waits for the parents to return.

Back Together

Session 1, Goal 4

Introduce children to the purpose of emotions and begin to build emotional awareness.

Psychoeducation About Emotions

As the parents rejoin their children, instruct the children to open their workbooks to Figure 1.2: *Normal, Natural, and Harmless.* Begin to provide some basic emotion education by introducing the idea that emotions are (1) normal, (2) natural, and (3) harmless, although they may feel very strong, overwhelming, or uncomfortable. Suggestions for introducing these concepts in a manner consistent with the Emotion Detectives theme include:

> *"A lot of the work we're doing in both of our groups is going to have to do with understanding and dealing with our strong emotions. So we're going to talk about emotions a lot (we call ourselves the Emotion Detectives for a reason)!"*

Encourage the children to volunteer to read aloud each of the words (normal, natural, harmless) for the group. Then, work to explain that emotions are normal, natural, and harmless. This may be done in the following way:

(1) Emotions are **normal**: Everyone experiences emotions, all the time.

> *"Every single one of us probably experiences lots of different emotions every day. That's just part of being human. Can anyone tell me an emotion he or she noticed having today?"*

(2) Emotions are **natural**: Every emotion has a purpose or a goal.

> *"Our emotions can feel pretty strong or intense. Emotions feel that way because they are always trying to get us to DO something. In this group, we are going to call the thing our emotion is trying to get us to do an Emotional Behavior. Think what would happen if you saw a lion trying to break down the door right now. What kind of emotion would you have? Why do you think you would be having that emotion (e.g., fear, etc.)?"*

Give children time to answer, and then point out the function of emotions. (For example, fear in truly dangerous situations tells us to run or fight the thing that makes us feel we are in danger.) You may also elicit examples of sadness or anger here and discuss the potential function of those natural emotions as well, if time permits or if the group experiences these more often.

> *"Our emotions have a purpose or a goal, even though we don't always realize it: they're trying to get us to DO something. In the case of the lion, our fear would be trying to protect us and get us out of danger. What emotional behaviors do you think we would do in order to protect ourselves in this situation?"*

Give the children time to answer before moving on.

(3) Emotions are **harmless**. Although emotions are often intense and sometimes make us feel uncomfortable, they are not *dangerous*, per se.

> *"Some emotions, like feeling sad, scared, or angry, don't always feel good. In fact, they make us pretty uncomfortable, and—because of this—we may want to get rid of those emotions as quickly as possible. However, our emotions are not actually dangerous; they are actually trying to help us or give us information in some way."*

Introducing Emotion Identification

At this point in the group, when the parents and children are back together and have been taught psychoeducational concepts, introduce Worksheet 1.4: *My Emotions at Home*. Have the children (or the parents of children who are unable to read) read the emotion words out loud. Then provide brief descriptions of the purpose of each emotion, along with examples. (For children who are unable to read, it is important to include them in as many ways as possible, such as having them provide examples of when they've experienced certain emotions.)

Happiness

We feel it when: We are pleased or joyous about something that happened or that we did.

The emotional behavior is: to keep doing whatever feels good, and often to tell someone else about it.

The purpose of this behavior is: to keep us doing things that we enjoy and are rewarding for us. Also, to share those activities/situations with other people.

Go through an example of happiness and its emotional behaviors (e.g., You are riding bikes with your best friend outside. What do you feel? What do you want to do?).

Anger

We feel it when: Someone has hurt or mistreated us or someone/something we care about, or we expect this is about to happen.

The emotional behavior is: yelling/screaming/fighting and so forth.

The purpose of this behavior is: to react and defend ourselves or whatever is being threatened.

Go through an example of anger and its emotional behaviors (e.g., You see a bully being mean to your sister. What do you feel? What do you want to do?).

Fear

We feel it when: We believe we are in danger.

The emotional behavior is: to run away or avoid the dangerous situation.

The purpose of this behavior is: to keep us safe!

Go through an example of fear and its emotional behaviors (e.g., You see a stranger near your home. What do you feel? What do you want to do?).

Sadness

We feel it when: We have had a disappointment or experience loss or think this may happen in the future.

The emotional behavior is: feeling tired, numb, wanting to sleep or rest, crying, and so forth.

<u>The purpose of this behavior is</u>: to help us rest up so that we can mourn for what was lost before we move forward; to withdraw from a situation that feels hopeless to avoid future discomfort.

Go through an example of sadness and its emotional behaviors (e.g., You find out your best friend is moving away. What do you feel? What do you want to do?).

To wrap up this content, again review emotional behaviors and their natural purposes (time permitting), including:

1. Happiness: to enjoy the good emotion and share with others
2. Anger: to defend ourselves or loved ones
3. Fear: to get away from danger
4. Sadness: to let our body rest

Emphasize that one major purpose of the UP-C is to recognize these emotional behaviors and start learning other, more helpful behaviors we might use when we feel strong or intense emotions that are leading to less helpful or less needed emotional behaviors.

Return to Worksheet 1.2: *My Goals for Emotion Detectives*

Redirect the children and their parents to Worksheet 1.2: *My Goals for Emotion Detectives*, introduced earlier in the session. Break off with parent/child dyads again to work on writing down two or three goals for each child that correspond to each core problem. You should review the SMART goal concept from Chapter 1 of this Therapist Guide and structure goals for each problem area with this concept as well as overarching UP-C treatment elements in mind. After 5 minutes, ask individuals to share one goal with the entire group.

Review Importance of Home Learning

Review the importance of completing home learning assignments once again. Address any barriers to home learning that might be raised by youth or parents (e.g., the child already has too much homework at school, not sure when to practice this, and so forth). This review might sound something like:

> *"Like we talked about before: home learning will help us become better Emotion Detectives. But without practice, we won't get better at these skills! Does anyone have any questions about this before I go over this week's home learning assignment and our reward system for home learning?"*

If you have not already, review the group reward (such as puzzle pieces) associated with home learning completion with both parents and youth:

"Home learning assignments are a team activity in this group. When you complete your home learning and bring it back, you get a puzzle piece. Everyone will get different pieces of the same puzzle. Once you get all of the puzzle pieces, you can put the puzzle together, and get the prize that is on the puzzle!"

Suggested Home Learning Assignment: My Emotions at Home

For home learning, assign *My Emotions at Home* (Worksheet 1.4) to be completed every night before bed. Each child checks off every emotion he or she experienced that day. In addition, once during the week, the child notes a specific emotion that he or she experienced that week and tries to identify the emotional behavior.

Conclude the session by allowing families to meet with their individual therapists (time permitting) to reflect on the session and provide answers to any initial questions the family might have.

Overall Parent Session 1 Goals

The main goal of this parent session is to introduce parents to the structure of treatment and to the three components of an emotion. A secondary but equally important goal for this first session is to build rapport among the parents and among parents and therapists.

- **Goal 1:** Introduce parents to the structure of treatment and the CLUES skills.
- **Goal 2:** Introduce parents to the three-component model of emotions.
- **Goal 3:** Discuss the cycle of avoidance and other emotional behaviors.

Parent Session 1 Content (Divided by Goals)

Parent Session 1, Goal 1
Introduce parents to the structure of treatment and the CLUES skills.

Getting to Know One Another

This is the first time that the parents come together in a group without their children. This is an excellent opportunity for the parents to get to know one another, openly discuss their child's struggles, and receive support from other parents who are experiencing similar parenting difficulties. Allow each parent(s) or caregiver several minutes to introduce themselves and to briefly explain why they are seeking treatment for their child at this time.

> **Therapist Note**
> *One important function of the parent UP-C group is to provide a forum for caregivers to support and empathize with one another's struggles. Many parents feel quite frustrated and discouraged by the time they begin treatment. They often believe that their child's difficulties are unusual, and they feel alone in their struggles. Parents typically feel relieved to hear that other children and parents are struggling with similar difficulties. Although it can be tempting to allot a significant amount of time to this supportive component of group, we have found that it typically works best to keep this part of the group brief and structured. There are many important skills to present in the parent group, and it is essential that parents learn these skills in order to support their children at home.*

Introduction to Treatment

Once parents and therapists have gotten an opportunity to know one another, emphasize the important role that caregivers play in helping their child to be successful in this treatment. You may wish to introduce the following points:

- **Attendance:** Because each skill in this treatment builds upon the previous one, it is important that caregivers **attend every session** of treatment. It is also helpful for the same caregiver or caregivers to consistently attend treatment each week so that at least one caregiver is getting the "full dose" of the treatment. It is helpful to prepare and hand out a copy of Figure 13.1: *Treatment Schedule* or something similar to every parent in the room.
- **Skills Acquisition and Practice:** Let caregivers know that part of the purpose of the parent group is for parents to learn the skills that their children are learning so that they can be "coaches" who are able

to prompt and support consistent use of skills at home. Parents may also be asked to apply skills to their own experiences, so that they can enhance their understanding of the skill and empathize with how difficult it is to use skills at times.

- ▪ **Parenting Strategies:** Emphasize that parenting an emotional child can be a frustrating and confusing experience. Parents often feel uncertain about how to help their child manage their strong feelings of sadness, anger, or anxiety. In this treatment, parents will also be learning about helpful strategies for parenting a child who experiences strong emotions so that they can become more confident in their ability to help their child manage these emotions. Let the parents know that although these strategies are helpful from your clinical experience and are based on research, they are the ultimate expert on their child! What works for one parent may not work for another.

If time allows, guide parents to read over *Getting Acquainted with Treatment* (p. 93 in workbook). Otherwise, instruct parents to read this over during the week and indicate if they have any questions about the treatment during the next session.

Introduction to the CLUES Skills

Ask the parents to turn to Figure 13.2: *CLUES Skills for Parents* and introduce the **CLUES skills**. Explain to the parents that children will be working to solve the mystery of their emotions during this treatment, and each letter of the CLUES acronym corresponds to a different set of skills that the children will be learning. Provide a very brief discussion of each skill, covering the following points:

1. **C**onsider How I Feel
   <u>Major Topics</u>: Learning about the purpose of an emotion, three parts of an emotion, and acting opposite of what emotions are telling you to do
2. **L**ook at My Thoughts
   <u>Major Topics</u>: Becoming more aware of thoughts and practicing flexibility in thinking
3. **U**se Detective Thinking and Problem Solving
   <u>Major Topics</u>: Challenging unhelpful or unrealistic thoughts, Problem Solving

4. **E**xperience My Emotions
   <u>Major Topics</u>: Present-moment awareness, situational emotion exposures

5. **S**tay Healthy and Happy
   <u>Major Topics</u>: Relapse prevention, celebrating accomplishments

Parent Session 1, Goal 2
Introduce parents to the three-component model of emotions.

Introduction to the Three Parts of an Emotion

During Session 2, children will be introduced to the three parts of an emotion (i.e., thoughts, body feelings, behaviors) as well as the concept of a trigger. Introduce the parents to the three-component model of emotions in this first session so that they can begin observing the different parts of their child's emotional responses over the course of the next week. The introduction to the three-component model of emotions in this session also prepares parents to begin to notice and track their own emotional responses to their child's strong emotions in the following session.

Ask parents to turn to Worksheet 13.1: *C for Parents*, and explain each component of an emotional experience. Provide examples of the emotional components, such as:

1. Getting invited to a party where your child doesn't know anyone (trigger)
2. Worrying that he will have to spend time with people he doesn't know and will have nothing to say (thoughts)
3. Getting sweaty palms and a racing heartbeat on the day of the party (body clues)
4. Telling you he doesn't feel well, and really doesn't want to go (behavior)

OR

1. Your child's friend sitting with another group of kids at lunch (trigger)
2. Thinking that his friend doesn't like him anymore (thought)
3. Eyes feeling watery and lump in throat (body clues)
4. Asking a parent to come pick him up and then isolating at home in his room (behavior)

Have parents each share an example of a time when their child felt anxious, sad, angry, or some other strong emotion. Ask them to discuss the trigger and to break down the emotional experience into its three component parts. (If time permits, you can also have the parents share an example from their own emotional experiences.)

Therapist Note

Explain to the parents that it may be difficult for their children to identify triggers at first. This may be because the trigger is an internal event (e.g., a thought or memory), an event that seems insignificant or minor to an outside observer, or because the child is not able to connect an event to the emotion he or she experiences. Parents can help their children generate ideas of what triggers might be present, and with practice both parties will improve in their ability to recognize the antecedents of emotional experiences.

Parent Session 1, Goal 3
Discuss the cycle of avoidance and other emotional behaviors.

Introduction to Emotional Behaviors

In this treatment, we refer to the action that an emotion wants us to take as an "emotional behavior." Introduce parents to this concept, emphasizing that emotional behaviors are not always maladaptive or ineffective. For example, it would be a good idea to run away if a speeding car were coming toward us or to take some time off from activities if a loved one passed away and we need to recover. However, using emotional behaviors when a situation does not call for it can get children stuck in a vicious cycle of emotional behaviors.

For example, **avoidance** is one of the most common emotional behaviors used by children with emotional disorders to manage distress. Emphasize that one reason why avoidance is such a common emotional behavior is that, in the short term, it reduces distress quickly because the child removes himself or herself from the situation or object that is causing the distress. Children learn that avoidance makes them feel better, so they continue to use it to manage their emotions.

However, this vicious cycle of avoidance has problematic long-term consequences. Introduce parents to these consequences by presenting the following scenarios:

1. What would happen if your child was feeling nervous and decided to avoid:
   a. First session of Emotion Detectives?
   b. Soccer practice?
   c. First day of school?
   d. Friend's birthday party?
2. What would happen if your child was feeling sad and decided to avoid:
   a. Riding a bike?
   b. Playing with friends?
   c. Doing homework?

Avoidance reduces an uncomfortable emotion very quickly, which "teaches" us that it was a successful coping strategy. But when we avoid situations, we never learn whether our feared or other negative outcome would have come true (for example, "no kids will like me"; "I'll get lost"; "I won't have fun"), and thus we cannot learn that the situation was inherently safe/rewarding. Therefore, we think the only successful way to cope with the situation is through avoidance. Finally, we may have missed out on important experiences during the first session/practice/social event, and thus feel as though we would be behind if we joined now.

During treatment sessions, you will teach children and parents to address and interrupt the cycle of avoidance. Parents can (and should) model brave behavior whenever possible, although this behavior may be difficult to do at first. Clarify that the parent group is a space to discuss successes and barriers to facing our emotions, rather than avoiding them.

Some children may not outright avoid situations that make them uncomfortable but may instead rely on behaviors (e.g., avoiding eye contact), objects (e.g., a stuffed animal), or people (e.g., a parent) to endure the distressing situations. These are called **safety behaviors** and are another type of emotional behavior because they help to reduce distress in the short term but can make it more difficult in the long term to endure the situation without using the safety behavior.

You may also wish to mention at this point that other children may not avoid situations that elicit strong emotions but instead may verbally or physically "attack" the situation or person that is making them angry or frustrated. Although the child is taking a more approach-oriented behavior to reduce distress, these types of aggressive behaviors often result in a

cycle of angry behaviors in the long term because the child never learns to experience uncomfortable emotions and generate more prosocial or adaptive methods for regulating them.

Suggested Parent Home Learning Assignment: C for Parents

Ask the parent to complete Worksheet 13.1: *C for Parents* in the workbook this week. In this home learning assignment, parents will attend to one time during which their child experiences a strong emotion and will identify the trigger and the three parts of their child's emotional experience.

Appendix 11.1: Weekly Top Problems Tracking Form

Weekly Top Problems Tracking Form		
CHILD:		PARENT:
1.		1.
2.		2.
3.		3.
Not at All a Problem	Somewhat a Problem	Very Much a Problem
0 1 2	3 4 5	6 7 8

	Child Ratings	**Parent Ratings**	
	1._____	1._____	What worked well this week?
Week 1	2._____	2._____	
	3._____	3._____	
	1._____	1._____	What worked well this week?
Week 2	2._____	2._____	
	3._____	3._____	
	1._____	1._____	What worked well this week?
Week 3	2._____	2._____	
	3._____	3._____	
	1._____	1._____	What worked well this week?
Week 4	2._____	2._____	
	3._____	3._____	
	1._____	1._____	What worked well this week?
Week 5	2._____	2._____	
	3._____	3._____	
	1._____	1._____	What worked well this week?
Week 6	2._____	2._____	
	3._____	3._____	

	1._____	1._____	What worked well this week?
Week 7	2._____	2._____	
	3._____	3._____	
	1._____	1._____	What worked well this week?
Week 8	2._____	2._____	
	3._____	3._____	
	1._____	1._____	What worked well this week?
Week 9	2._____	2._____	
	3._____	3._____	
	1._____	1._____	What worked well this week?
Week 10	2._____	2._____	
	3._____	3._____	
	1._____	1._____	What worked well this week?
Week 11	2._____	2._____	
	3._____	3._____	
	1._____	1._____	What worked well this week?
Week 12	2._____	2._____	
	3._____	3._____	
	1._____	1._____	What worked well this week?
Week 13	2._____	2._____	
	3._____	3._____.	
	1._____	1._____	What worked well this week?
Week 14	2._____	2._____	
	3._____	3._____	
	1._____	1._____	What worked well this week?
Week 15	2._____	2._____	
	3._____	3._____	

CHAPTER 12   UP-C Session 2: Getting to Know Your Emotions

C Skill: Consider How I Feel

MATERIALS NEEDED FOR GROUP

- For Each Child Group Session:
  1. Detective CLUES kits for each child
  2. Poker chips
  3. Puzzle
  4. Prize box
  5. Large piece of paper or whiteboard to record children's answers for any group activities
- For Session 2 Only:
  6. Large emotion thermometer
  7. UP-C Workbook Chapter 2
     a. *The Emotion Thermometer* (Figure 2.1)
     b. *C for Children* (Worksheet 2.1)
     c. *Cycle of Emotions and Behaviors* (Figure 2.2)
     d. *Rewards List* (Worksheet 2.2)
- For Home Learning:
  8. *Solving the Mystery of Our Emotions: Before, During, and After* (Form 2.1)
- Assessments to Be Given at Every Session:
  9. *Weekly Top Problems Tracking Form* (Use the same form started during Session 1 for each child, found in Appendix 11.1 at the end of Chapter 11 of this Therapist Guide)

■ For Parent Group Session:
10. UP-C Workbook Chapter 13
   a. *Sample Double Before, During, and After* (Figure 13.3)
■ For Parent Home Learning:
11. *Double Before, During, and After* (Worksheet 13.2)

Therapist Preparation

In preparation for this session, you should create a large thermometer with markers and butcher paper. The butcher paper should be long enough for each child client to stand beside it when it is laid out (approximately 10–12 feet). On the butcher paper, draw a large thermometer or similar scale, with numbers marked 0 through 8 along the side (to indicate the intensity or strength of the emotion). This scale will then be used for the *Emotion Thermometer* activity later in the session. If you are short on time or working with older youth, you can print out a large picture of a thermometer and adjust the activity described below to the picture's smaller appearance.

Overall Session 2 Goals

The main goal of this session is to provide education about the structure and function of emotions. The child group members will begin to practice identifying and rating the intensity of their emotions, as well as breaking emotions down into their component parts (e.g., thoughts, body clues, behaviors). Children also learn to understand the course of their emotional experiences by examining what happens *Before, During, and After* a given emotion. The cycle of avoidance and other emotional behaviors are also covered.

■ **Goal 1:** Learn to identify and rate the strength or intensity of different emotions.
■ **Goal 2:** Continue to normalize emotional experiences.
■ **Goal 3:** Introduce the three parts of an emotional experience.
■ **Goal 4:** Help children to understand the cycle of avoidance and other emotional behaviors.
■ **Goal 5:** Identify rewards children would like to earn during treatment for new, helpful behaviors.

Session 2, Goal 1

Learn to identify and rate the strength or intensity of different emotions.

While the Group Is Together

As you welcome back the group for the start of the second session, circulate and assist parents and children by obtaining severity ratings for each of their three top problems and continue to praise and encourage children as they work toward their goals. These ratings should be entered on the same *Weekly Top Problems Tracking Form* (Appendix 11.1 at the end of Chapter 11 in this Therapist Guide) begun during Session 1. Also check that each child has completed the home learning assignment. Encourage any children who have not completed the assignment to do so next time. For those children who have completed the assignment, distribute one puzzle piece to each.

Briefly review content introduced in the UP-C Session 1 (e.g., the Emotion Detectives theme, the introduction of varying types of strong or intense emotions, and the idea that these emotions are prompting us to do some helpful and some less helpful behaviors). After this brief review, if conducting groups simultaneously, the parents leave the room for the parent group. If conducting the child group independently, parents move to the waiting area.

Child Group Alone

Emotion Thermometer Activity

Review with the children that last week the group talked about the fact that emotions are normal—that everyone has them all the time. Then explain that, even though everyone has emotions, different kids are scared of or sad or angry about very different things. Explain that the group is going to play a game to practice identifying how each group member feels when faced with different situations or things. Remind the child group members that everyone is different, so each group member might have different answers. There are, in fact, no right or wrong answers in this game!

Introduce the concept of an emotion thermometer using the *Emotion Thermometer* (Figure 2.1) as a guide. You may choose to introduce the idea of an **emotion thermometer** in the following way:

> *"Just like a normal thermometer goes up when it is hot, the number on the emotion thermometer goes up as our emotions get stronger. We might feel stronger emotions at different times or when we have different thoughts. Look at what Jack tells us here! When Nina is about to go on a roller coaster, she feels scared at a 4. But when he goes on a roller coaster, Jack feels scared at a 0. Jack is scared of bugs, though; his emotion thermometer goes up when he sees a bumble bee!"*

Next, bring out the large *Emotion Thermometer* that you created, lay it on the floor in the middle of the room, and explain to the group that they will be using it to take the "temperature" of their emotions, from cold/none (0), to cool/low (2), to warm/medium (4), to hot/a lot (6), to very hot/very much (8). One at a time, present a potentially emotionally evocative situation to the group such as:

1. Eating ice cream
2. Seeing a friend get hurt
3. Going to the dentist
4. First day of school
5. Losing a game (e.g., checkers, kickball)

Ask the children to report (by standing next to the large thermometer) how strongly they would feel the emotion in that situation or *how high/hot their "temperature" would be* on the thermometer. All children in the group may rate their emotional intensity at once by having multiple children standing next to the same number or different numbers that represent their impression of the emotional intensity they would have in response to the trigger presented. You can also join this activity to demonstrate a range of responses to each scenario. Make sure to point out similarities and differences across ratings of intensity. Use this as an opportunity to discuss the normative experience of emotions, what emotions children would have in the scenarios presented, as well as how each group member experiences such situations differently.

Session 2, Goal 2

Continue to normalize emotional experiences.

Review with the children that emotions are normal, natural, and harmless. A review of this idea might sound something like:

*"Last time we talked about our feelings and how they always have a purpose. Emotions tell us something about what is going on around us. When an emotion feels uncomfortable or icky, it feels that way because the emotion wants us to do something, like get away, rest, fight, or get help. The emotion does not want to be ignored because it is trying to get us to **do something**. But sometimes we feel these strong emotions even when there is nothing truly wrong or dangerous happening around us."*

Alarm Game

The alarm game is used to allow children to begin to differentiate between situations that are truly threatening (**true alarm**) and those that just feel threatening but are not actually (**false alarm**). Explain that our brains have an alarm system that goes off when it seems that something very bad or very dangerous is happening. The problem is that for some kids, their alarm system is too sensitive and goes off too easily or too strongly. This is called a false alarm. It may help to use the analogy of a car alarm that seems to go off whenever anyone or anything gets near it, even though nobody is trying to break into the car. Similarly, sometimes our fear alarm goes off when nothing truly dangerous is happening, our sadness alarm goes off when nothing very bad or terrible just happened to us, or our anger alarm goes off when we don't actually need to defend ourselves. Provide the following instructions and examples for this activity:

*"I want you to listen closely to some stories and help me decide which situations are actually dangerous, very bad, or causing a real problem for the person. If the story is describing something that is actually very bad or threatening, then it is a true alarm. On the other hand, if Jack and Nina just **feel** like the situation is very bad or dangerous, even if things are probably going to be fine, then it is a false alarm. You decide: is it a true or false alarm?"*

Examples:

- *Jack is going to the store and sees a car coming around the corner really fast! He gets scared that he is going to get hit, so he runs out of the way.* True or false alarm? (True)

- *Nina is going to a birthday party and is worried that she is wearing the wrong kind of clothes. She is afraid that everyone will laugh at her, so she decides not to go.*
  True or false alarm? (False)

- *Jack is playing tag during recess and he falls. He doesn't really hurt himself, but he gets a grass stain on his shirt and skins his knee. He gets really upset and angry at himself and cannot calm down. He goes to the nurse and asks to go home.*
  True or false alarm? (False)

- *Nina sees some kids talking and laughing across the street. She believes that they are laughing at her. She feels really sad because she feels like no matter what she does, other kids just don't like her. She goes back to her house and spends the rest of the day alone in her room.*
  True or false alarm? (False)

- *Jack trips in the hallway over another kid's foot. The other kid says sorry right away and that it was an accident. Jack gets very angry. He thinks the other kid must have done it purposely and yells at the other kid.*
  True or false alarm? (False)

- *Nina walks into class and another kid walks up to her and calls her a mean name. This kid is not nice to Nina a lot of the time and has called her mean names in the past. Nina feels really sad and decides to tell the teacher.*
  True or false alarm? (True)

After completing the alarm game, reflect with the children about what is different between true and false alarms, and how they can tell the difference. Emphasize that true alarms occur when there is true danger or something is really wrong in our lives, and the strong emotions that we feel help prepare us to get to safety, rest up, defend ourselves, or get help. False alarms occur when our bodies want us to avoid something even though there is no real danger or harm occurring. Sometimes, we also feel alarms in our bodies more strongly or quickly than expected given the amount of actual danger present. We can look more closely at the "parts" of our reactions to strong emotions to help us tell if we are dealing with a true or false alarm.

Session 2, Goal 3
Introduce the three parts of an emotional experience.

The Parts of an Emotion

To segue from the alarm game to discussing the three parts of our emotional responses, you might state:

> *"Even if we are having a false alarm, we might be feeling scared, anxious, angry, or sad, just the same as we would for a true alarm. Either way, it can be really helpful to look at the different parts of our emotions. Doing this can help give us even more clues as to what might keep strong or uncomfortable emotions going, even when they could be false alarms. Let's look at your workbook to help understand more about what I mean."*

Direct children to *C for Children* (Worksheet 2.1). Explain the idea that, even though emotions can be overwhelming and confusing, as detectives, group members can take a closer look and begin to realize that there are several parts of an emotion. Children should be told that, by beginning to recognize when they experience strong emotions as well as the parts of these reactions, they can begin to figure out why their emotions feel so strong and how to deal with them more effectively. This discussion might sound something like:

> *"Most of the time our emotions are a big mystery to us. When an emotion starts, everything begins to happen so fast. Often our emotions feel so strong that it's really hard to imagine that they have different parts. But, by looking at these emotions closely and breaking them down, we might be able to figure out what we can do to help!"*

Triggers

Next, introduce the concept of a **trigger**, or the situation, person, place, thought, or thing that seems to be leading us to feeling a strong emotion. Remember as you present this material that triggers may be external to the child or internal (thoughts, physical sensations). This might sound something like:

> *"Before every strong emotion there is a trigger, and this trigger is what we think is leading us to feel this strong reaction. For instance, if you're scared because there is a lion trying to break down your door, the lion is the trigger. It is the thing that leads you to feel scared. A trigger might be a situation like riding on an elevator, but it could also be hearing some news, seeing something, thinking about certain things, or even just having a conversation with someone. The trigger does NOT have to be something outside of our bodies. Sometimes a trigger can also be a*

thought we had or a feeling in our bodies, like our heart beating faster or a sad thought. There are many, many more possible triggers. And sometimes they are easier to identify than others. The trigger might be obvious, like a lion, or not so obvious, like remembering something someone said earlier today or even just our breathing feeling faster than normal.

Here is a trick for figuring out the trigger:

- *If you think of a sentence about an emotion*
- *Like: I was (scared/happy/sad/surprised/angry) because . . .*
- *Whatever comes after the '**because**' is probably part of the trigger."*

You might then present an example (e.g., angry/frustrated because you just lost a game or your friend won't share something with you) and ask the children to identify the trigger. You would then ask the children to brainstorm about possible triggers for the situation provided. As time permits, you can further personalize this information with situations more relevant to your child clients until the children clearly understand that the trigger is a big factor leading to strong emotions and subsequent responses to them.

The Three Components of Emotions

Draw three circles (on paper, whiteboard, or chalkboard, for example) and write one of the following titles above each circle: (1) **thoughts**, (2) **body clues**, and (3) **behaviors** while the children follow along in their workbooks using Worksheet 2.1: *C for Children*. Then explain each of these parts of the emotion/emotional reaction to the children. After explaining each component of an emotional reaction, ask children to identify the component within an example (e.g., being scared in an elevator, being angry after getting a bad grade, being sad about a friend moving away). This might be done in the following way:

*"**Thoughts** are what we think. A thought is something that the person is thinking or saying to herself that leads to feeling the emotion or makes the emotion stronger. The thought might be about something that happened in the past, something that is happening right now, or something that might happen in the future. A thought can also be described as the words in a thought bubble above a character's head in a comic or cartoon. Examples of thoughts that can be related to strong emotions include:*

Fear: That snake is going to bite me.

Sadness: I am never going to get to play with that toy again now that it's broken.

Anger: My sister is so mean to me at dinnertime.

Body clues *are what we feel in our bodies. Body clues refer to the things that we feel in different parts of our bodies while we are experiencing an emotion. Examples of body clues for different emotions include:*

Fear: nausea, dizziness, heart racing, fast breathing

Sadness: tightness in the throat, fatigue, headache, crying

Anger: feeling warm, tense or tight muscles

Behavior *is what we do. The behavior refers to the action that we take (or may want to take) as a result of experiencing an emotion. Examples of behaviors related to emotions are:*

Fear: escape/running away

Sadness: lying down or crying

Anger: yelling, throwing something."

Therapist Note

Remind the children that the purpose of emotions is to get us to do something (usually to reduce the severity of the thoughts and body clues).

The following is an additional example of the three components of an emotion:

*"It's Friday after school. Nina has a big book report to give in class on Monday, but she doesn't like talking in front of other people. Nina hasn't started working on the project yet. Every time she starts working on the project, she worries that the kids will laugh at her on Monday, and she's worried that she will sound stupid (these are her **thoughts**). When Nina thinks about the report on Monday, she feels her muscles and stomach tense up (these are her **body clues**). To try and make these feelings go away she decides to watch some TV to get her mind off of the project and the kids at school (this is the **behavior**). This is one example of what might happen when you know about an event that's going to occur and you're thinking ahead about what it will be like."*

Explain that, unlike in that example, sometimes the emotion can build up really quickly. You can provide the following example to illustrate this:

"Imagine you have to go to the dentist for a regular checkup. The dentist tells you, 'You have a big cavity, and I am going to fill it right now!' Your emotion might feel really strong, REALLY fast:

a) *Trigger: The dentist tells you he is going to fill your cavity.*

b) *Thoughts: Your thoughts might be, 'Oh no, this is going to hurt; I don't want to do this.'*

c) *Body clues: You may notice your hands getting sweaty and your stomach turning over and over.*

d) *Behavior: You might look for your mom or tell the dentist you don't have time to do it right now and will have to schedule it another time."*

Session 2, Goal 4

Help children understand the cycle of avoidance and other emotional behaviors.

Using Figure 2.2: *Cycle of Emotions and Behaviors*, introduce the cycle of avoidance and other emotional behaviors, like aggression. This might sound something like:

> *"As we've seen, each **emotion has three parts**. Often, we have a strong emotion like feeling sad, angry, or afraid because it's helpful to us, and the behavior that the emotion is telling us to do keeps us safe or protects us in some other way. But sometimes, like we learned in the alarm game, our emotional behaviors don't help us. Instead they sometimes keep us from doing things we enjoy, like going to a party or spending time with other kids who we like, or emotional behaviors may get us into trouble.*
>
> *Many times, our emotions seem to be telling us that we need to do something to avoid the situation that is making us feel nervous or sad. Does anyone know what 'avoid' means? (Pause for response). To avoid is to get away or stay away from a situation, sometimes because the strong emotions we have feel really yucky or upsetting. We'd rather be home or with our parents or another place where it feels safer or where we feel protected.*
>
> *Avoiding seems like a really helpful thing to do in order to feel better in the short term. For example, if we don't go to the party, we don't have to spend all day worrying that someone might make fun of us or feeling sad that we may not have that many people to talk to. The problem is that avoiding (or escaping from, or even sometimes distracting ourselves from) a particular trigger doesn't allow us to actually figure out what might REALLY happen in that situation. For instance, are we SURE that people would make fun of us at the party or do we know for sure that there wouldn't be more or new people to talk to? Probably not. What else could happen? It's hard to know until we try it out.*
>
> *Instead of making us want to avoid a situation, sometimes our emotions may make us want to do things like fight or yell in the situation that is making us feel*

*the emotion. For example, if your mom asks you to turn off your videogame in the middle of an important part to do your homework, you might feel really angry at her. Your anger might be so strong that you act on it right away by yelling or slamming the door to your room. This is a different type of **emotional behavior**, and often when we're angry it feels really hard to stop ourselves from acting on some of these behaviors. However, right now, would yelling or slamming your door be helpful or not helpful to you?*

Let's think about emotional behaviors like avoiding or yelling in the long term. If we never go to any parties because we don't want anyone to think something bad about us, what would happen? How do you think your mom would react to you yelling and slamming the door? What might happen if you keep doing that over time? Emotional behaviors may make us feel better right now, but they make us feel worse or cause more problems for us later on, and we don't learn how to deal with them in a more helpful way as they are happening.

But our work together here in Emotion Detectives will help us to pick more helpful behaviors, so that we act in ways that work out for us better in the long run. So you are on the right track!"

At this point, work with individual children to fill in the three-component model on *C for Children* (Worksheet 2.1) for at least one personally relevant emotional situation until the parents return.

Back Together

Session 2, Goal 5

Identify rewards children would like to earn during treatment for new, helpful behaviors.

Rewards Lists

Break into parent/child dyads, and hand out Worksheet 2.2: *Rewards List*. Instruct parents and children to brainstorm appropriate rewards for engaging in new, more helpful actions and/or brave behaviors. This might include a discussion about how the children will be working hard to change emotional behaviors by **acting opposite** or doing things differently when they feel a strong emotion, which takes a lot of bravery and effort and can be difficult to do without some good rewards.

> **Therapist Note**
>
> *Opposite action will be covered more fully in Chapter 13 (Session 3 of Module C). Thus, only a brief discussion of this concept should be introduced in relation to reward here.*

Work with each family to identify a minimum of five rewards for new, more helpful actions and/or brave behavior that can be used in treatment. In general, rewards ideally should be low to no cost and can include special times, privileges, and activities. Examples might include an ice-cream cone, getting to pick where the family goes to dinner (or what they eat at home), getting to pick a movie to rent, going to the park with a parent, getting a small toy or token, or reading a book with mom or dad. For children who want to incorporate screen time as a reward, suggest to families that this reward be clearly scheduled to follow the desired helpful or brave behavior and not be given freely before the behavior has been completed.

> **Suggested Home Learning Assignment: Solving the Mystery of Our Emotions: Before, During, and After**
>
> As a last component of Session 2, review the home learning assignment for the upcoming week. Children complete the home learning assignment described on *Solving the Mystery of Our Emotions: Before, During, and After* (Form 2.1). Instruct the children to pick an emotion they experience over the upcoming week and to use their *Solving the Mystery of Our Emotions* form to identify the Before (the trigger), the During (the three parts of their emotional response or experience), and the After (the consequences of the emotional behavior). For the After, instruct children to identify all the consequences of using the emotional behavior they can think of, including both short-term and long-term ones. It may be helpful to walk each child and parent through completing this home learning assignment, using the emotional experience they already identified on their *C for Children* worksheet. Let children and parents know that children are expected to track one emotional experience each week for the rest of treatment using this form.

Overall Parent Session 2 Goals

The main goal of this session is to introduce parents to the idea that the parenting behaviors they use in response to their child's strong emotions may accidentally maintain or even amplify their child's distress, despite good intentions to help their children in emotional situations. Parents are introduced to the *Double Before, During, and After* (*Double BDA*, Worksheet 13.2) as a means of tracking their own emotions and parenting behaviors in response to their child's strong emotions. Toward the end of the session, you will provide an overview of one common emotional parenting behavior (criticism) and its opposite parenting behavior (praise/positive reinforcement) in preparation for the creation of rewards lists at the end of the session.

- **Goal 1:** Introduce parents to Worksheet 13.2: *Double Before, During, and After.*
- **Goal 2:** Introduce parents to four emotional parenting behaviors and their opposite parenting behaviors.
- **Goal 3:** Discuss providing positive reinforcement as an opposite parenting behavior for criticism.

Parent Session 2 Content (Divided by Goals)

Parent Session 2, Goal 1

Introduce parents to Worksheet 13.2: Double Before, During, and After (Double BDA).

> **Therapist Note**
> *You should begin this session and each subsequent one with a **brief** check-in regarding major changes in child symptoms/functioning over the past week, as well as a review of home learning assignments. Typically, you should limit this check-in to no more than 10 minutes in order to leave adequate time to cover new content.*

Emotional Parenting Behaviors

In this session, you will be introducing parents to the idea that some behaviors and parenting strategies they use to manage child distress—hereafter referred to as **emotional parenting behaviors**—may not be optimally effective and may even backfire, resulting in increased distress. When beginning this discussion, we suggest that you first align with the families over their struggle to parent their children as best they can.

You should normalize the struggles parents face when parenting a child with an emotional disorder, and you should be sure to praise parents for attempting to support their child and manage their child's behavior as best they can.

An effective way to begin this discussion may be to use Worksheet 13.1: *C for Parents*, which you just reviewed, to highlight how mysterious and distressing children's emotional responses can be for parents. Depending upon the examples shared by parents, you may wish to highlight some of the following points: (1) how difficult it can be to identify or understand triggers for children's emotions; (2) how quickly emotional experiences can escalate; (3) how difficult it can be to encourage "approach behaviors" when children have a strong desire to avoid; and (4) how confusing it can be to know how to respond to somatic symptoms of distress. Given how mysterious children's emotional experiences can seem to parents, and given how little insight children often have into their own emotions, it is no wonder that parents often feel confused about how best to manage their child's distress! Naturally, parents often act in these situations from a desire to lessen their child's distress, but some of the strategies used by parents unintentionally limit the child's interaction with upsetting situations or stimuli, thereby accidentally reinforcing the child's emotional disorder symptoms over time.

Double Before, During, and After Worksheet

Introduce parents to Figure 13.3: *Sample Double Before, During, and After*. For further guidance on how to introduce this figure to parents, see "Goal 1" in Module-P of the UP-A Therapist Guide (Chapter 9 of this book). After you discuss the sample form with the parents, ask them to complete Worksheet 13.2: *Double BDA* during the session, using the same emotional experience they broke down on the Worksheet 13.1: *C for Parents* home learning assignment. After parents have completed the *Double BDA*, ask them to share their emotional reactions, parenting behaviors, and short- and long-term consequences of those behaviors. As parents share, pay particular attention to times when they respond in a manner that limits their child's distress in the short term but reinforces future use of avoidance or other emotional behaviors to manage emotions. You should gently point out these responses while also normalizing the frustration, anxiety, sadness, or anger experienced by parents.

Parent Session 2, Goal 2

Introduce parents to four emotional parenting behaviors and their opposite parenting behaviors.

Four Emotional Parenting Behaviors

Now that parents have begun to identify how some of their behaviors and responses to their child's emotions may be counterproductive in the long term, it is helpful to introduce parents to four types of emotional behaviors that may be particularly ineffective in managing their child's strong emotions. Ask parents to turn to Table 13.1 in the parent portion of the UP-C workbook, titled *Common Emotional Parenting Behaviors and Their Opposite Parenting Behaviors.*

Therapist Note

Before beginning this discussion, it is important to note that some parents are quite sensitive to discussions of how they can adjust their parenting behaviors to manage their child's symptoms more effectively and promote more independent coping. Some parents may become defensive during this conversation because they feel their parenting behaviors are being criticized, and indeed they may be "primed" to react in this way due to numerous suggestions and even criticisms of their parenting they have received in the past from family members, teachers, or friends. Some parents may feel misunderstood or invalidated because they do believe that they have tried everything, and none of it has worked!

To facilitate an open discussion of emotional parenting behaviors, it can be helpful to reinforce the following points:

1. These four emotional parenting behaviors are extremely common (even in parents of children without emotional disorders) and often arise out of well-intentioned efforts to reduce the child's distress.

2. All parents can benefit from learning more effective ways to manage their child's distress. The strategies discussed in this treatment are not ones that come naturally to parents, and they are helpful for all parents to learn.

3. Parenting is overwhelming, exhausting, and anxiety-provoking at times. Parents are allowed to have their emotions too, and there will naturally be times when parents act in ways to minimize their own emotional responses to child distress. Parents are not expected to use

these strategies perfectly by the end of treatment, and we encourage parents to be aware of their limits.

Provide a brief overview of each of the four emotional parenting behaviors listed in Table 13.1, discussing examples of each behavior and short- and long-term consequences as necessary. Briefly review each of the four opposite parenting behaviors, emphasizing that these will be addressed in more depth throughout treatment.

Parent Session 2, Goal 3

Discuss providing positive reinforcement as an opposite parenting behavior to criticism.

Criticism

Point out that all the parents in the room are there because there may be things that are not going very well for their child right now, and there are problems that need to be addressed in order to improve their child's functioning and quality of life. These problems will be addressed in this treatment; however, especially early in treatment, it is important to focus on *things that are going well* for their child or ways in which their child is coping effectively. Often, children with emotional challenges think that they "can't do anything right." This can be a result of unrealistic or unhelpful thinking (which we will discuss further in UP-C Sessions 5 and 6), but children may also believe this because teachers, friends, coaches, and even parents at times focus on the things that are going wrong rather than on the things that are going right. Children with emotional disorders may also be especially sensitive to perceived criticism and may be more likely to interpret ambiguous expressions or statements as being critical.

Increasing Positive Reinforcement

Explain to parents that we would like them to begin practicing paying more attention to (i.e., reinforcing) times when their child is being successful or attempting to use skills, and paying less attention to or even ignoring times when their child is being disruptive or annoying or worrying excessively. Often parents pay too much attention to these types of behaviors in an effort to reduce them or because it is difficult for them to tolerate their child's distress. Point out, however, that attention can accidentally or paradoxically increase the problem behavior or emotion, even if the parent perceives the attention as being negative or corrective. Attention is a powerful reinforcer, and children who are not receiving positive attention will often prefer negative attention to no attention at all. By providing more positive attention to skills use and ignoring minor misbehaviors, parents encourage children to continue to engage in positive behaviors and increase their sense of self-esteem or self-efficacy.

Discuss that there are many ways for parents to attend to and reinforce their child. Brainstorm ideas with the parents, making sure to highlight the following reinforcement methods: looking in the child's direction, smiling, nodding, verbal praise (e.g., "Great job talking to your teacher even though it was difficult"), and rewards (both tangible and intangible).

Explain to parents that when the group comes back together in a few moments, parents and children will spend some time together generating a Rewards List. The purpose of this Rewards List is to identify reinforcements that parents and therapists can use throughout treatment to encourage brave or more helpful behavior in situations where children experience strong emotions. Reassure parents that these rewards are *not* intended to be costly and that they and their child are encouraged to generate examples of non-monetary rewards (e.g., watching a movie on a school night, getting to stay up late one night, choosing what's for dinner, activity alone with a parent without other siblings present). Reassure parents that rewards can be phased out after their child is successfully approaching or coping with a situation.

Suggested Parent Home Learning Assignment: *Double BDA*

Ask each parent to complete at least one *Double BDA* (Worksheet 13.2) for home learning, focusing on an emotional experience their child has in the upcoming week.

CHAPTER 13

UP-C Session 3: Using Science Experiments to Change Our Emotions and Behavior

C Skill: Consider How I Feel

MATERIALS NEEDED FOR GROUP

- For Each Child Group Session:
  1. Detective CLUES kits for each child
  2. Poker chips
  3. Puzzle
  4. Prize box
  5. Large piece of paper or whiteboard to record children's answers for any group activities
- For Session 3 Only:
  6. iPhone/iPod/musical device (song to dance to) + speakers
  7. UP-C Workbook Chapter 3
     a. *Acting Opposite* (Worksheet 3.1)
     b. *Parts of a Science Experiment* (Worksheet 3.2)
     c. *The Emotion Thermometer for Happy* (Figure 3.1)
     d. *Nina's Emotion and Activity Diary* (Figure 3.2)
     e. *List of Activities* (Worksheet 3.3)
     f. *My Activities List* (Worksheet 3.4)
- For Home Learning:
  8. *My Emotion and Activity Diary* (Worksheet 3.5)
  9. *Solving the Mystery of Our Emotions: Before, During, and After* (Form 2.1; use the same form started after Session 2)
  10. *Acting Opposite Plans* (Form 3.1) (optional)

Assessments to Be Given at Every Session

11. *Weekly Top Problems Tracking Form* (Use the same form started during Session 1 for each child, found in Appendix 11.1 at the end of Chapter 11 of this Therapist Guide)

For Parent Group Session:

12. UP-C Workbook Chapter 13
    a. *10 Ways to Reinforce Your Child* (Worksheet 13.3)

For Parent Home Learning:

13. *Double Before, During, and After* (Worksheet 13.4)
14. *10 Ways to Reinforce Your Child Worksheet*, bottom part (Worksheet 13.3)

Therapist Preparation

In preparation for this session, choose a child-appropriate, upbeat song, and bring equipment to play the song during session.

Overall Session 3 Goals

The main goal of this session is to teach children the skill of acting opposite to what their emotional behavior may be telling them to do, and then apply this skill in a "science experiment" focused on sadness. Although you will be devoting some time at the beginning of this session to a discussion of acting opposite in the context of other emotions, we focus on sadness primarily because most children can relate to the experience of feeling bored or sad at some point, and it is relatively easy for them to see how changing their behavior changes this emotion. This session also helps set the stage for situational emotion exposures for other emotions later in this treatment. For further discussion of the rationale for emotion-focused behavioral experiments *and options for initiating exposure work following this session rather than waiting until later in treatment*, see UP-A Module 3 (Chapter 3 in this book).

- **Goal 1:** Learn about the concept of acting opposite.
- **Goal 2:** Introduce the idea of using science experiments to help with emotional behaviors and acting opposite.
- **Goal 3:** Review the connection between activity and emotions and identify enjoyable activities.
- **Goal 4:** Teach children how to track their emotions and activities in the context of a science experiment.

Session 3, Goal 1

Learn about the concept of acting opposite.

While the Group Is Together

As you welcome back the group for the start of the third session, circulate and assist parents and children in providing severity ratings for each of their three top problems and continue to praise and encourage children as they work toward their goals. These ratings should be entered on the same *Weekly Top Problems Tracking Form* (Appendix 11.1 at the end of Chapter 11 in this Therapist Guide) begun during Session 1. Also check that each child has completed the home learning assignment. Complete a brief review of last session's assignment so that each child goes over his or her *Solving the Mystery of Our Emotions: Before, During, and After* (Form 2.1) together in the group. Ask the children to briefly explain the Before, During, and After for their emotional experience. For those children who have completed the home learning activities, distribute one puzzle piece to each.

Child Group Alone

As you continue to welcome child group members to today's session, remind them of the three parts of their emotional response to triggers. Explain that the focus of today's group session will be on the "behavior" part of that response. Then introduce the idea of **acting opposite**, or differently, from the thing that our emotion normally wants us to do. You might introduce this in the following way:

"You may remember that we all talked about how every emotion or strong feeling we have has an emotional behavior that goes along with it. Like when we feel sad, we sometimes feel like we want to go lie down and rest. Sometimes when we feel a strong emotion, especially ones like fear or anger, we go and do something right away, without stopping to think about whether there is anything else we could do—like, we may run away if we are afraid. And sometimes this is definitely the

most helpful thing we can do in the moment. But sometimes doing something **different** *would actually help us even more—or at least help us more in terms of learning how to deal with our strong emotions."*

Ask the children to turn to Worksheet 3.1: *Acting Opposite* in their workbooks and to work together to think about whether they ever noticed the thing that their strong emotion wanted them to do but they did something else instead. Allow them to share. This can initially be a difficult concept for children to grasp, so you may share appropriate examples if children have difficulty. Examples might include being nervous to speak up in class but deciding to volunteer to share first, or feeling sad on a Saturday but deciding to call a friend to hang out.

"Doing something different from what your emotion wants you to do is called 'acting opposite.' As we have been discussing, sometimes our emotions are actually false alarms, telling us that a situation is really bad or really dangerous when it actually isn't. When this happens, our emotions may be telling us to do more than we need to do or something we don't need to do altogether. Acting opposite is a tool we can use to see if some other behavior is more helpful to us than the one our emotion wants us to try out first. In your workbook on the page that says 'Acting Opposite' at the top, Nina has given us an example of what acting opposite might be like for angry emotions!"

Lead the children in a discussion of opposite actions for at least three or four different emotions. Some examples include:

- *Sadness*: going for a walk; calling a friend
- *Anxiety*: approaching the situation that is making you anxious
- *Anger/frustration*: calmly expressing your opinion, apologizing

Have children write down some of their ideas for ways to act opposite in the boxes on Worksheet 3.1: *Acting Opposite*. Explain to the children that, this week, they will be working on acting opposite when feeling sad, down, or bored. However, you can encourage them to act opposite during other times too when they notice that their emotional behaviors are not really helping them out that much.

Session 3, Goal 2

Introduce the idea of using science experiments to help with emotional behaviors and acting opposite.

Begin by asking the children if they notice a connection between their emotions and the activities they do in an average day or week:

"What kind of emotion do you feel when you're stuck inside during recess on a rainy day? How about when you go outside for recess? What emotion do you feel when you are doing an activity you really enjoy, such as art or sports or dance? What kinds of things do you do or play with to make you feel most happy?".

Therapist Note

Do not feel pressured to make sure the participants fully understand the link between emotions and activity at this point, as they will be given the opportunity to make this link for themselves during the next activity and in subsequent sections. Simply ask the children to brainstorm ideas of different ways their emotions might be linked to activity as an introduction to the next section.

Science Experiments to Help with Emotional Behaviors

To introduce the connection between emotion and activities, ask the children to participate in the first **science experiment** to see what might happen if they try out a new or different behavior. The concept of using science experiments to explore the idea of acting opposite can be introduced to children as follows. You should have children write down the parts of a science experiment and how each part might apply to a science experiment on emotions on Worksheet 3.2: *Parts of a Science Experiment* as you review them with the group:

"What is a science experiment? Has anyone ever done a science experiment before? (Wait for examples from the group). Great! Well, Jack is going to help us think about all the parts of a science experiment today, and we will work together to think about how each part might work for a science experiment about emotions!

Any science experiment starts with (1) a question. In the case of our emotions, one question might be, if I do something different than I normally do when I feel sad, angry, or afraid, how would that feel? The second step in a science experiment is to (2) make a guess about what could happen. This is sometimes called a hypothesis. So, if I was feeling afraid at a party and I normally would stay home or avoid that party, something different I could try would be to go for 10 minutes and see if it is better than I thought it might be. I might guess that it would feel hard for me at first, but then get easier or feel less scary the longer I stayed. The next steps in a science experiment are to (3) try out my experiment and (4) watch how it goes. Did everything turn out the way I guessed it would? Or were there any surprises?

Finally, depending on how the experiment went, I might want to (5) try my experiment again, making any changes needed to make sure it goes even better the next time. So, if I didn't feel better right away when I went to the party and decided to leave anyway, maybe I need to ask myself, did I stay long enough to feel better? Did I look for friends or family who could have made it even more fun? Maybe I should try again. If the experiment did go well, I learned that my new, different behavior could help me feel better and that I should practice it even more often!"

You can tell group members that they are going to try a science experiment here in session to see how they feel when they change their activity or what they are doing. Tell them to pay close attention to their feelings in their body, and any emotions they experience, during this science experiment.

Begin the experiment by asking the children to turn to Figure 3.1: *The Emotion Thermometer for Happy* in their workbooks. Have them use the thermometer as a guide to rate their level of happiness on a 0-to-8 scale, with 0 = not happy; 2 = a little happy; 4 = medium happy; 6 = very happy; or 8 = very, very happy. Record the children's ratings on the board or on a large piece of paper.

Therapist Note

While some children may relate to the "happy" terminology on Figure 3.1, others may respond better to prompts regarding increased feelings of calmness or excitement. For children who do not appear to understand the idea of increasing feelings of "happiness," you may consider prompting them to indicate whether they experienced increased feelings of calmness or excitement following the group activity.

Tell the children that you will be trying out one science experiment on emotions together. To demonstrate how activity can change emotions, you and the children will dance to an upbeat song to see if doing the opposite of what sad makes us want to do (lay around) makes us happier. Use Worksheet 3.2: *Parts of a Science Experiment* as a guide as you go through the parts of a science experiment using dancing as an example. ("Dancing" is not required, but instruct the children to keep moving until the song is over.) This might be done in the following way:

"Okay, so we said that any science experiment starts with (1) a question. In this experiment, we are going to ask whether doing an activity changes our emotion level on the happy thermometer. We will try this out by having a mini dance party today! The second step in a science experiment is to (2) make a guess about what could happen. What does everyone think might happen to our happiness level when we dance? How do you think it might change? (Provide children time to answer, but if they don't, mention that you think it might make you feel happier

to dance to a fun song.) The next steps in a science experiment are to (3) try out my experiment and (4) watch how it goes. So, let's try it out!"

Dance to an approximately two-minute child-friendly song with the children. After the song/activity ends, have the children re-rate their emotion on the emotion thermometer from 0 to 8. Notice whether participants feel better when sitting around prior to engaging in the activity, or after they dance/run. Ask children to reflect on why they think their emotion level changed (or stayed the same). You might approach this discussion in the following way:

"Did everything turn out the way we guessed it would? (Collect feedback from the children). Depending on how it went for us, we might want to (5) try our experiment again, making any changes needed to make sure it goes even better the next time. If this experiment went well for us, we learned that our new, different behavior could help us feel better and that we should practice it even more often! If not, we might try something else fun to change our happiness level next time."

Therapist Note

Children with social anxiety or shyness may struggle with the use of dance as a science experiment, as it may bring up fears of negative social evaluation or inhibition overall. This is not meant to be an intense exposure task, and thus the activity can be modified to address these concerns (e.g., having children dance facing the wall or running in place instead of dancing) or replaced entirely by having the children run down the hallway in a race with each other or with you, instead.

Therapist Note

Note that, on occasion, some children may not report an increase in their emotional intensity rating after engaging in this activity, and on occasion children may report that they feel a little worse. Should this occur, take it as an opportunity to point out that we all enjoy different things. Some kids may enjoy dancing and that makes them feel better, while for others this kind of activity may bring up other emotions (e.g., slightly increased anxiety). Let the children know that one thing about all good science experiments is that we can change them at times to get the best outcome, so if one child doesn't respond as happily to this particular experiment, he might if the activity is a more enjoyable one for him (like playing soccer or talking with a friend).

Session 3, Goal 3
Review the connection between activity and emotions and identify enjoyable activities.

Demonstrate the Link Between Activity and Emotion Over Time via an Example

Introduce *Nina's Emotion and Activity Diary* (Figure 3.2). This might sound something like:

> *"You all remember one of our Emotion Detectives, Nina. Nina has actually been feeling really down in the dumps lately. She has been feeling really tired, really sad, and worried about school and the future. Nina asked her therapist what she could do to feel better.*
>
> *Her therapist suggested that Nina come up with a list of fun activities in session and track which activities she participated in over the course of the week in her Emotion and Activity Diary (direct attention to the diary; Figure 3.2). She also kept track of her emotion rating each day."*

While looking at Nina's diary, have children (who are able) read out the *type and number* of activities and the emotion rating for each day and report whether they see a trend between the types of activities Nina does, or the amount of activity and her emotion ratings. Encourage any children who have difficulty reading to say the number of activities that Nina engaged in, or to brainstorm other fun or enjoyable activities Nina could do.

You can ask several follow-up questions, such as:

1. What kind of activities did she engage in?
2. Which ones made her happy?
3. Which activities (or lack of activities) made her less happy?
4. What was the result of Nina's science experiment? Did doing more or less activities change how happy she was?

Introduce Enjoyable Activities

Introduce the *List of Activities* (Worksheet 3.3). Discuss the range of activities that children can engage in to change their emotion when they are feeling an intense emotion like sadness, in particular, and have the children begin to think about how different types of activities may be better in different situations. This discussion might begin as described below:

> *"One of the things we learned from looking at Nina's diary is that the number and type of activities she did each day had an impact on how sad or down she felt. This is true for most of us. Knowing about this link between our activities*

and the intensity of an emotion like sadness allows us to choose activities that we enjoy in order to help us feel better and use science experiments to try out new behaviors that can help. Let's talk about all the different types of activities we can choose for science experiments we might do about our own activities and emotion this week."

List types of activities that most people enjoy (i.e., helping others, learning new things, doing things with people, and moving our bodies) using Worksheet 3.3: *List of Activities* as a guide. Work together as a group to come up with at least one activity in each category that someone might like (can be general ideas or can be specific to each group member).

Session 3, Goal 4

Teach children how to track their emotions and activities in the context of a science experiment.

Discuss the idea that sometimes science experiments like using activity to make us feel better when we are down or upset can be hard at first:

"It may feel difficult to jump up and run a mile, or play soccer, start an art project, or do homework when we are feeling sad, down, tired, or bored. We may just want to sit on the couch and watch TV or play videogames. We might just want to play on the computer. We might just want to sleep.

But we just learned that these active, engaging, and healthy activities could help to change our emotions and help us feel happier and less sad. Remember: this is what acting opposite is all about! So, the most important time to try to do these activities is exactly when we're feeling sad/bored/tired/down. And remember that this is only your first try at this science experiment this week. Part of a science experiment is sometimes to tweak or change it after we see how it goes the first time in order to make it a success. And that's okay too!"

Explain to the children that this week they will be conducting a science experiment to see if doing an activity when they are feeling sad or down helps to improve their sad-, down-, or boredom-related emotions. Discuss the importance of considering both (1) fun, enjoyable, and exciting activities and (2) activities that can be done without much preparation or assistance. Also emphasize the importance of having a plan to engage in this experiment during the most critical moments; have the children try to identify the times of day or situations when they believe they will be most vulnerable to sadness or boredom, and help them address potential barriers to engaging in activities during these times. This discussion of barriers might be introduced as follows:

> *"Let's say you've made a great list of things to do, and then one day this week your friends just aren't being nice and you are feeling down in the dumps. So, you open up your activity list and decide: I want to go practice rock climbing. But your parents are busy and can't take you to a rock climbing gym. Plus, it can be really expensive to rock climb. It can be tough when you can't drive, or you don't have money and you just don't have access to all the fun things you would do if you could.*
>
> *So, you need a plan for this type of science experiment! Some of these activities will have to be planned ahead of time. It can be a good idea to plan them for a time when you are usually bored or feel down—not for times when you feel afraid (these are not meant to be distractions; we want to face our fears, not avoid them!). Think back over the past week and try to remember the times when you were most bored or sad. Was it after school when there was nothing to do but watch TV? How about on weekend mornings before your parents woke up?*
>
> *Other activities might be easy to do 'at the drop of a hat.' Make sure you and your parents put plenty of these 'fun but easy' activities on your list so you can be sure to find something to do if you can't get a ride somewhere.*
>
> *Finally, there may be activities on your list that are kind of difficult, like learning a new skill or getting better at something you already do. Sometimes these are the hardest to pick up and do, because we don't want to do hard work when we're sad."*

Ask the children to focus on why they might want to engage in these types of activities for their science experiment this week, especially more challenging ones (e.g., focusing on learning something new or getting better at something they already know how to do, which can make them feel good about themselves; if they practice and stick with it, they can accomplish all kinds of things).

Next, emphasize the importance of consistent practice. This discussion might sound something like:

> *"Finally, let's talk about a big word: **consistency**. Sometimes we start new activities or experiments but then give up on them rather quickly. Maybe we decide it would be fun to play the guitar or better for us get up a little earlier each morning to practice our spelling. But, after a few days or weeks, we realize that practicing something new can also be hard work. An important thing to remember is that this skill is really about continuing to try and get up, get out, and do stuff! Even if we practice a little less one day or try a different song to practice another, the fact that we continue to try at all is most important!*

234

Finally, remember your science experiment rules. If it's not working, don't give up! Try to revise the plan and try again. Eventually, these kinds of experiments will lead to fewer unhappy days and more happy ones."

Continue to Work on Lists of Activities for the Children in the Group

Have the children use the *List of Activities* (Worksheet 3.3) and *My Activities List* (Worksheet 3.4) to generate a full list of activities, including those that are easy to do and ones that may require planning. Work with each child to come up with a plan for how/when to engage in difficult activities this week.

Therapist Note

Note that some children, instead of engaging in too little activity, may actually be overscheduled with activities. Sometimes, these children find that this high activity load actually worsens their mood because they have little time for relaxation, they are not necessarily enjoying all the activities they are engaging in, the activities are too high pressure, and so forth. With such children, it may be helpful to focus on activities that personally give them the most enjoyment, rather than just increasing activity overall. This might involve assisting a child with identifying activities he does that he truly enjoys, activities he does that he does not enjoy, and finally activities he may want to engage in instead of those he is currently doing. You may want to coordinate with the parents of such children at the end of session to have a conversation about which activities are valuable, enjoyable, and worth continuing to pursue.

Back Together

Tell parents that the children learned about science experiments today and that children will be doing their own science experiments at home to figure out if activities change how happy they are each day during the week.

Then, note that children can use *Nina's Emotion and Activity Diary* as an example. Tell parents and children that, next session, the whole group will talk about whether or not doing more enjoyable activities made each of the children's emotions change! This might be done in the following way:

"Okay, kids, as you may remember, earlier today we looked at Nina's Emotion and Activity Diary. In this diary, Nina wrote down each day how strong her emotions

felt, the type and number of activities she did, and any link she noticed between her activities and her emotions. This week, you will get a chance to do your own diary (Worksheet 3.5). At the end of each day, right before you go to bed, write down your overall emotion rating for the day, the type and number of activities you did, and anything you noticed about the link between your activities and your emotions. Parents, you may need to help your kids remember to fill out the diary each evening, and your kids may also need your help remembering what activities they did. Kids, two times this week when you are feeling sad/bored, you should do a science experiment by choosing to do an activity from your My Activities List. Try to notice and write down how acting opposite affected your mood at the bottom of My Emotion and Activity Diary. Next week, bring these diaries back so that we can talk about what you noticed.

In addition to your diary, we also want you to continue to log one emotional experience on the form you used last time (Form 2.1: Solving the Mystery of Our Emotions: Before, During, and After)."

Suggested Home Learning Assignment: *My Emotion and Activity Diary* and *Solving the Mystery of Our Emotions: Before, During, and After* (with option of assigning ongoing opposite action experiments)

The primary home learning assignment for this session is *My Emotion and Activity Diary*. Children should also add another entry to their *Solving the Mystery of Our Emotions: Before, During, and After*. For any children who have more substantial problems with emotional disorder symptoms that could benefit from continued practice with opposite action (e.g., OCD symptoms, sadness, anger), you may choose to assign these children to more continuously track opposite action practice each week using Form 3.1: *Acting Opposite Plans*.

Therapist Note

Note that there are important skills to come in the UP-C Sessions 4 through 8 that will support the conduct of further and more challenging science experiments, including exposure work. We will focus more on science experiments as they relate to fear, anxiety, and avoidance behavior specifically starting in UP-C Session 9. Therefore, while one can definitely choose to focus on exposure activities starting at this point in treatment versus sadness-related experiments or following sadness-related experiments, particularly if providing UP-C in an individual therapy format, please consider the child's and the family's readiness for exposure before you move in this direction.

Overall Parent Session 3 Goals

The main goal of this session is to introduce parents to the concept of using science experiments to see what happens when we take different "opposite" actions from those that have been maladaptive during emotional states. Parents will learn how to support their child this week as he or she begins to engage in a series of opposite action science experiments for sadness and withdrawal. Toward the end of the session, parents are introduced to Worksheet 13.3: *10 Ways to Reinforce your Child*, and you will help parents plan how they will reinforce their child for acting differently from what his or her emotions are telling him or her to do this week.

- **Goal 1:** Introduce parents to the idea of using science experiments to act opposite of emotional behaviors.
- **Goal 2:** Discuss how parents can support their children in completing science experiments for sadness.
- **Goal 3:** Introduce parents to Worksheet 13.3: *10 Ways to Reinforce Your Child*, and help parents create a reinforcement plan for the week.

Parent Session 3 Content (Divided by Goals)

Parent Session 3, Goal 1

Introduce parents to the idea of using science experiments to act opposite of emotional behaviors.

> **Therapist Note**
> *You should begin this session and each subsequent one with a brief check-in regarding major changes in child symptoms/functioning over the past week, as well as a review of home learning assignments. Typically, you should limit this check-in to no more than 10 minutes in order to leave adequate time to cover new content.*

The first goal of this session is to introduce parents to a few new terms they will encounter in this session and in subsequent ones. The first of these terms—"acting opposite"—involves acting differently or opposite from an emotion's predominant action-related urges. Remind the parents that, as discussed in Session 1, all emotions have an action urge associated with them—that is, the emotion is trying to get us to do something such as reduce the emotion we are experiencing and/or remove ourselves from the emotion-eliciting situation. This can be a good thing during times when acting on the emotion is adaptive or effective, or helps keep us safe. You may wish to solicit examples from parents of times when acting on an emotion is adaptive or beneficial. However, often our emotions are providing us false information about a situation and telling us to do more than we need to do or something we don't need to do at all. If we always act on the emotion, we will never figure this out. In these situations, parents will be encouraging their child to act opposite of what the emotion is telling the child to do, which will actually *reduce* strong or unhelpful emotions in the long term.

With the parents, discuss examples of action urges and opposite actions for three or four different emotions, including sadness, anxiety, anger, and any other emotions that the children in the group tend to experience frequently. Have parents turn to Table 13.2: *Common Emotional Behaviors and Their Opposite Actions* in Chapter 13 of the parent workbook to guide this discussion. It may also be helpful to encourage parents to consider times when they acted opposite to an emotion's action-related urge and discuss the outcome.

Explain to parents that, in this treatment, we will be encouraging their child to act opposite or differently from what an emotion is telling the child to do in all kinds of ways, and we will also be giving their child the skills to do this. In this session, we will be encouraging their child to act opposite by asking him or her to conduct a science experiment for sadness and withdrawal. Just like with any other science experiment, the children will use science experiments in this session as a way of gathering information to test whether their thoughts about something are true. When children feel sad, they often engage in emotionally driven behaviors such as isolating from others, sleeping, lying around, or watching television. Children who are depressed often think that participating in activities that are more active, social, or engaging will just make them feel worse. In our science experiments this week, we will test these beliefs or hypotheses by asking children to engage in greater levels of enjoyable and personally meaningful activities to see if their emotion changes.

Therapist Note

As an optional activity, you may ask parents to participate in a "dance party," similar to the one the children completed in the child component of this session. Have parents rate their mood before and after dancing to an upbeat song, and discuss any changes they notice in their mood as a result.

Parent Session 3, Goal 2

Discuss how parents can support their children in completing science experiments for sadness.

Explain to parents that, this week, children will be completing two main tasks for home learning: (1) monitoring their emotion and activity levels each day by completing a daily emotion and activity diary and (2) engaging in two science experiments where they will see what happens when they choose to do an activity that is different from what their emotion is telling them to do when they are feeling down, sad, or bored. To illustrate what a completed emotion and activity diary looks like, it may be helpful to show parents a copy of *Nina's Emotion and Activity Diary* (Figure 3.2 in the child portion of the workbook). Explain that each child will be completing his or her own diary that looks just like Nina's in order to simply observe how his or her own emotion and activity levels are connected. Additionally, explain that the children are beginning to create lists of fun or enjoyable activities in the child group, focusing on four different types of activities: helping others (service activities), learning new things (mastery activities), doing things with people (social activities), and moving our bodies (physical activities). Children can use this list (in addition to activities suggested by parents) to select activities for their science experiments this week.

Emphasize to parents the importance of helping their child to identify a range of activities from each category. Parents should be sure that children identify at least some activities that are inexpensive (or free), that are easy to do, and that can be performed independently in case a parent is not available to help. In the case of mastery activities, parents should also help their child to identify realistic goals that he or she is capable of accomplishing. Finally, emphasize the importance of planning activities ahead of time so that children are not "stuck" when a down mood hits:

> "To set your children up for success, you can help by ensuring that they have a range of activities on their list. We want to make sure that your child has ideas for activities that might be easy to do 'at the drop of a hat.' Together, we will make sure that your children have plenty of these fun but easy activities on their lists so they can be sure to find something to do, even things around the house, if nobody is available to assist them or they can't get a ride somewhere.
>
> You can also facilitate science experiments by helping your child plan activities ahead of time. It can be a good idea to plan science experiments for a time when

your child is usually bored or feels down—not for times when your child feels afraid (these are not meant to be distractions; we want to face our fears, not avoid them!). For this week, you can draw upon your own knowledge of your child and your observations to help him or her identify a time when it may be effective to engage in a science experiment. After your child completes the emotion and activity diary this week, you can use it in the future to help your child to identify patterns. If you notice that there are specific times that seem to generate boredom or sadness (such as after school when there is nothing to do, or before you wake up on the weekends), encourage your child to engage in an opposite action science experiment during these times to see what happens when he or she acts differently from what the emotion is telling him or her to do.

Finally, there may be activities on the list that are kind of difficult, like learning a new skill or getting better at something your child already does. Sometimes these are the hardest activities to pick up and do, because we don't want to do hard work when we're sad. However, it can be important to engage in these activities to build a sense of mastery and accomplishment."

To build empathy for how difficult it can be for their children to act differently from what an emotion is telling them to do, explain to the parents that it is often really tough to get up and engage in an activity when we are bored, tired, or feeling down or sad. You may wish to draw upon parents' own experiences by asking them to offer examples of times when they had difficulty engaging in an activity, even though they knew it would positively impact their emotions. Parents can facilitate science experiments by explaining why they might want to do these activities when feeling down, and how good they'll feel after they do them.

Parent Session 3, Goal 3
Introduce parents to Worksheet 13.3: 10 Ways to Reinforce Your Child, and help parents create a reinforcement plan for the week.

Check in with the parents about their reactions to the Rewards List their child created during the previous session, addressing any concerns the parents may have about the rewards their child selected or about rewarding their child in general. Suggest that, because engaging in opposite actions for sadness and withdrawal can be difficult, this week may be a good time to consider reinforcing their child for his or her efforts. If parents have difficulty understanding why they need to reward their child for engaging in activities that are supposed to be enjoyable, remind them that when their child is feeling down or sad it is often difficult for the child to see the inherently reinforcing qualities of these activities. Inertia can also make it very difficult to act opposite to emotional behaviors. Encouragement in the form of rewards or other reinforcements can be very helpful during these times!

Ask parents to turn to *10 Ways to Reinforce Your Child* (Worksheet 13.3) in the parent workbook. Review this worksheet and suggest that parents practice using as many different types of reinforcement this week as possible. Assist them in creating a plan for how they will reinforce their child for engaging in science experiments this week.

Suggested Parent Home Learning Assignment: *Double BDA* and *10 Ways to Reinforce Your Child*

Ask each parent to continue to complete at least one *Double BDA* for home learning (Worksheet 13.4). Parents should also complete the bottom portion of *10 Ways to Reinforce Your Child* (Worksheet 13.3), noting different methods of reinforcement they use during the week and how their child responds to reinforcement.

CHAPTER 14 UP-C Session 4: Our Body Clues

C Skill: Consider How I Feel

MATERIALS NEEDED FOR GROUP

- For Each Child Group Session:
  1. Detective CLUES kits for each child
  2. Poker chips
  3. Puzzle
  4. Prize box
  5. Large piece of paper or whiteboard to record children's answers for any group activities
- For Session 4 Only:
  6. Large roll of paper and art supplies for "body drawing"
  7. C badge
  8. UP-C Workbook Chapter 4:
     a. What Are Body Clues? (Figure 4.1)
     b. Becoming a Body Detective (Figure 4.2)
     c. Finding Your Body Clues (Worksheet 4.1)
     d. How to Body Scan! (Figure 4.3)
     e. Monitoring How My Body Feels (Form 4.1)
- For Home Learning:
  9. *Finding Your Body Clues at Home* (Worksheet 4.2)
  10. *Solving the Mystery of Our Emotions: Before, During, and After Worksheet* (Form 2.1; use the same form started after Session 2)

- Assessments to be Given at Every Session
  11. Weekly Top Problems Tracking Form (Use the same form started during Session 1 for each child, found in Appendix 11.1 at the end of Chapter 11 of this Therapist Guide)
- For Parent Group Session:
  12. UP-C Workbook Chapter 13
     a. *Empathizing with Your Child's Struggle* (Worksheet 13.5)
- For Parent Home Learning:
  13. *Double Before, During, and After* (Worksheet 13.6)
  14. *Empathizing with Your Child's Struggle*, bottom part (Worksheet 13.5)

Therapist Preparation

In preparation for this session, prepare a large piece of paper (approximately 5 feet long) for each child. Also have markers and other drawing supplies available (in preparation for the "Body Drawings" activity). Alternatively, a body drawing figure is available in the UP-C workbook (Worksheet 4.1: *Finding Your Body Clues*), if a large roll of paper is unavailable or not desired. At the end of the session, the children will receive their first "CLUES" badge, indicating that they have completed the C skill. Typically, badges are letter-shaped stickers or construction-paper letters that the children can put on their CLUES kits to monitor their progress. This should be a celebrated accomplishment for the child and family and noted by you as such.

Overall Session 4 Goals

The primary goal of this session is to teach the children and their parents about the physiological sensations (or **body clues**) that arise along with strong emotions. To that end, participants engage in a number of activities during this session to hone their skills at detecting body clues (e.g., body scanning, body drawings, and sensational exposures). These activities are designed to build both awareness and tolerance of physiological sensations and to discourage avoidance and other unhelpful emotional behaviors in response to uncomfortable sensations that may arise when experiencing strong emotions.

- ▪ **Goal 1:** Describe the concept of body clues and their relation to strong emotions.
- ▪ **Goal 2:** Learn to identify body clues for different emotions.
- ▪ **Goal 3:** Teach the skill of body scanning to develop awareness of body clues.
- ▪ **Goal 4:** Help the children practice experiencing body clues without using avoidance or distraction.

Session 4 Content (Divided by Goals)

Session 4, Goal 1

Describe the concept of body clues and their relation to strong emotions.

While the group is together

As you welcome back the group for the start of the fourth session, circulate and assist parents and children in providing severity ratings for each of their three top problems and continue to praise and encourage children as they work toward their goals. These ratings should be entered on the same *Weekly Top Problems Tracking Form* (Appendix 11.1 at the end of Chapter 11 in this Therapist Guide) begun during Session 1. Also check that each child has completed the home learning assignment. Complete a brief review of last session's assignment so that each child goes over her *My Emotion and Activity Diary* (Worksheet 3.5) and her *Solving the Mystery of Our Emotions: Before, During, and After* (Form 2.1) together in the group. For those children who have completed the home learning assignments, distribute one puzzle piece to each.

> **Therapist Note**
> *During home learning activity review, you may need to remind parents not to answer for their child but to assist if the child has trouble explaining a situation.*

Introducing Body Clues

Start out by reminding children about the three parts of an emotion, letting them know that the focus of today's session will be on the "feelings" part of an emotion. Have children turn to Figure 4.1: *What Are Body Clues?* in their workbooks. Using this figure as a guide, explain to the children that we will call the feelings in our bodies during emotions "body clues" because they can provide important clues to what emotions we might be feeling. This group session will focus on teaching the children to become better "body detectives," or to better understand the types of physical sensations that might be experienced before, during, and after a strong emotion like sadness, fear, or anger. Toward the end of the session, the children will be participating in some science experiments to see what happens when they do activities to bring up strong physical sensations in their bodies.

Introduce the children to the idea that although body clues often feel uncomfortable and sometimes even scary, body clues are actually telling us important information and can even help us to survive. Review the **fight-or-flight system** as one example of how our body clues help keep us safe. The fight-or-flight response is a reaction in our bodies that occurs when we believe we are being attacked or threatened in some way. When we experience this reaction, our brains tell a part of our nervous system (the sympathetic nervous system) to release some chemicals into our body so that we can attack or flee from the threat.

Review some examples of clues our bodies give us that we are experiencing a fight-or-flight response, including:

- Heart beating faster
- Breathing faster
- Food moving through the body more slowly
- More blood flowing to our legs and big muscles
- Less blood flowing to our head
- Shaking
- Dry mouth

You may choose to describe the fight-or-flight response in the following way:

"The purpose of these body changes is to (1) get more blood to your muscles and away from other parts of your body that don't need it as much; (2) to give your body extra

energy; and (3) to give you extra speed and strength—all to run away or fight off
an attacker! The human body is pretty amazing in this way. These amazing body
changes are really helpful when you're in a dangerous situation, but sometimes you
might feel these body clues when there is nothing really threatening around, like with
a false alarm. During this session, you will be learning more about what YOUR
body clues are in these types of situations and about what to do when you experience
uncomfortable body clues when nothing really bad or dangerous is happening."

Introduce the idea that two kids might both feel very sad or anxious, but they may notice very different body clues. Body clues can also be mysterious because one feeling could have many different causes. For example, if your stomach feels funny, causes could include:

- Hunger
- Illness
- Anxiety/Worry
- Anger
- Sadness

If your hands are sweaty, causes could include:

- Physical activity
- Temperature
- Illness
- Anxiety/Worry

Tell children to open their workbooks to Figure 4.2: *Becoming a Body Detective*. Explain that now that the children have learned about body clues—the feelings in our bodies we might have when we are feeling sick, hungry, or an emotion—they are ready to become body detectives. Using Figure 4.2 as a guide, explain (1) that body detectives are Emotion Detectives who are really good at knowing when they are feeling body clues and (2) they are also good at understanding what emotions different body clues might tell them they are having. Tell the children that body clues can give them important information about what emotions they might be experiencing, but each child needs to become aware of these body clues first. Connect the idea of becoming more aware of body clues to the overall themes of becoming an Emotion Detective and conducting a science experiment to better understand and do helpful things when feeling strong emotions. This might be accomplished by saying:

"Today, we are going to be doing some science experiments to better understand
how our body reacts to different things and situations around us, including times

when we feel a strong emotion. *As we do these science experiments, we can think of ourselves as **body detectives** who are trying to solve the mystery of why our body acts the way it does!"*

Work with the children as a group to read through the list of different emotions provided in Figure 4.2. Then, have children share which body clues on the list they have experienced. Finally, instruct the children to write down which body clues they experience the most often at the bottom of the page.

Session 4, Goal 2

Learn to identify body clues for different emotions.

Body Drawing Activity

Explain to the children that they will begin by identifying the clues that their bodies give them when they are experiencing different emotions. Use either the body drawing provided in Worksheet 4.1: *Finding Your Body Clues* in the workbook or use a large piece of paper and trace the outline of each child's body onto it, allowing the children to personalize and decorate their body drawings with markers and crayons. Ask the children to identify specific parts of their bodies where they experience body clues for different emotions, and have them mark their body drawing with examples. Before doing so, go through the following prompts and have children generate ideas about where in their bodies they may experience body clues related to the following situations and emotions:

General example:

Jack is in class about to give a big presentation.

- *Where does he feel nervous?*
- *Maybe excited?*

Personal examples:

- *You feel sad about a pet passing away. Where do you feel it? What do you feel?*
- *Your best friend comes back from a long vacation and you're really excited to see him. Where do you feel it? What do you feel?*
- *Your sister went into your room even though you told her not to, and you're really angry. Where do you feel it? What do you feel?*

> **Therapist Note**
>
> *You may wish to encourage children to color-code the body clues they have for different strong emotions (e.g., red for anger, blue for sadness, and green for anxiety).*

> **Therapist Note**
>
> *Some children struggle, even with the standard prompts provided, to come up with ideas about what body clues they experience. It may be helpful in these cases for youth to consider specific situations or things that make them feel a strong emotion and complete their body drawing for these more specific examples. Another option is for you to generate ideas about your own body clues in various situations, if the child still appears unable to complete this task using her own examples.*

Session 4, Goal 3

Teach the skill of body scanning to develop awareness of body clues.

Body Scanning Activity

Body scanning is a type of present-moment awareness skill similar to those that will be introduced in Session 8. In this session, body scanning is introduced both as a means of building awareness of body clues and as a means of "sticking with" and approaching, rather than avoiding, body sensations. Like other present-moment awareness skills, a primary goal of body scanning is to *notice, say something about*, and *experience* any sensations that are occurring and to stay present while watching these sensations reduce naturally. Introduce this activity by explaining body scanning as follows:

> *"Often there is so much else going on when we feel a strong emotion that it is hard to pay attention to just the clues in our bodies! When we want to pay attention to those clues we can practice something called body scanning. When we body scan, what we are doing is noticing our body sensations, saying something about them to ourselves, and experiencing them. This might feel uncomfortable at first, especially if we are used to trying to get rid of or ignore body clues. But it is important to pay attention to our body clues because we can't figure out what to do about our emotions if we don't know that they are there in the first place!"*

Have children turn to Figure 4.3: *How to Body Scan!* in their workbooks. Using the figure as a guide, begin by teaching the children the skill of body scanning in a neutral context. Instruct the children to focus on the clues in their bodies by closing their eyes and becoming aware of their bodies. Then, guide children through the following steps:

"Starting at the tip-top of your head, slowly move down your body. Notice any parts of your body that feel tight and uncomfortable. Make sure you move down all the way to your toes.

As you notice each body clue, rate how strong each one is on a 0-to-8 scale.

Say something to yourself about what each body clue feels like.

Experience each body clue by sticking with the feeling, even if it is uncomfortable. Notice how your body clues change over time.

After you have practiced experiencing your body clues, now rate again how strong each one is. What do you notice?"

After practicing body scanning, engage the children in a discussion of the different body clues they noticed and how these body clues changed over time.

Session 4, Goal 4

Help the children practice experiencing body clues without using avoidance or distraction.

The last goal of Session 4 involves helping children to realize that, although body clues can feel uncomfortable, they are not harmful and can be tolerated. Activities that introduce uncomfortable physical sensations are used to help demonstrate this. Such activities are called "sensational exposures" because they are used to help children confront and deal with uncomfortable physical sensations, and can be framed to children as science experiments used to help them notice things about their body clues (i.e., that, even if they feel uncomfortable, they are not harmful, and go away on their own). This concept might be introduced in the following way:

"We often have body clues when we are afraid, sad, or angry. We need to understand that these yucky body clues can be experienced without danger, and that we do not need to escape them in order to be safe. For example, when I'm feeling short of breath, I do not have to get away as soon as possible even if I feel like I need to. When my body feels heavy, I can get up and do something anyway, even if I feel like I cannot do anything else. When my face is really hot, I do not need to yell at someone even if I feel angry and like I do need to yell. We will do practice exercises that may cause you some feelings (like sweaty palms, heart racing)

that are similar to feelings you would have if you were angry or anxious. Also, I want you to understand that you don't need to DO anything to change these physical sensations—they will go away on their own! Remember, the feelings you experience while doing these science experiments are normal, natural, and cannot hurt you."

Tell the children that you are going to work as a group to do a science experiment sort of like you did last session with acting opposite, but this time, to make ourselves feel body clues and see if body feelings do come and go on their own without having to do anything to make them go away.

Practice Sensational Exposures

As a group, do at least three of the following sensational exposures (science experiments):

- Shake head from side to side for 30 seconds.
- Run in place for 1 minute/50 jumping jacks.
- Hold breath for 30 seconds.
- Spin for 1 minute.
- Wall sit for 30 seconds.
- Place head between knee for 30 seconds and then lift head (to an upright position) quickly.

Use body scanning before and after sensational exposures to allow children to pay close attention to sensations in their bodies in a non-judgmental way. Have them fill out *Monitoring How My Body Feels* (Form 4.1) for each sensational exposure. Then allow the physical sensations that occurred as a result of the exposure to lessen. Encourage the children to just let the feelings pass. When the sensations are down by half (on a 0-to-8 scale) from their initial intensity, tell the children to raise their hands.

Ask the children to volunteer the physical sensations they experienced, the intensity of those sensations (on 0-to-8 scale), and the anxiety (or other emotion) they felt on a 0-to-8 scale before, during, and after each exercise.

Discuss the fact that, just as the body clues we made ourselves feel in this experiment started out strong during and right after the exposure and then lessened over time, the same occurs when we approach emotional situations we have been avoiding. We might initially feel rather intense anxiety, sadness, or anger, but these emotions will often reduce naturally if we give them a chance and stay in the situation.

Back together

As the parents rejoin the group, let children know that they have now earned their first badge—the C badge—for completing the "Consider How I Feel" section of treatment and learning how to solve the mystery of feelings that happen in their bodies. Give each child the C badge, and allow them to affix the badge to their CLUES kit or place it in the kit.

> **Suggested Home Learning Assignment:** *Finding Your Body Clues at Home* and *Solving the Mystery of Our Emotions: Before, During, and After* (with option of assigning ongoing opposite action experiments)
>
> *The primary home assignment for this session is completing* Finding Your Body Clues at Home *(Worksheet 4.2). Children should practice body scanning by completing one of the science experiments learned during session and draw the body clues they experience during this exercise on the human figure outline. In addition, families should log one emotional experience on the* Solving the Mystery of Our Emotions: Before, During, and After *form.*

As with all sessions, you may conclude by checking in with your individual families, as time permits.

Overall Parent Session 4 Goals

The main goal of this session is to build parent awareness of the somatic component of emotional experiences. You will teach the parents to perform a body scan—a present-moment awareness exercise—so that they are able to help their children identify somatic components of emotions. Also review the concept of somatization, or expressing emotional experiences as physical experiences. Parents learn to identify times when their children may be expressing emotions as somatic complaints and learn the steps for expressing empathy for their children when they are struggling with strong emotions.

- **Goal 1:** Introduce parents to the concept of somatization and help them to identify when their children are expressing emotions through somatic complaints.
- **Goal 2:** Teach parents how to perform a body scan.
- **Goal 3:** Introduce parents to sensational exposures and practice sensational exposures in session.
- **Goal 4:** Teach parents how to express empathy when their child is struggling with a strong emotion.

Parent Session 4 Content (Divided by Goals)

Parent Session 4, Goal 1

Introduce parents to the concept of somatization and help them to identify when their children are expressing emotions through somatic complaints.

Therapist Note

Remember to begin this session and each subsequent one with a brief check-in regarding major changes in child symptoms/functioning over the past week, as well as a review of home learning. Typically, you should limit this check-in to no more than 10 minutes in order to leave adequate time to cover new content.

Explain to the parents that this week their children will be learning more about the "body clues" component of an emotional experience (what we call *feelings* or *somatic sensations* in this treatment). Emphasize that children vary tremendously in the extent to which they are aware of and are able to identify body clues: some children struggle to identify any somatic sensations, while other children may be overly aware of what is happening in their bodies. Encourage parents to consider which of these descriptions is more like their child. For the child who is relatively unaware of the somatic aspects of his or her emotions, the activities in this session will help build greater awareness of body clues. For children who are overly aware of body sensations, the activities in this session will help them learn how to observe their body sensations more objectively and recognize that these sensations do decrease with time.

Some parents find that when their children are experiencing a strong emotion, they are not always able to say that they are feeling anxious, depressed, or irritable. Often, their children express these emotions as somatic complaints. For example, a child who is feeling anxious about attending school might complain of frequent headaches or nausea in the morning, while a child who is struggling with sadness or depression might tell a parent that she is feeling tired or experiencing muscle aches. This may be because the child is not aware of the emotion he or she is experiencing, or it may be because the child does not know how to describe the emotion. In this session and throughout treatment, children will learn to become better at both identifying and expressing the emotions they are feeling.

Ask the parents to identify any frequent somatic complaints their children seem to experience. The following are somatic complaints commonly experienced in children with emotional disorders:

- Stomachaches
- Nausea
- Vomiting
- Headaches
- Muscle aches
- Fatigue
- Dizziness

Discuss how confusing it can be for parents when their children complain of these somatic symptoms. Many of these complaints also appear in children who are physically ill, and it can be difficult to tell if a child is experiencing physical illness (such as a cold or the flu) as opposed to strong emotions. Explain to parents that one way to distinguish between physical illness and strong emotions is to notice patterns in the timing of somatic complaints. If a child regularly experiences somatic symptoms before or after a particular event (e.g., before school, before soccer games, after arguing with friends), there is a good chance that these somatic symptoms are strongly related to the triggering event. Parents can help their children become more aware of the connection between triggers and somatic symptoms by pointing out any patterns they observe in these symptoms (e.g., "I notice you often feel nauseated at the end of the weekend"), and exploring possible emotion-related triggers for these sensations (e.g., "Do you think you might be feeling nervous about returning to school tomorrow?").

Invite parents to reflect upon any patterns they have noticed in their child's somatic symptoms. You should also emphasize that just because a somatic symptom is related to an emotion, it doesn't mean that the child is *not* experiencing nausea, muscle aches, and so forth. Emotion-related body sensations can be just as uncomfortable as illness-related sensations! It may also be relevant to mention here that in children with physical conditions or medical illnesses, strong emotions can often make their symptoms worse.

Parent Session 4, Goal 2

Teach parents how to perform a body scan.

Instruct parents that, next time their child complains of a somatic symptom, they can be "detective sidekicks" and help their child identify other body clues to the emotions he or she may be feeling. Body scanning is a form of nonjudgmental awareness in which the children will practice paying attention to their body clues in a more objective way—like a scientist or detective—without doing anything to get rid of those physical sensations. Explain that when children practice body scanning, they are **noticing** the sensations, **saying something about them** to themselves or out loud, and **experiencing** them without trying to make them go away.

Explain to the parents that they will now be learning how to practice body scanning themselves so that they can assist their children with the exercise. Using an explanation and script similar to that used with the children in Goal 3 of this session, guide the parents through body scanning in a neutral context. After practicing body scanning, encourage parents to describe body sensations they noticed, as well as whether they had the urge to *do* something to get rid of any of those body sensations. Discuss whether it was difficult for the parents to sit with and attend to those body sensations without doing anything to try to make them go away.

Engage the parents in a discussion of helpful times to practice body scanning with their children over the next week. If their children are experiencing somatic symptoms (e.g., stomachache, headache, nausea), parents may wish to use body scanning to encourage their children to describe these sensations in a more objective manner and to help them notice other body clues for emotions they may also be experiencing. Parents may also wish to encourage their children to do a body scan if it seems that they are experiencing a strong emotion such as sadness, anger, or anxiety but are unable to recognize it as such.

Parent Session 4, Goal 3

Introduce parents to sensational exposures and practice sensational exposures in session.

Let the parents know that in today's session, their children will be participating in some activities that introduce uncomfortable physical sensations in order to help them realize that, although body clues can feel uncomfortable, they are not harmful. These activities are called **sensational exposures** because they expose children to uncomfortable physical sensations, with the goal of helping them learn that they can tolerate these sensations and that they will eventually reduce over time. These exposures are conducted as yet another type of "science experiment," as children are encouraged to make a hypothesis or guess about how strong their body clues will be and their reaction to them, do an experiment to bring on these body clues, and see if their hypothesis was correct.

Emphasize that sensational exposures may sometimes be distressing for children because they are not used to simply noticing their uncomfortable physical sensations without acting on them or doing something to reduce them. It is important for parents to be aware of this and, if they notice their child experiencing distress during sensational exposures at home, they should encourage their child to sit with the uncomfortable physical sensations rather than trying to escape from them. It is natural for parents to want to do something to minimize their child's distress but, if they do this during sensational exposure practice, they will end up reinforcing the same problematic cycles of emotional behaviors that brought their child to treatment in the first place. The goal of sensational exposures is to understand that uncomfortable body clues are not dangerous. When children feel shortness of breath or dizziness, they do not need to lie down or get away as fast as possible, and when their bodies feel heavy, they can get up and do something anyway even if they feel like they cannot.

As a group, practice two or three sensational exposures with the parents. You may wish to choose the same sensational exposures the children will be completing in their group session, although this is not necessary. The purpose of this practice is both to teach parents how to do sensational exposures, so that they can facilitate practice at home, and to build parent empathy for how difficult it can be to sit with uncomfortable physical sensations without doing anything to get rid of them. Encourage the parents to use body scanning before and after sensational exposures to pay close attention to the sensations in their bodies in a nonjudgmental way. Have the parents rate the intensity of their physical sensations on a 0-to-8 scale immediately after the exposure, and tell them to raise their hands when their sensations are down by half. You may wish to bring a copy of the *Monitoring How My Body Feels* (Form 4.1) to show the parents or have them turn to this form in the child section of the workbook.

Parent Session 4, Goal 4

Teach parents how to express empathy when their child is struggling with a strong emotion.

It is natural for parents to feel frustrated and impatient when their children are frequently experiencing strong emotions, especially when these emotions are accompanied by high levels of somatic distress or by avoidance and other emotional behaviors. Parents often believe that one effective way to address high levels of emotion is to minimize or even deny symptoms (e.g., "Your stomach doesn't really hurt;" "There's nothing to be angry about;" "This isn't that hard to do"). Parents who use these kinds of statements (and all parents *do* use these statements from time to time) often do so because they believe that if they minimize these symptoms, their child will follow suit and be less bothered by them. Although this strategy may work occasionally, it can often make children more confused and doubtful about their own internal experiences due to the discrepancy between what they are feeling and what their parent says they are feeling. These statements are also often perceived as criticism and can make children feel wrong, incompetent, and invalidated.

Emphasize the importance of expressing empathy when children are experiencing strong emotions. Expressing empathy means acknowledging a child's emotional experience and expressing that you understand why the child is feeling that way, given the situation or trigger. Let parents know that expressing empathy *does not* mean that they agree with the way the child is expressing it, or believe that the emotional response is in proportion to the trigger. In fact, an important part of expressing empathy involves encouraging the child to identify and use appropriate coping skills.

Review Worksheet 13.5: *Empathizing with Your Child's Struggle.* Cover each step of expressing empathy with the parents, using role-play as needed.

CHAPTER 15

UP-C Session 5: Look at My Thoughts

L Skill: Look at My Thoughts

- For Each Child Group Session:
  1. Detective CLUES kits for each child
  2. Poker chips
  3. Puzzle
  4. Prize box
  5. Large piece of paper or whiteboard to record children's answers for any group activities
- For Session 5 Only:
  6. Printouts of three or four optical illusions
  7. L badge
  8. UP-C Workbook Chapter 5
     a. *What Are Snap Judgments?* (Worksheet 5.1)
     b. *Thinking Traps and Emotion Detectives* (Figure 5.1)
     c. *L for Children* (Worksheet 5.2)
     d. *Match the Thought to the Trap!* (Worksheet 5.3)
     e. *Steps to Being a Flexible Thinker* (Worksheet 5.4)
- For Home Learning:
  9. *L for Children at Home* (Worksheet 5.5)
  10. *Solving the Mystery of Our Emotions: Before, During, and After* (Form 2.1; use the same form started after Session 2)
- Assessments to Be Given at Every Session:
  11. *Weekly Top Problems Tracking Form* (Use the same form started during Session 1 for each child, found in Appendix 11.1 at the end of Chapter 11 of this Therapist Guide)

■ For Parent Group Session:
  12. UP-C Workbook Chapter 14
     a. *L for Parents* (Worksheet 14.1)
     b. *Understanding Learned Behaviors* (Worksheet 14.2)
     c. *Guidelines for Creating a Reinforcement System at Home* (Figure 14.1)
     d. *Guidelines for Creating an Effective Behavior Management System at Home* (Figure 14.2)
■ For Parent Home Learning:
  13. *L for Parents* (Worksheet 14.1)
  14. *Understanding Learned Behaviors* (Worksheet 14.2)

Therapist Preparation

At the end of Session 5 the children will receive their second CLUES badge, indicating that they have completed the L skill. Typically, badges are letter-shaped stickers or construction paper letters that the children can put on their CLUES kits to monitor their progress. This should be a celebrated accomplishment for the child and his family and noted by you as such.

Overall Session 5 Goals

The main goal of this session is to introduce the idea of *flexible thinking* to both parents and children. Specifically, this session teaches children to recognize that their initial negative or threatening interpretation of an ambiguous situation may not necessarily be realistic or accurate. This is a difficult concept for both parents and children to grasp, so it is important that it be introduced slowly and with many examples.

■ **Goal 1:** Introduce the concept of flexible thinking.
■ **Goal 2:** Teach children to recognize common "thinking traps."

Session 5 Content (Divided by Goals)

Session 5, Goal 1
Introduce the concept of flexible thinking.

As you welcome back the group for the start of the fifth session, circulate and assist parents and children in providing severity ratings for each of their three top problems and continue to praise and encourage children as they work toward their goals. These ratings should be entered on the same *Weekly Top Problems Tracking Form* (Appendix 11.1 at the end of Chapter 11 in this Therapist Guide) begun during Session 1. Also check that each child has completed the home learning assignment. As you begin Session 5, it may also be a good time to reflect on any progress in top problems to date individually with each family, as time permits. Encourage the children and parents who have made any progress regarding top problems to keep up the hard work, and work to overcome any barriers to progress as needed. Ask any children who have not completed the home learning assignments to do so next time (or to complete them briefly during the top problems review). For those children who have completed their home learning assignment, distribute one puzzle piece to each. Briefly review content discussed during the previous session and encourage each child to share his or her home learning assignment (Worksheet 4.2: *Finding Your Body Clues at Home*) with the group.

Therapist Note

During top problems and home learning review, you may need to remind parents not to answer for their child but to assist if the child has trouble explaining a situation. If the child has difficulty discussing top problems or home learning content, encourage the child to say as much as he or she is initially comfortable with and remind parents and children that comfort discussing these topics should gradually increase over the course of treatment.

Child Group Alone

Optical Illusions Activity

An extensive discussion of the rationale for the optical illusions activity and a selection of recommended optical illusions, along with their likely interpretations, appear in Chapter 5 and Table 5.1, respectively, of this Therapist Guide. Review this material before engaging in this UP-C session, if possible, in order to fully understand the purpose of this exercise.

Select three or four optical illusions (from the list in Table 5.1) and distribute or show each optical illusion, one at a time, to the children. Ask them to examine each picture and pay attention to their first impression of or the first thing that "pops into their mind" about the picture. Then, ask whether there may be something else to see within the picture or a different interpretation other than their initial one. You can use the following questions to guide this discussion:

- What is the first thing you think of or see when you look at this picture? (Take this opportunity to point out that the children may differ in what they see first. We can each have different *automatic interpretations* of the same situation.)
- Does anyone see anything else in the picture?
- If you didn't see another picture at first, how long did it take before you were able to see something else in the picture?
- Once you saw one thing in the picture, was it hard to see something else?

Begin to discuss the concept that, in any given situation, more than one guess or interpretation can be true. However, we often assume that our first interpretation is the most accurate one, without thinking about other possibilities.

Instruct children to turn to Worksheet 5.1: *What Are Snap Judgments?* in their workbooks. Using this worksheet as a guide, ask the children whether this concept could also apply to emotional situations. Snap judgments happen in many everyday situations all the time. For example, if a child sees two children talking together closely on the playground, he can interpret that situation in many different ways. He can think that the other children are talking to each other about something that has nothing to do with him or he can think that they might be talking about him.

Explain to the children that when we are feeling a strong emotion, we are especially likely to focus on just one guess about or interpretation of a situation and not think about what else could be true. And what we focus on is not usually the happier guess about what could be true! In other words, when we are feeling a strong emotion, we are much more likely to think those two children might be talking about us!

Note that, in these cases when we experience strong emotions, it can be difficult to see any other interpretation but our *snap judgment* (such as

Jack thinking that the kids were laughing at him, when maybe they were laughing at a funny joke that had nothing to do with Jack at all):

"We assume that our snap judgment must be true, and the more we think that it is true, the worse we feel. To help get unstuck, we have to learn about and get really good at recognizing some common snap judgments. If we recognize them more easily, we'll be better at remembering to look for other possibilities."

Next, present these additional ambiguous vignettes (also provided on Worksheet 5.1 in the workbook) to demonstrate how emotional situations can also be seen from multiple points of view:

"Jack walks by a group of kids laughing. He thinks that they must be making fun of him."

"Jack waves to his friend across the hallway, but his friend doesn't wave back. He thinks his friend must be angry at him."

"Jack strikes out during a baseball game. He thinks he must be a terrible player."

For each of these situations, ask the children to identify and write down the following on Worksheet 5.1:

- Jack's first interpretation or explanation of the situation
- Other possible interpretations or explanations of the situation

As you discuss, casually reinforce the idea that it is common and normal for there to be multiple interpretations of a given situation that may be true and that our job as "Emotion Detectives" is to start thinking about how our emotions might lead us to use or believe in our initial snap judgments too much.

Session 5, Goal 2
Teach children to recognize common "thinking traps."

Introducing Thinking Traps

Review the concept that everyone uses shortcuts in thinking or snap judgments that can make our daily lives easier, because they allow us to act quickly in a situation without spending too much time thinking about what we should do. You may choose to further explain the concept in the following way:

"We have certain ways of looking at what's going on around us that make it simpler to live. These are like shortcuts for our brain, and they can be really

*helpful. When we feel strong emotions our brains often jump to an explanation of what's happening, even if we haven't yet figured out the clues to tell us what's going on. Sometimes these snap judgments or shortcuts get us into trouble because we haven't completely thought through the situation, and they can lead us to make the wrong conclusion. This is why we call them **thinking traps**.*"

Next, direct children to *Thinking Traps and Emotion Detectives* (Figure 5.1) in their workbook, and introduce common thinking traps by describing each thinking trap character. This might be done in the following way:

*"Jumping to conclusions: **Jumping Jack**. In this thinking trap, you think the chances that something bad will happen are much higher than they really are. An example is: On the news, you hear about a house getting robbed, and you feel that there is a high chance that your house will get robbed too.*

*Mind reading: **Psychic Suki**. In this thinking trap, you think you know what other people are thinking about a situation, even when you don't have any facts to support that idea. An example is: Your best friend forgets to say goodbye to you, and you assume that she or he no longer likes you.*"

*Thinking the worst: **Disaster Darrell**. In this thinking trap, you believe that the worst possible thing has happened or will happen, and that you will be unable to cope. An example is: You think that doing poorly on a test will lead to failing out of school.*"

*Ignoring the positive: **Negative Nina**. This thinking trap leads to focusing on the negative parts of a situation while minimizing or ignoring the positive aspects. An example is: Instead of focusing on the fun parts about going to camp, you focus on the negatives (being away from your parents, having to meet new people).*"

Direct the children to Worksheet 5.2: *L for Children*. Work with the children to read through the examples given for each thinking trap and direct the children to write down one example of when they might have experienced each thinking trap. Allow the children to share their examples with the child group.

If time permits, playing a game with the four thinking traps can improve children's retention of and ability to apply the thinking traps. Ask the children to turn to Worksheet 5.3: *Match the Thought to the Trap!* Have children draw lines on Worksheet 5.3 connecting each thinking trap character in the left column to the most likely thinking trap thought they might have in the right column (Key: *Psychic Susan: C; Jumping Jack: B; Disaster Dan: D; Negative Nina: A*). To make this activity more engaging, you might choose to split group members into two teams to work on the assignment, and have teams compete to finish the game first.

Instruct children to turn to Worksheet 5.4: *Steps to Being a Flexible Thinker*. Using this worksheet as a guide, explain that we want children in the Emotion Detectives program to be able to climb out of their thinking traps, and in order to do this we need to practice using three steps. Re-introduce Jumping Jack's thinking trap example from Worksheet 5.3, also reprinted on Worksheet 5.4, to help children walk through the first two steps of flexible thinking. This might be done in the following way:

> "*The first step is to have them become experts at identifying the thinking traps. Can anyone tell us which thinking trap Jack is stuck in here? Let's all write it down.*"

Review as a group that the trap is Jumping to Conclusions.

> "*The second step is to become more flexible by looking for what else might be true.*"

Have the children practice thinking of alternative interpretations of the thinking trap.
Then, note that the third step is to use Detective Thinking to find evidence, which will be discussed during the next session in more detail.

You may choose to provide a short introduction to Detective Thinking in the following way:

> "*Next time, we're going to use our Emotion Detective skills to look for clues that will tell us whether our thinking trap thought is true or not. Then, we'll learn about different ways to look at tough situations that are based on the facts and the evidence. For today, we just want to learn that sometimes we do fall into those traps. Everyone does! It's important to learn to notice our thinking traps and realize that sometimes they aren't always the truth; something else might also be true.*"

If time permits, solicit examples from the children of times when they were thinking about a situation in a way that was not realistic or helpful, and have the other children help identify the thinking trap that they were falling into. Children can write down their own examples on Worksheet 5.2: *L for Children*.

Back Together

At the end of this session, tell the children that they have now earned their second badge—the L badge—for completing the "Look at My Thoughts" section of treatment. Explain that this badge shows that they have learned how to notice when they might be falling into a thinking trap and to understand that there is more than one way to think about different situations. Give each child the L badge, and allow them to affix the badge to their CLUES kit or place it in the kit.

As with all sessions, you may conclude by checking in about progress or concerns with your individual families, as time permits.

Suggested Home Learning Assignment: *L for Children at Home* and *Solving the Mystery of Our Emotions: Before, During, and After* (with option of assigning ongoing opposite action experiments)

The home learning for this week is to fill out personal examples of thinking traps on Worksheet 5.5: *L for Children at Home*. During a quiet period at home, have children work with their parents to choose times when they have fallen into each of the thinking traps on the worksheet. Children should also add another entry to their *Solving the Mystery of Our Emotions: Before, During, and After*.

Overall Parent Session 5 Goals

The main goal of this parent session is to introduce parents to the concept of cognitive flexibility, emphasizing that their child's first interpretation of a situation may not be the most realistic or accurate. Parents learn about the four thinking traps covered in the child component of this session so that parents can help their children identify distortions in their thinking. This session also covers an additional emotional parenting behavior (inconsistency) and its opposite parenting behavior (consistent reinforcement and discipline).

- **Goal 1:** Introduce parents to the concept of cognitive flexibility.
- **Goal 2:** Introduce parents to the four common thinking traps covered in the child group.
- **Goal 3:** Discuss the emotional parenting behavior of inconsistency and its opposite parenting behavior, consistent reinforcement and discipline.

Parent Session 5, Goal 1

Introduce parents to the concept of cognitive flexibility.

Therapist Note

Remember to begin this session and each subsequent one with a brief check-in (no more than 10 minutes) regarding major changes in child symptoms/functioning over the past week, as well as a review of home learning assignments.

Flexible Thinking

Introduce the idea that over time and with experience, we develop ideas about the world or **heuristics** that we internalize in order to help us navigate our environment. A simple example of a heuristic is a stoplight. We know that red means "stop" and green means "go" without having to consciously think about it. This makes driving much easier. Ask the parents to imagine how difficult it would be if they had to stop and consider the meaning of a red or green or yellow light every time they got to a stoplight! While these **automatic interpretations** or snap judgments, as we are calling them in the child group, can be very useful, they can also get us into patterns that can be problematic. This can happen when the heuristic we learn isn't accurate, or when we apply it to situations where the heuristic doesn't fit or is inappropriate.

Optical Illusions

Use a variety of optical illusions (the same or similar to those presented in the child group) to explore automatic interpretations. Ask the parents to look at these images and describe or write down what first comes to mind. Ask each parent to then share his or her first impressions. Note the discrepancy between different responses, emphasizing that one interpretation is not right or wrong. For whatever reasons, people focus their attention on different elements of their environment, and *shifting our attention is more difficult than maintaining our focus.* In these situations, there are multiple "alternative interpretations," but these alternatives can often be difficult to see because our initial "automatic interpretations" are so powerful.

Relate these ideas to emotions, explaining that the emotions we are experiencing can "bias" or influence what we focus on and/or how we interpret the environment. Emphasize that snap judgments are even more common during emotional situations. This makes sense because, when we are in situations that are truly threatening or dangerous, it is important that we act quickly on our emotions to get to safety or communicate our needs. In these "true alarm" types of situations, quickly identifying the threat is important to our survival, and there is no need to spend much time thinking about our interpretation. However, in "false alarm" situations—where nothing truly dangerous or threatening is happening but our emotions are telling us differently—acting on our automatic interpretations can get us into trouble. As time permits, ask parents to share examples of times when their strong emotions biased their perceptions or interpretations of a situation.

Parent Session 5, Goal 2

Introduce parents to the four common thinking traps covered in the child group.

Thinking Traps

Ask parents to turn to Worksheet 14.1: *L for Parents* in the workbook. Discuss that there are some typical cognitive distortions or "thinking traps" that we all fall into from time to time. When these lead us into uncomfortable and emotionally charged reactions, we need to recognize and address them. A few examples of thinking traps include:

- *Jumping to conclusions*—overestimating the likelihood that something will happen.

> **Therapist Note**
> *A good way to distinguish this from the "thinking the worst" trap below is to suggest that this thinking trap can lead to both good and bad conclusions (e.g., if a child sees a pamphlet for Disney World on the kitchen table, he assumes his family is going on a trip there). Another way to distinguish these thinking traps is to suggest that "thinking the worst" involves*

*automatically jumping to the **very worst** possible scenario, while "jumping to conclusions" does not necessarily mean that you are thinking about the worst thing that could happen. Use examples to further illustrate these distinctions as needed.*

- *Mind reading*—the belief that you know what someone else is thinking, even when you have limited or no evidence.
- *Thinking the worst*—the tendency to think that the worst possible outcome is going to happen. Often this goes hand in hand with the "jumping to conclusions" trap mentioned above, which would be jumping to the worst conclusion.

Therapist Note

Another important aspect of the "thinking the worst" thinking trap to emphasize is that, when people think the worst, they often believe that they would not be able to cope with their feared outcome if it were to occur. In reality, people often have no evidence that they would be unable to cope, and they sometimes overlook evidence of times when they have successfully coped with the same or similar outcomes in the past.

- *Ignoring the positive*—the tendency to focus on the negative aspects of a situation while ignoring the positive.

Therapist Note

Use an example in which someone receives both praise and criticism for a presentation, but when asked how it went, she only describes the criticism.

Ask the parents to share examples of thinking traps that they themselves have fallen into, and follow up by asking them to provide examples of when their children fell into thinking traps. Emphasize that while children fall into thinking traps, their thoughts aren't always wrong; rather, there is usually another explanation as well. Emphasize that more than one thing can be true.

Parents often fall into thinking traps about their child or their child's strong emotions. Ask if the parents have ever jumped to conclusions about (1) their child's behaviors and (2) their child's capabilities. Parents should be encouraged to challenge their own thoughts in addition to helping their children challenge theirs.

Parent Session 5, Goal 3

Discuss the emotional parenting behavior of inconsistency and its opposite parenting behavior, consistent reinforcement and discipline.

Types of Reinforcement and Punishment

Introduce the concepts of *reinforcement* and *punishment* as methods for shaping children's behavior so that they are more likely to do the things that we want them to do. Describe the concepts of positive reinforcement, negative reinforcement, positive punishment, and negative punishment. Parents may find it helpful to turn to Worksheet 14.2: *Understanding Learned Behaviors* as you introduce the different types of reinforcement and punishment. As you explain these concepts, emphasize that reinforcement is something that is used to increase a desired behavior, while punishment is used to decrease an undesirable behavior.

- *Positive reinforcement* refers to providing praise, attention, or rewards for behaviors and actions that the parent would like to see again. For example, if a child who often delays starting her homework sits down to begin studying soon after school, a parent might note, "Julia, I love how you are getting started with your homework right away today." Remind parents that they have already begun to practice increasing their use of positive reinforcement.
- *Negative reinforcement* refers to the introduction of an unwanted stimulus (e.g., yelling) that only goes away when the child engages in the desired behavior (e.g., sitting down to begin her homework).
- *Positive punishment* refers to the introduction of an unwanted stimulus (e.g., yelling) after a child has engaged in an unwanted behavior (e.g., using her phone when she is supposed to be focusing on homework).
- *Negative punishment* refers to the removal of a reinforcer (e.g., TV time, game time, dessert) after a child has engaged in an unwanted behavior (e.g., using her phone when she is supposed to be doing homework).

Ask the parents to reflect on what type of behavior management strategy they use the most, as well as on what type they use the least. Explain that this treatment focuses most heavily on increasing positive reinforcement, although use of negative punishment and other discipline strategies will be briefly reviewed during this session.

Emotional Parenting Behavior: Inconsistent Reinforcement and Punishment

Check in with the parents briefly about their efforts to reward or reinforce positive behaviors, attempts to use skills, and effective coping. Ask parents to describe the types of behaviors they have been attempting to reinforce, as well as any changes they have noticed in their child as a result of using more frequent reinforcement. Ask parents to also reflect on and discuss what gets in the way of their ability to provide consistent praise and discipline. Some parents of children with emotional disorders may provide insufficient praise when their child approaches or effectively manages situations that might not appear to be difficult for the average child but are extremely difficult for a child who struggles with strong emotions. Parents may also sometimes fail to notice and praise the small steps their child may be making, especially if the child is still experiencing significant struggles. However, by not noticing and responding to times when the child is successful, parents may inadvertently reduce the chance that the child will continue to approach or use effective coping in such situations in the future.

On the other hand, parents may be reluctant to discipline their emotional child (e.g., by removing privileges) for naughty or inappropriate behaviors. Sometimes this is due to the parents' own strong emotions. Parents may feel overwhelmed and be somewhat reluctant to implement punishments for misbehavior due to anticipation that their child may become upset or dysregulated if they were to do so. Other parents may feel guilty for punishing their child, which may cause them to avoid delivering the punishment in the first place or to prematurely retract the punishment. Still other parents may be reluctant to punish misbehavior if they feel that the child's difficulty with regulating emotions has contributed to the misbehavior. However, failure to consistently discipline naughty or inappropriate behavior, no matter the cause, can maintain the behavior by teaching the child that it is acceptable or that he can sometimes get away with it.

Opposite Parenting Behavior: Consistent Discipline and Punishment

Consistent Reinforcement

When attempting to increase brave or compliant behaviors, creating a reinforcement system can be an effective way to ensure that reinforcement is being provided consistently. When praise and rewards are consistent, children learn that they will experience a desirable outcome when they do things that are difficult. This association makes it more likely that children will continue to engage in previously avoided situations and attempt to use the tools in their detective kits to cope with their emotions effectively.

Have parents turn to Figure 14.1: *Guidelines for Creating a Reinforcement System at Home*. Using this figure as a guide, discuss the ways in which consistent reinforcement is provided in this treatment (e.g., puzzle pieces for home learning assignment completion, tokens or poker chips for desirable behaviors in group). Explain to parents that, when their child begins to complete situational exposures, both the parents and children will be planning rewards that the children can earn for each step of the exposure plan they complete. This is one example of a reward or reinforcement system. Explain that when children begin to complete exposure steps, it is important to provide rewards as soon as possible after completion of the exposure to increase learning and the likelihood that the child will continue to demonstrate brave or appropriate behavior when approaching exposures. *Specific, labeled praise* and *enthusiasm* about the child's behavior should be used in the moment to acknowledge successes.

In the meantime, parents may wish to develop reinforcement systems at home so that they can more consistently reward their child for using skills, approaching difficult situations, or demonstrating good behavior. This can be accomplished by creating a token system (e.g., a jar that can be filled with marbles or other objects that can be cashed in for a larger reward) or a reward chart. Let parents know that if they choose to do this, it is important to focus on a maximum of two or three behaviors at a time and to consistently and immediately reinforce the behaviors (e.g., by putting a sticker on the chart or a marble in the jar).

Consistent Behavior Management

Below is information about several behavior management strategies you may wish to address with parents during this session. It should be emphasized that poor consistency in the use of behavior management skills may actually worsen problem behaviors over time, and thus parents must be able to fully commit to consistent usage. Instruct parents to turn to Figure 14.2: *Guidelines for Creating an Effective Behavior Management System at Home*. Discuss the following important aspects of the figure:

1. *Creating Appropriate House Rules:* Parents with few or no overt rules regarding aggression or defiance may wish to begin by establishing just one clear, behaviorally grounded house rule (e.g., no hitting) and enforce this rule every time it is broken. Once an initial rule is established and maintained, others can be added gradually over time. We strongly encourage families to think about whether they have clearly discussed any house rules with their children and, if not, to start with one or two rules maximum that can be clearly presented and have clear consequences if broken.

2. *Using Effective Commands:* The way in which parents ask their children to do something matters! Some parents want their child to do something but state it as a question or request, leaving room for their child to refuse. Parents may also give up easily when their child doesn't do something right away and step in and do it themselves. This teaches children that they don't actually have to comply with their parent because the parent will take care of it for them. Explain that when giving commands, it is important to do so clearly and consistently. Introduce the following rules for effective commands:
   a) Gain the child's attention (e.g., "Emily, please look at me").
   b) Once attention is gained, use a firm (but not angry) voice requesting that the child do something.
   c) Issue only one command at a time and provide a brief interval for compliance to occur (e.g., "Emily, turn off the computer").
   d) After a brief wait, if compliance does not occur, re-issue the command. If compliance does occur, a reward should be given.
   e) If an additional prompt does not result in compliance, a consequence warning may be given (e.g., "If you don't turn off the computer, you will lose screen time for the night").
   The parent should be prepared to praise and/or reward any compliance behavior and provide the stated consequence if compliance does not occur.

3. *Response Cost Procedures:* As noted in the "effective commands" section above, one strategy for delivering consequences involves the removal of a preferred activity or item for a specified period of time. Typically, this timeframe should be brief (i.e., no more than one day),

and the parent should make sure to clearly state a command AND a warning before removing privileges.

Ask the parents to pay attention to how they are reinforcing and disciplining their child this week and to practice being more consistent.

Suggested Parent Home Learning Assignment: *L for Parents* and *Understanding Learned Behaviors*

Ask all parents to complete Worksheet 14.1: *L for Parents* by providing an example of both one of their own and one of their child's thoughts for each thinking trap. Also ask parents to complete Worksheet 14.2: *Understanding Learned Behaviors* by providing an example of a time during the week (or in the past) when they use each type of reinforcement and punishment.

CHAPTER 16 | UP-C Session 6: Use Detective Thinking

U Skill: Use Detective Thinking and Problem Solving

MATERIALS NEEDED FOR GROUP

- For Each Child Group Session:
  1. Detective CLUES kits for each child
  2. Poker chips
  3. Puzzle
  4. Prize box
  5. Large piece of paper or whiteboard to record children's answers for any group activities
- For Session 6 Only:
  6. Clues for mystery game
  7. UP-C Workbook Chapter 6
     a. *Mystery Game–Clues* (Worksheet 6.1)
     b. *U for Children* (Worksheet 6.2)
     c. *Detective Thinking Practice* (Worksheet 6.3)
     d. *When to Use Detective Thinking* (Figure 6.1)
- For Home Learning:
  8. *U for Children at Home* (Worksheet 6.4)
  9. *Solving the Mystery of Our Emotions: Before, During, and After* (Form 2.1; use the same form started after Session 2)
- Assessments to Be Given at Every Session:
  10. *Weekly Top Problems Tracking Form* (Use the same form started during Session 1 for each child, found in Appendix 11.1 at the end of Chapter 11 of this Therapist Guide)

- For Parent Group Session:
  11. UP-C Workbook Chapter 15
      a. *U for Parents* (Worksheet 15.1)
      b. *Using Reinforcement to Encourage Independent Behavior* (Figure 15.1)
- For Parent Home Learning:
  12. *U for Parents* (Worksheet 15.1)—optional
  13. *Encouraging Independent Behaviors* (Worksheet 15.2)

Therapist Preparation

At the beginning of this session, the children will be working together to use Emotion Detective skills to solve a non-emotional mystery. We provide a number of suggestions for this mystery under "Goal 1" of the session. Prior to the session, you will want to choose a mystery for the children to solve and make any initial requisite preparation. Depending on the mystery you choose, you may require access to a computer or other materials. It may also be helpful to consider where and how children can locate clues for solving the mystery in case you need to guide the children toward helpful evidence.

Overall Session 6 Goals

The main goal of this session is to present the skill of cognitive reappraisal to children and families, hereafter referred to as Detective Thinking (e.g. coming up with an idea or a "best guess" of what might happen in a situation that elicits strong emotions, gathering facts and clues to find out whether this best guess is likely to be true, going over the clues, and coming to a final decision about what might happen and how likely the initial best guess is to be true). This skill is first taught through a non-emotional activity (the mystery game), wherein the children try to solve a fun mystery using the Detective Thinking steps. The idea of this game is to present the concepts that (a) some situations may appear vague or unclear and (b) we can use our powers of observation and the collection of factual information, especially when we are not feeling overwhelmed by strong emotions, to better understand what could be true in these situations.

Children then learn how to apply Detective Thinking strategies to personally relevant emotional situations, treating their emotional thought as a guess and gathering evidence to see what else might be true. This skill is harder for children to do when they are at the height of an emotional situation, so with parents and wherever possible with children, it is helpful to reinforce the idea that it is ideal to solve mysteries often and to use Detective Thinking *before* emotions feel too strong or overwhelming.

- **Goal 1:** Introduce the concept of detective thinking in a non-emotional way using the "mystery game."
- **Goal 2:** Apply the skill of Detective Thinking to increasingly emotional and personally relevant examples.

Session 6 Content (Divided by Goals)

Session 6, Goal 1

Introduce the concept of detective thinking in a non-emotional way using the "mystery game."

While the Group Is Together

As you welcome back the group for the start of the sixth session, circulate and assist parents and children in providing severity ratings for each of their three top problems and continue to praise and encourage children as they work toward their goals. These ratings should be entered on the same *Weekly Top Problems Tracking Form* (Appendix 11.1 at the end of Chapter 11 in this Therapist Guide) begun during Session 1. Also check that each child has completed the home learning assignment. Ask any children who have not completed the home learning assignment to do so next time (or to complete them briefly during the top problems review). For those children who have completed their home learning assignment, distribute one puzzle piece to each. Briefly review content discussed during the previous session and encourage each child to share his or her home learning assignment (*L for Children at Home*) with the group.

Mystery Game—Clues

Present the goal of the mystery game. The purpose of this game is to present a challenging new skill (Detective Thinking or cognitive reappraisal) in a manner that is accessible to young children through use of a non-emotional practice opportunity. In presenting the idea of the mystery game to children, you might say the following:

> *"We will be using our Emotion Detective skills to solve mysteries today. Eventually, we want to solve the mystery of our emotions! But it's sometimes easier to practice a new skill before our emotions feel very, very strong. So, we are going to play a fun **mystery game** altogether that will introduce new detective skills to us. This game is kind of like when we looked at those pictures (of optical illusions) in the last session and tried to guess what else could be happening. Only this time we are going to work together as a group to find clues around us that could tell us more about what is truly happening in a certain situation and help us solve the mystery."*

Ask the children what steps detectives use to solve mysteries. Help them generate something similar to the following list of steps and write them down on a whiteboard or chalkboard for the children to remember:

- First we define or describe what the mystery is.
- Next we take our best guess about what the answer to the mystery might be.
- Then we look for evidence or gather clues to see if our guess is true, or if something else might be true. We look for facts (ask people questions, look online, and so on). We look for alternatives (what else could be true?).
- Then, when we've found all the clues, we go back to our original guess and see if our guess was right.

Next, solicit ideas from the group for what mysteries the group could try to solve together in a short amount of time (10–15 minutes) within the clinical setting you are currently in, or introduce one of the mystery game options listed below.

How to Structure the Mystery Game

In essence, you want to pick a mystery that (a) is something the children won't immediately know the answer to already; (b) has some way to be solved; and (c) can be solved by seeking clues or facts in the physical setting you are in during session. The options for the particular mystery to be solved with child clients are infinite, but some options include the following:

- Identify how many people work in a given building or on the floor you are occupying
- Find out how many people in a given work space have children or go to a certain school
- Identify how many things are for sale in a given business
- Find out how many different species of a certain animal or bug there are on Earth (if using a computer)
- Find out when the building you are in was built
- Find out how many people live in a specific city, country, continent, or the world
- Figure out how much people weigh in space
- Identify how many rooms there are in a given building or on a given floor you are occupying
- Place an object or objects in a closed box with a small opening that is large enough for children to stick their hand in but small enough so that children cannot see what is in the box. Then, have the children generate ideas about what is in the box based on both clues provided by you and clues generated from evidence-gathering (e.g., shaking the box, putting a hand inside the box).

Using Worksheet 6.1: *Mystery Game—Clues*, first have the children attempt an initial guess about what the answer to the mystery could be. Then, work in small groups or as one larger group with the therapist(s) to fill in as many clues as possible to help solve the mystery. Clues could be obtained by asking other people for factual information, by conducting a guided review of information online, or by reviewing posted signs or other information accessible in your setting.

Once the group reconvenes, give children a moment to fill in their "best guess" on the worksheet as to what the answer to the mystery is (you should already know the correct answer). Praise and encourage all children for participating and looking for evidence no matter if their solution was correct or not. Emphasize how more than one answer can be correct, noting that how you get information (e.g., either by asking an expert or looking information up on a directory) can lead to different conclusions:

> "Even though we first came up with a guess to solve the mystery, our first guess doesn't always turn out to be true after we gather all the clues. This is why it

is important not to always believe our first thought or snap judgment about a situation is true—it might just be a thinking trap!"

Further Debrief After the Mystery Game

Ask the children to guess why we tried to solve this mystery again. Remind them that many situations in the real world require us to look for clues to understand what might be really happening around us. Emotions, especially very strong ones, clog up our ability to see what is happening around us clearly. But a skill called **Detective Thinking**, especially when we practice it a lot, can help us to almost automatically use this skill every time we start to feel worried, sad, or angry.

Session 6, Goal 2

Apply the skill of Detective Thinking to increasingly emotional and personally relevant examples.

Introducing Detective Thinking

Direct children to *U for Children* (Worksheet 6.2). Introduce Detective Thinking by going through the steps on the worksheet with the group, emphasizing that thinking traps arise really quickly and that Detective Thinking allows us to slow down and figure out what else might be true. This might be done in the following way:

"Thinking traps can come up anytime and get us into trouble. Sometimes, they make us think that something bad or scary might be true or is about to happen. Because of this, thinking traps sometimes lead to emotions of anxiety, sadness, or worry. We're going to use our new mystery-solving skills to help get us out of thinking traps! Just like when we solved the last mystery together, we will use steps to gather some clues and help us think slowly and carefully about how likely it is that our thinking traps are true—like a detective."

Then, instruct children to follow along on their copies of *U for Children* as you describe each step of Detective Thinking on the worksheet. You might say:

*"It is very important that whenever we use Detective Thinking we follow some special steps. We call these steps the **Stop, Slow, Go steps**, because these steps help us slow our thinking down enough to gather clues and think about whether*

*our thinking trap is likely to be true. First comes **Stop**. This means that before we enter a situation that makes us feel a strong emotion, we stop to ask ourselves **what is the situation** or **what is going on here** that is making us feel a strong emotion. Next, we ask **what is the thought** that is leading us to feel this strong emotion (e.g., sadness, anger, worry, or fear). Next, we need to ask ourselves **what is our best guess of what is going on** and **how likely is it to happen (0–100 percent)**.*

*After we figure out what is going on in our minds and around us, we can move to the **Slow** part of Detective Thinking. We are going to slowly, calmly, and carefully look for **evidence or clues**. Just like with our previous mystery, we will gather clues to figure out how likely it is that our best guess is right and whether there might be something else that could also be true.*

In order to gather clues, we might ask ourselves some important questions like:
- *What is the thinking trap?*
- *What's happened in this situation in the past?*
- *Have I coped with (or dealt with) this situation before and survived?*
- *Am I 100 percent sure that my thought is true?*
- *What else could be true?*
- *Is there anything good about this situation?*
- *If my thought is true, can I cope with it?*

*After we finish gathering clues, we are ready for the **Go** step! We have to **check our best guess** by asking ourselves yet again **how likely it is to happen (0–100 percent)** now that we have all the evidence or clues in front of us. A lot of times, when we get stuck in thinking traps, it is easy to feel like something is definitely going to happen and will be really bad if it does happen, even if those things are not really true. But once we gather clues and think carefully about the situation, we are often able to become more **flexible thinkers** and become less sure about a scary, angry, worried, or sad thought being true.*

*Finally, we should ask ourselves to think about all the clues we have in front of us and what we think is really most likely to be true in the current situation. Once we better understand that, we can tell ourselves some things that might help us get through this situation or future ones like it. So, the last step here is to ask ourselves **what are our coping thoughts?***

Then, if time permits, spend a few minutes walking the children through the steps using an example that you generate (e.g., I walk into a room and two girls are laughing; what might be going on?).

Detective Thinking Practice

Ask the children to turn to Worksheet 6.3: *Detective Thinking Practice*, and explain to them that the Emotion Detectives would like their help solving more mysteries! These mysteries will be focused on thinking traps. Read and work through examples on the worksheet. Begin by introducing Darrell's situation. This might be done in the following way:

> *"Okay! Now that we have learned to be great mystery-solvers, let's help our Emotion Detective friends solve a couple of their own emotion mysteries. First, we have Darrell. He says that he got in a fight with his best friend on the way here. He doesn't even remember what it was about and he can't believe it really happened! He mentions here that he thinks they will probably never talk to each other again, and that, if they stop talking, he won't be able to hang out with their other friends either."*

Ask the children if anyone has ever had a fight with a friend or worried about losing a friend or even being worried that a friend is just mad at them. These types of questions can help children relate to Darrell's situation. Next, mention to the children that Darrell has started filling out his Detective Thinking worksheet with his Stop, Slow, Go steps but that he needs their help to finish, because he feels pretty stuck in his thinking trap. Ask the group to either split up or work as a whole to help Darrell become a more flexible thinker.

After completing Darrell's form with the group, introduce Jack's situation. You may choose to transition to Jack in the following way:

> *"Great job helping Darrell climb out of his thinking trap and learn to be a more flexible thinker! I wonder if we can help one more detective with his thinking trap too? Okay, so here is what Jack is having some trouble with. He says his mom was*

10 minutes late picking him up from soccer and he was feeling sure that she had been in an accident and was probably hurt."

Again, inquire whether the children can relate to Jack in this situation because they have been worried about something bad happening to someone they love. Direct their attention to the worksheet once again and note that, like Darrell, Jack was a really awesome detective and started filling out the worksheet on his own. Then, ask the children if they can help him fill in the rest and come up with some coping thoughts as a whole group or in smaller groups.

During this activity, try to encourage the children to generate as many answers and best guesses to Detective Thinking questions as possible. Then, working as a group, try to decide which thoughts seem most accurate. Emphasize again the fact that more than one explanation of a situation could be true. Make sure to remind children that the goal of this activity is to help the detectives get out of their thinking traps, which can make them feel like they can only see a situation in one way. We want them to become more flexible thinkers who are able to think about situations in many different ways and find helpful coping thoughts, even when they feel stressed out!

Back Together

As you welcome parents back to the room, instruct the children to turn to Figure 6.1: *When to Use Detective Thinking* in their workbooks. As a group, work with the parents and children to go over times when it is most helpful to use this skill. Emphasize that we may fall into thinking traps even before we enter situations or deal with things that we think are going to be hard or make us feel really stressed. Invite the children and parents to share whether they have experienced thinking traps in any of the situations presented in Figure 6.1.

Next, instruct each parent–child dyad to work together to identify an upcoming situation the child may be worried about or a hypothetical "ambiguous" situation that could arise based on the child's current areas of difficulty or strong emotions. Have the parent and child discuss how they can use Detective Thinking to search for clues and identify more helpful coping thoughts.

> **Suggested Home Learning Assignment:** *U for Children* and *Solving the Mystery of Our Emotions: Before, During, and After* (with option of assigning ongoing opposite action experiments)
>
> The home learning for this week is to fill out Worksheet 6.4: *U for Children at Home* with a personal example. During a quiet time at home, have the children work with their parents to practice Detective Thinking. Specifically, with help from their parents, have children complete each step of Detective Thinking for one thinking trap experienced during the week. Children should also add another entry to their *Solving the Mystery of Our Emotions: Before, During, and After*.

Overall Parent Session 6 Goals

The main goal of this parent session is to teach parents the skill of cognitive restructuring (referred to as "Detective Thinking" in this treatment) so that they can support their child's use of the skill at home. Parents are introduced to the steps of Detective Thinking and are asked to practice applying the skill to emotional thoughts relevant to adults and to their own child's experience. Parents also learn about the emotional parenting behavior overcontrol/overprotection and its opposite parenting behavior, healthy independence-granting.

- **Goal 1:** Introduce parents to the concept of Detective Thinking.
- **Goal 2:** Practice Detective Thinking with parents, using examples relevant to adults and children.
- **Goal 3:** Introduce parents to the emotional parenting behavior of overcontrol/overprotection and its opposite parenting behavior, healthy independence-granting.

Parent Session 6 Content (Divided by Goals)

Parent Session 6, Goal 1
Introduce parents to the concept of Detective Thinking.

> **Therapist Note**
> *Remember to begin this session and each subsequent one with a brief check-in (no more than 10 minutes) regarding major changes in child symptoms/functioning over the past week, as well as a review of home learning assignments.*

Reviewing Flexible Thinking

Review the discussion of flexible thinking from last week's session. Reiterate that ambiguous situations may be interpreted in many different ways (referencing the optical illusions) and that it is often difficult to shift our attention from what we see as "fact" and consider different interpretations. Further, when we experience a strong emotion, we are even more likely to quickly narrow in on one interpretation of a situation, without considering other possibilities, and act on that interpretation. In other words, we get stuck in a "thinking trap." However, we tend not to recognize how our current emotions may be impacting our interpretations of events, and it is often difficult to see that other possible interpretations of the situation may be just as accurate or realistic. The more we fall into the same thinking traps, the more stuck we become, leading us to interpret similar situations in the same unhelpful or inaccurate ways over and over again.

Tell the parents that their children will be learning a skill in this session to help them think more flexibly about emotional situations. Emphasize that, although this skill may lead their children to more "positive" interpretations of situations, the primary goal is not to promote positive thinking. Rather, we want their children to be able to entertain multiple interpretations of a situation so that they can decide what is the most realistic or helpful way to think about the situation.

Introducing Detective Thinking Steps

Ask parents to turn to Worksheet 15.1: *U for Parents* in the parent workbook. Explain that Detective Thinking is a step-by-step process for teaching their child to consider his or her interpretation of an emotional situation as a detective would—in other words, as a guess to be tested against the evidence. Examining all the evidence for a given thought helps children to think more flexibly about emotional situations and to consider what else might be true. At the end of the process, the goal is for their child to arrive at a more realistic, accurate, or helpful interpretation or thought about the situation. As discussed already, this thought may or may not be positive. In many emotional situations, an unpleasant outcome is not impossible and may even be likely. However, the realistic outcome, even when unpleasant, is often not as bad as it may initially seem, and children often underestimate their ability to cope with such outcomes.

Teach parents the steps of Detective Thinking as they are laid out on the *U for Parents* worksheet. Tell the parents that "Stop, Slow, Go" is a handy phrase that helps children to remember these steps.

Explain that we refer to the first step of Detective Thinking as the **Stop** step because we want children to learn to stop themselves when they are approaching an emotional situation or feeling a strong emotion and figure out what they are thinking, *before* they act on a given interpretation of the situation. The goal of this step is for children to identify their thought and how likely they believe it to be true, before they have gathered any evidence.

During the **Slow** step, children are taking their time to gather evidence for their first thought or "snap judgment" by considering what else could be true and what else has happened to themselves or others in the past in that same situation. Children should also be encouraged to think about how they would cope with their feared outcome if it does indeed turn out to be true. In summary, the overall goal of this step is to slow down the child's thinking about an emotional situation to create time for flexible thinking.

Finally, in the **Go** step, children are asked to re-evaluate the likelihood of their original thought or hypothesis, given all the evidence, and to come up with a more realistic or helpful coping thought that takes all the evidence into account. We call this step the Go step because we want children to proceed and act on their emotion only after they have gone through the steps of evaluating their initial interpretation.

Explain to parents that although Detective Thinking can be used whenever a child or parent realizes that strong emotions are influencing the child's thoughts about a situation, Detective Thinking is often most effective when used *before* entering or engaging with an emotional situation. When we are at the height of a strong emotion, especially if that emotion is very intense, it is often difficult to recognize the influence our emotions are having on our thoughts. It may also be difficult to remember to use a skill, let alone to recall the steps involved. When used *before* an upcoming emotional situation, though, Detective Thinking can reduce the intensity of the child's emotions ahead of time and help prevent emotional behaviors. Let parents know that when they and children reunite at the end of this session, they will be completing a worksheet together to identify good times for their child to use Detective Thinking.

Parent Session 6, Goal 2

Practice detective thinking with parents, using examples relevant to adults and children.

Therapist Note

During this session, it is crucial for parents to practice using Detective Thinking in the parent group so that they understand the skill well enough to immediately begin to support their child in using it at home. We often find it helpful for parents to practice using the skill for their own emotional thoughts, in addition to their child's emotional thoughts, as this deepens their understanding of the skill and their ability to use it flexibly. However, if you do not have time in session for parents to practice Detective Thinking on both adult-relevant and child-relevant emotional thoughts, you may assign one of these practices for home learning.

Detective Thinking Practice with Adult-Themed Emotional Thoughts

Emphasize to parents that Detective Thinking is a useful skill for anyone to practice, including adults and children and even those without an emotional disorder. After all, we all experience strong emotions from time to time, and strong emotions increase our likelihood of making snap judgments or falling into thinking traps. For this reason, we feel it is helpful in this treatment for parents to practice using Detective Thinking for their own emotional thoughts or for emotional thoughts typical of other parents or adults.

Engage parents in one or both of the following activities, as time permits:

- **As a group, practice Detective Thinking for a typical adult emotional thought.** Examples of such thoughts are provided below, but you may prefer to solicit examples from the group.
  - Your spouse is late coming home from work. You assume he or she got into a car accident.
  - Your last performance review at work was excellent. However, you feel like a failure for not being named employee of the year.

- Your child got detention for the second time this quarter. You assume that her teacher must think you're a bad parent.

■ **Ask each parent to identify a recent emotional thought and complete the steps of Detective Thinking independently.** After all the parents finish, ask them to discuss their experiences with the exercise and to reflect upon any steps that were difficult.

Detective Thinking Practice with Child-Themed Emotional Thoughts

As time permits, ask one of the parents to volunteer one of his or her child's recent emotional thoughts—one that he or she believes may be a thinking trap. Have the parent describe the situation and the thought the child experienced. Role-play with that parent (who can pretend to be the child) to model how the parent might guide the child through the steps of Detective Thinking at home. If desired, you can encourage parents to make the Detective Thinking process difficult during this role-play, particularly if they expect their child will be resistant to the process; this allows parents to help anticipate barriers to completion and to see examples of how to address difficult questions or responses.

Parent Session 6, Goal 3

Introduce parents to the emotional parenting behavior of overcontrol/overprotection and its opposite parenting behavior, healthy independence-granting.

Therapist Note

Although the topic of overcontrol/overprotection and its opposite parenting behavior is ideally presented fully to all parents of children with emotional difficulties, time could be short for this topic if the Detective Thinking discussion was extensive in the group. If pressed for time, consider presenting the concept of overcontrol/overprotection briefly along with the rationale for encouraging independent behavior as an opposite action, with further discussion about this topic in Session 7 following review of the related home learning assignment.

Emotional Parenting Behavior: Overcontrol/Overprotection

Explain that parents have a natural impulse to care for and protect their children, particularly when their children are distressed. This natural impulse is useful and adaptive when a child is in an unsafe or new situation and *requires* the assistance of parents to survive or effectively navigate the situation. However, children with emotional disorders experience distress more frequently or intensely than other children, often in response to situations that are not truly dangerous or threatening (e.g., false-alarm situations). Explain that many parents will step in and do things for their child in these types of situations to quickly reduce their child's distress, or alternatively will help their child avoid situations that elicit strong emotions. We call these parenting behaviors **overcontrol** or **overprotection**, meaning that parents are attempting to control or protect their child from situations that are not inherently dangerous and that their child could navigate on his or her own. Remind parents that these actions are quite natural and arise from a healthy and protective urge to reduce their child's distress. However, they can have unintended negative consequences and get children stuck in problematic cycles of emotional behaviors.

Review with the parents the following three unintended consequences of overcontrol/overprotection:

- First, when parents step in to control or protect their child from a situation, the child often gets the message that there is something about the situation that should be feared or avoided. Otherwise, why would the parent be stepping in?
- Second, parental overcontrol/overprotection reduces a child's sense of self-efficacy, or sense that he or she is a capable individual who can be successful in coping with all kinds of situations. When children don't practice doing things on their own and learning from their mistakes, they may come to believe that they are incapable of doing things on their own.
- Finally, overcontrol/overprotection reinforces a child's use of avoidance or other emotional behaviors. Children learn that they can continue avoid situations that elicit strong emotions because their parents will allow them to do so or will step in and take care of these situations for them.

Opposite Parenting Behavior: Healthy Independence-Granting

Explain to parents that we want them to begin allowing their children to assume more independence in areas where the parents have historically been overcontrolling or overprotective. This can be very difficult at first for both the parents and the children, as children may initially appear more distressed when parents back off from protecting their child from experiencing uncomfortable emotions. Parents in turn may struggle with seeing their child in distress and *not* rushing in to do something to protect their child or immediately reduce distress. Parents also struggle at times to know what situations or tasks their child is capable of approaching independently, particularly if a parent has been stepping in to rescue the child from these situations or tasks for a very long time.

Introduce parents to the concept of **shaping**, a procedure for helping children successively approximate independent performance of age-appropriate activities. Shaping involves successively encouraging or rewarding each step closer toward a desired behavior. For example, if a parent has always arranged play dates for the child, calling a friend to invite him over to play may be very difficult for the child. The parent may wish to start by praising or rewarding the child's attempt to find out the friend's number, then praise the child for texting or calling the friend to say "hello," and then later praise or reward the child for calling the friend to ask about his plans this weekend.

Explain that parents can also use some of the parenting behaviors they have learned already, such as positive reinforcement and planned ignoring, to encourage their child's independent coping. These strategies can be used in the following ways:

- **Reinforce** the child's attempts to use coping skills or solve problems independently, regardless of the outcome. By reinforcing these behaviors through praise or rewards, the parent increases the likelihood that the child will use these skills again in the future when difficult situations or emotions come up.
- Practice **planned ignoring** of minor displays of distress or requests for help. By ignoring crying, whining, or reassurance-seeking in false-alarm situations, the parent is encouraging the child to deal with these situations more independently. In contrast, when the parent runs to the child's aid, the child does not get an opportunity to practice independently using skills to cope with the problem.
- These two strategies are often powerful when combined. Even if a child is behaving inappropriately in a situation, parents can still look out for and reward aspects of their child's behavior that are desirable or effective. For example, if the child is whining about having to attend a birthday party but continues to walk toward the car, the parent can choose to ignore the whining and praise the child for getting into the car anyway. This is called **differential**

reinforcement. You might direct parents to Figure 15.1: *Using Reinforcement to Encourage Independent Behaviors* for additional guidance regarding the implementation of these strategies at home.

Suggested Parent Home Learning Assignment: *Encouraging Independent Behaviors* **and** *U for Parents*

Ask each parent to complete both parts of Worksheet 15.2: *Encouraging Independent Behaviors*. This worksheet asks parents to identify three areas to promote greater independence, as well as how they might use shaping principles to shape their child's behavior in one of these areas. You may also wish to ask parents to complete the *U for Parents* worksheet using one of their own or one of their child's emotional thoughts from the upcoming week.

CHAPTER 17 | UP-C Session 7: Problem Solving and Conflict Management

U Skill: Use Detective Thinking and Problem Solving

MATERIALS NEEDED FOR GROUP

- For Each Child Group Session:
  1. Detective CLUES kits for each child
  2. Poker chips
  3. Puzzle
  4. Prize box
  5. Large piece of paper or whiteboard to record children's answers for any group activities
- For Session 7 Only:
  6. A large stuffed animal or other similar object
  7. U Badge
  8. UP-C Workbook Chapter 7
     a. *Problem Solving Steps* (Figure 7.1)
     b. *Problem Solving Game* (Worksheet 7.1)
     c. *Problem Solving Practice* (Worksheet 7.2)
- For Home Learning:
  9. *Problem Solving at Home with Others* (Worksheet 7.3)
  10. *Solving the Mystery of Our Emotions: Before, During, and After* (Form 2.1; use the same form started after Session 2)
- Assessments to Be Given at Every Session:
  11. *Weekly Top Problems Tracking Form* (Use the same form started during Session 1 for each child, found in Appendix 11.1 at the end of Chapter 11 of this Therapist Guide)

- For Parent Group Session:
  12. UP-C Workbook Chapter 15
      a. *Problem Solving Steps* (Figure 15.2)
      b. *Problem Solving Steps Practice* (Worksheet 15.3)
- For Parent Home Learning:
  13. *Shaping Detective Thinking and Problem Solving at Home* (Worksheet 15.4)

Therapist Preparation

In preparation for this session, obtain a stuffed animal or similar object for use during a non-emotional example of Problem Solving during session. At the end of the session, the children will receive their third "CLUES" badge, indicating that they have completed the U Skill. Typically, badges are letter-shaped stickers or construction paper letters that the children can put on their CLUES kits to monitor their progress. This should be a celebrated accomplishment for the children and their families and noted by you as such.

Overall Session 7 Goals

The main objective of this session is to teach the children Problem Solving, a series of steps children can use to get out of situations where they feel "stuck" or unable to come to a good solution. This is an extension of the "flexible thinking" work accomplished in Sessions 5 and 6 of the UP-C, as children will be encouraged to use their powers of observation and flexible thinking strategies to generate possible actions that can be taken in difficult circumstances. Similar to the structure of Session 6, Problem Solving skills are first introduced in this session by having the children engage in a non-emotional activity in which they have to work together to solve a fun or silly "problem" (e.g., trying to get a stuffed animal from one side of the room to the other without using their hands or arms). Later these same steps are applied to more emotional situations and other types of problems, including those in which there is a higher degree of interpersonal conflict (e.g., between siblings, at school, or with parents).

- **Goal 1:** Introduce Problem Solving with a non-emotional example, or the "Problem Solving game."
- **Goal 2:** Practice Problem Solving using increasingly personally relevant scenarios.

Session 7, Goal 1

Introduce Problem Solving with a non-emotional example, or the "Problem Solving game."

While the Group Is Together

As you welcome back the group for the start of the seventh session, circulate and assist parents and children in providing severity ratings for each of their three top problems and continue to praise and encourage children as they work toward their goals. These ratings should be entered on the same *Weekly Top Problems Tracking Form* (Appendix 11.1 at the end of Chapter 11 in this Therapist Guide) begun during Session 1. Also check that each child has completed the home learning assignment. Ask any children who have not completed the home learning assignment to do so next time (or to complete it briefly during the top problems review). For those children who have completed their home learning assignment, distribute one puzzle piece to each. Briefly review content discussed during the previous session and encourage each child to share his or her home learning assignment (*U for Children at Home*) with the group.

Child Group Alone

Introducing Problem Solving

Why Do We Teach Problem Solving to Children?

This section of treatment continues along the same theme as the previous sessions in terms of focusing on the idea of practicing flexible thinking. Children who often experience strong emotions, including anxiety, depression, or anger, often think rigidly and inflexibly about emotional situations, not only making the same unhelpful interpretations over and over but also having difficulty recognizing alternative things to do to solve a problem, even if what they have been doing to solve problems in the past has repeatedly been ineffective. It is important to help children distinguish between Detective Thinking and Problem Solving. For instance, in the previous session focusing on Detective Thinking, children learned to be flexible thinkers by trying to think logically about different ways they might interpret a given, ambiguous situation. In this session, **Problem Solving** is introduced as an *additional Emotion Detective skill* for thinking more flexibly, but about how one might *deal with* a given situation rather than how one might think about a given situation alone.

Explain to the children that Detective Thinking is most useful when the situation itself is not truly dangerous or bad, but when our false alarm might be going off telling us that there is danger when there is not, or when there is nothing that can be done to change the current situation. Children can use Problem Solving in addition to or instead of Detective Thinking when they might need to come up with some *helpful things to do* in a tough situation. When there are ways that the children can act to solve a problem or things they can do to improve a situation, we also want them to be able to *think flexibly* about different ways of solving the problem, rather than quickly jumping to conclusions and getting stuck in one solution. You might choose to explain this concept in the following way:

> *"Problem Solving is another type of Emotion Detective skill you can use to help you get out of situations where you may feel stuck or may be having trouble coming up with ways to deal with a problem. It is not Detective Thinking because with Problem Solving we are trying to come up with helpful things we can do to solve a problem, and with Detective Thinking we are trying to change the way we think about something that might not truly be dangerous or that we can't really change."*

Explain to the children that Problem Solving involves a few steps and that you will be practicing as a group by doing a fun activity. Tell the group that before you do the fun game to practice the Problem Solving steps, you first need to make sure the children know what all the steps are. Instruct the children to turn to Figure 7.1: *Problem Solving Steps* in their workbooks. Using this figure as a guide, go over the steps of Problem Solving with the group, making sure to emphasize both the non-emotional and emotional examples of each problem. If time permits, you can also write these steps on a whiteboard or chalkboard as children follow along:

- *Define the problem*—Objectively and clearly identify what the current problem could be. Take it slow and try to be clear and simple in your description of the problem at present.
- *Brainstorm solutions*—Come up with at least three to five options for what you could do to solve the problem.
- *List the pros and cons for each solution*—Identify at least one good thing and one not-so-good thing about each solution you listed.
- *Pick a solution and try it out*—Given what you have learned so far, what is your best option? Try it out and watch what happens!
- *How did it work?*—Did your pick go as well as you thought it would? Was it helpful?
- *If the first choice doesn't work, try another solution, and so on.*—If your first pick worked, great! But it might take trying two or three different solutions before you find the right one. Like any good detective, you want to watch what happens carefully and decide if you need to try again.

Emphasize the Steps of Problem Solving Using a Non-emotional Example

The purpose of this game is to present Problem Solving in a way that is accessible to young children through use of a non-emotional practice opportunity, similar to that introduced during the previous session for teaching Detective Thinking.

Ask the children to turn to Worksheet 7.1: *Problem Solving Game* in their workbooks. Then, explain that you will all be working together to figure out how to solve a silly problem. Explain to the children that often, when learning a new skill, it can be easier to practice with a fun example first before trying to use the skill to deal with tougher emotions. In presenting the idea of the Problem Solving game to children, you might explain:

"We will be using this new Emotion Detective skill, Problem Solving, to solve problems today. Soon, we will want to solve problems that have to do with emotions! But, like we talked about last time with Detective Thinking, it's sometimes easier to practice a new skill before our emotions feel very, very strong. So, we are going to play a fun **Problem Solving game** *as a group that will help us learn this new Emotion Detective skill. This time we are going to work together as a group to figure out how to solve the problem of moving a toy across the room without using our hands."*

Have the children work together to use the steps listed on Worksheet 7.1: *Problem Solving Game* to solve the silly problem of getting a toy or stuffed animal from one side of the room to the other without using their hands (e.g., "Kermit the frog is stuck on a lily pad! We need to help him get over to the island [on the other side of the room] without using our hands"). Write the Problem Solving steps on the whiteboard or chalkboard or have children fill in Worksheet 7.1 as a group as they strategize about how to solve this fun problem. Once the options have been clearly laid out, along with pros and cons, let each child who wishes to do so pick a strategy to try out and then decide as a group which might be the best option.

Therapist Note

During the brainstorming section, encourage children to come up with at least one wacky or silly solution. This relieves the pressure of only coming up with "good" solutions and may also help children become more open-minded and flexible about other options they wouldn't have otherwise considered (e.g., in the above example, having the children move Kermit across the room by blowing on him).

Session 7, Goal 2

Practice Problem Solving using increasingly personally relevant scenarios.

Problem Solving Practice

Introduce Worksheet 7.2: *Problem Solving Practice*. Reinforce the Problem Solving steps by having the group work together to help solve Jack's problem:

- Jack wants to play videogames but he isn't allowed to until his grades get better.

Have the children follow along the worksheet, allowing individual children to volunteer reading aloud portions of Jack's defined problem, brainstormed solutions, and list of pros and cons for each solution. Then, work as a group to choose which solution Jack should try first.

Explain that, although Jack's problem had to do with studying, school, and grades, a lot of other children use Problem Solving for problems with other people, including family, friends, and other kids. Introduce the concept of conflict management via Problem Solving as follows:

"When we have problems or arguments with our parents, siblings, friends, or people at school, our first response is often to get really angry or upset with the other person."

Ask the children for examples of things that they have done when feeling really angry or upset with another person, such as

- Slamming doors
- Yelling
- Crying
- Fighting back

Let the children know that they can use Problem Solving in these types of situations so that they don't react so strongly and do something they might later regret. Emphasize that it may be difficult to remember and follow the steps of Problem Solving during the height of the emotion, so it is important to go through the Problem Solving steps before problems with other people come up. This way, the children don't have to spend time brainstorming different solutions in the moment, and they can immediately put their plan into action rather than lashing out or losing control.

Direct the children's attention back to Worksheet 7.2 and read over Nina's situation together:

- Nina has been feeling angry with her best friend because she did not invite Nina to a party.

Have the children attempt to work through Nina's problem together as a group by defining the problem, brainstorming solutions, listing the pros and cons for each solution, and picking the best solution to try out. Then, if time permits, you can have the children pick a personally relevant example generated from one of the group members to try to work through as a group.

Therapist Note

Generally you should allow the child to generate the solutions; however, some children may have difficulty generating solutions or may frequently miss some possibilities. At these times, you may wish to help the child, noting that during periods of high emotion it can be difficult to pick any solution except the one that we think we need to do to reduce our uncomfortable emotional experiences.

Wrap up the group by telling children the following:

"Today we learned a lot about different problems that kids get into all the time. The important thing to remember is that it is okay to have problems sometimes. We just need to use our Problem Solving skills to help us get out of them in the best way.

<u>We can't change what other people do:</u>

- *Your sister may still steal your toys.*
- *Your parents might still yell at you.*
- *Your friends might still be mean sometimes.*
- *You might sometimes not know how to study or you might get a bad grade.*

But we can change how we react! By using Problem Solving skills we can work on managing our own reactions, and this might even change the way other people react in the future."

Suggested Home Learning Assignment: *Problem Solving at Home with Others* and *Solving the Mystery of Our Emotions: Before, During, and After* (with option of assigning ongoing opposite action experiments)

The home learning for this week is to fill out Worksheet 7.3: Problem Solving at Home with Others using a personal example. During a quiet time at home, have children work with their parents to practice Problem Solving using this worksheet as a guide. Children should also add another entry to their Solving the Mystery of Our Emotions: Before, During, and After.

Make sure to hand out the "U" Badge to the children at the end of the session.

Overall Parent Session 7 Goals

The main goal of this parent session is to continue to promote the goal of flexible thinking about emotional situations through Problem Solving. Problem Solving is a strategy for generating and evaluating multiple solutions to a problem before deciding how to act. Just as children who struggle with strong emotions tend to interpret emotional situations quickly without considering alternatives, these children also tend to get stuck in the same solutions for day-to-day problems and have difficulty seeing other possible solutions. Parents learn the steps of Problem Solving and how to support their child in using them. Build upon the discussion of healthy independence-granting introduced in the previous session by explaining how parents can prompt children to use Detective Thinking and Problem Solving as opposite parenting behaviors to reassurance and accommodation.

- **Goal 1:** Introduce parents to the steps of Problem Solving, another Emotion Detective skill for developing cognitive flexibility.
- **Goal 2:** Discuss the application of Problem Solving to interpersonal conflict situations.
- **Goal 3:** Review parents' efforts at healthy independence-granting, pointing out how parents can promote independent use of Detective Thinking and Problem Solving as alternatives to reassurance-seeking and accommodation.

Parent Session 7 Content (Divided by Goals)

Parent Session 7, Goal 1

Introduce parents to the steps of Problem Solving, another Emotion Detective skill for developing cognitive flexibility.

Therapist Note

Remember to begin this session and each subsequent one with a brief check-in (no more than 10 minutes) regarding major changes in child symptoms/functioning over the past week, as well as a review of home learning assignments. For this session, we recommend reviewing U for Parents (Worksheet 15.1) at the beginning of the session and incorporating a review of Encouraging Independent Behaviors (Worksheet 15.2) into the discussion of Goal 3 near the end of the session.

Brief Review of Detective Thinking

Briefly review the purpose and steps of Detective Thinking with the parents, particularly if you have not already done so during home learning review. Remind them that emotional situations often lead us to make *snap judgments* that are not always realistic, accurate, or helpful. Detective thinking is a way of slowing down our thinking so that we can look for evidence to test these snap judgments before acting on them. Emphasize to parents that it is important for children to arrive at a coping thought, or alternative interpretation of the situation, at the end of Detective Thinking. If children are completing Detective Thinking before entering an emotional situation (which is ideal!), they can use their coping thought when in the situation to think more realistically and reduce distress.

Orient parents to the fact that they and their children are currently in the "U" skill of treatment ("Use Detective Thinking and Problem Solving"). Remind parents that the purpose of this section of treatment is to teach the children to think more flexibly. Children who struggle with strong emotions of anxiety, depression, or anger often think rigidly and inflexibly about emotional situations, making the same unhelpful interpretations over and over or trying to solve problems in the same ineffective ways. With Detective Thinking, children learned to be more flexible in how they are interpreting or thinking about a given situation. In this session, children will be learning **Problem Solving**, yet another Emotion Detective skill for thinking more flexibly. Emphasize to the parents that Detective Thinking is particularly useful when the situation itself is not the problem (e.g., a child is overestimating the likelihood of something negative happening, like the plane crashing on the way to a vacation), or when there is nothing that can be done to change the situation (e.g., when a child needs to endure something that might cause anxiety, sadness, or anger, like a performance for a socially anxious child). When either one of these conditions occurs, it is often most helpful to change the way we are thinking about the situation by using Detective Thinking. This is sometimes referred to as a **secondary control** strategy. In contrast, **Problem Solving** is a **primary control** strategy that is useful when the situation itself is the problem and may be able to be changed (e.g., a child is not sure how to most effectively study for an upcoming test, or would like to figure out how to resolve a conflict with a peer or teacher). When the situation or approach to the situation can be changed, we want children to be able to think flexibly about different ways of solving the problem rather than quickly jumping to and getting stuck in one solution.

Problem Solving

Ask the parents to turn to *Problem Solving Steps* (Figure 15.2) in the parent workbook. Go through each step with the parents one by one, highlighting the following points about each step:

- Define the problem:

  "Before your child can solve a problem, he or she needs to figure out exactly what the problem is. The way your child describes the problem will influence the kinds of solutions he or she comes up with. Therefore, it is important to really get to the heart of the issue, and to be as simple, concrete, and specific as possible."

- Brainstorm solutions:

  "At this point, your child should generate as many solutions as possible, without putting any kind of judgment on them as good solutions or bad solutions. The point here is to generate, generate, generate! It may be especially helpful to come up with some wacky or unrealistic solutions, as these ideas may help reduce the pressure to only come up with good solutions. Additionally, it might help you and your child become more creative with generating solutions."

- List the pros and cons for each solution:

  "Now is the time for your child to start weighing each solution. For each of the solutions your child has generated, make a pros and cons list, or the good things and bad things about each solution. Try to encourage and help your child come up with at least one pro and one con for each solution, ideally more."

- Pick a solution and try it out:

  "Based on the lists your child has generated of pros and cons for each solution, help your child pick a solution to try out. This will most likely be one that has more pros than cons, but should also be a realistic and manageable solution. It may also be helpful to consider whether some of the pros and cons for each example should be weighted differently. For example, punching somebody to communicate anger may cause severe harm to that person, so this would be a pretty serious 'con.' Even if it is the only 'con,' it is probably severe enough to disqualify this solution from being the first choice."

- If needed, go through the Problem Solving steps again:

  "Help your child figure out whether the solution he or she picked worked. If so, great! If not, why not? If it sort of worked, what were the good parts, and what were the bad parts? Based on what your child learns by trying this semi-successful solution, can he or she identify the next solution to try or even come up with a new solution?

If the first solution doesn't get your child unstuck, help your child pick a different one from the list, modify the solution he or she already tried out, or pick a new solution entirely."

Emphasize to the parents that Problem Solving is a process they may need to follow several times before finding an optimal solution. Often the first solution chosen by their child will not be as successful as their child thought it might be—in fact, it might be entirely unsuccessful. This can be very discouraging! In addition to assisting their child with completing the Problem Solving steps, parents should check in with their child after he or she has tried a solution to see how it worked out. Parents should *positively* emphasize the importance of perseverance and effort when solving problems and encourage their child to continue to try out different options until he or she discovers one that works.

Lead the parents in Problem Solving practice during the session, using either a hypothetical example of a typical adult problem or a problem volunteered by one of the parents. Take the parents through the Problem Solving steps for whichever example you select, one at a time. Parents can use Worksheet 15.3: *Problem Solving Steps Practice* to write down each of the steps identified by the group. Examples of possible adult problems for this exercise include:

- You were planning to take your child to the zoo today, but at the last minute your boss asked you to work on an important project.
- You and your spouse are having a disagreement about where to take the family on vacation this year.
- Your child is assigned to a teacher who you believe to be the worst in the grade level, and you are concerned that your child's performance will suffer.
- You are frustrated because your friend cancelled plans with you for the third weekend in a row.

After working through an adult problem, discuss the parents' experiences using the Problem Solving steps as a group. Discuss any steps that seemed challenging or confusing to parents. Ask parents to volunteer examples of current problems with which their child is struggling and may benefit from using the Problem Solving steps.

Parent Session 7, Goal 2

Discuss the application of Problem Solving to interpersonal conflict situations.

Children with emotional disorders often struggle with interpersonal interactions and conflict due to their strong emotions. Provide parents with several examples of this, including the following:

- Children with anxiety may struggle to stick up for themselves when being bullied or taken advantage of by a friend.
- Children with depression may need to repair friendships due to engaging in problematic isolation and withdrawal from friends.
- Children who struggle with anger may be quick to fight with friends and say things they later regret.
- Children with anxiety may have difficulty meeting new kids after switching schools.
- Children with depression may fail to turn in school assignments due to being too tired and down to complete them.

Although it may be helpful for parents to encourage their child to use Detective Thinking in these situations if they notice their child falling into thinking traps, it is also important to note that all of these problems do have *many possible solutions.*

Emphasize that the Problem Solving steps may be used to help children manage conflict situations or difficult interpersonal interactions with family members, friends, or peers at school. Ask parents to think of a time when their child had an interpersonal difficulty with someone else and how he or she resolved the problem. Ask parents to reflect on whether the use of the Problem Solving steps might have been helpful, and how parents can attempt to help their children implement these steps before such an event occurs again. Emphasize that the best time to discuss these strategies is outside of the emotional situation.

Parent Session 7, Goal 3

Review parents' efforts at healthy independence-granting, pointing out how parents can promote independent use of Detective Thinking and Problem Solving as alternatives to reassurance-seeking and accommodation.

In this final section of Session 7, begin by checking in with the parents about their attempts to shape more independent behavior during the past week. This may be a good time to briefly review *Encouraging Independent Behaviors* (Worksheet 15.2).

In addition to the independent behaviors parents have been promoting during the past week, explain that Detective Thinking and Problem

Solving (the U skills) are two strategies children can use to cope with their emotions and problems more independently. When feeling strong emotions, children often ask for excessive reassurance or recruit parents or others to solve their problems for them. This results in children becoming overly dependent upon others to regulate their emotions or solve problems.

Explain to the parents why excessive reassurance is a form of overprotection and encourage them to shape their child's use of Detective Thinking instead of providing reassurance. To initiate this discussion, ask parents what they typically say when their child is expressing worry, fear, hopelessness, or pessimism about a situation. Address the different responses parents may provide, but highlight the fact that many parents tend to attempt to reassure their child that the situation will turn out okay or that nothing bad is going to happen. In fact, many children actively and frequently seek reassurance from their parents and may explicitly ask their parents to tell them that everything is going to be okay. Many parents feel better after providing reassurance because they naturally wish to help their child feel better, and some children may temporarily appear less emotional after receiving reassurance.

Explain to the parents, however, that providing reassurance is yet another way that they attempt to protect their children from negative outcomes or control their child's thinking about a situation. *The more reassurance parents provide, the more their child becomes dependent upon that reassurance and less able to independently evaluate whether the feared outcome is realistic.* Reassurance-seeking becomes an emotional behavior that the child turns to whenever he or she is feeling distressed about a situation. Some children even come to believe that things will *only* be okay if their parent reassures them that they will.

Parents also may fall into the trap of becoming overly involved in solving problems for their child. This trap is easy to fall into for a number of reasons. First, when a child is facing a problem, a parent is often easily able to determine what approach will likely work best for the child. Parents may feel it saves time and distress to simply tell their child what to do, rather than waiting for the child to figure it out. Parents may also be concerned that if they allow their child to solve his or her own problems, he or she may end up choosing the wrong solution, leading to more distress or further problems. All parents want to protect their children from suffering, so it is quite natural for parents to step in and tell the child what to do in these situations or take care of the problem for him or her.

Explain to the parents that, just as children can become dependent on parents to provide reassurance that a situation will turn out okay, children may also become dependent on parents to solve problems for them. The more parents solve problems for their children, the less practice children get at solving them on their own, and the more dependent they become on parents. This may also negatively impact a child's sense of self-efficacy and exacerbate his or her natural tendency to be relatively inflexible in his or her approach to solving problems. Plus, sometimes children learn best from making mistakes, and if parents prevent their children from making mistakes, they limit opportunities for their child to learn.

Encourage parents to promote independence over the next week by encouraging their child to practice Detective Thinking whenever he or she seeks excessive reassurance, and by prompting children to go through the Problem Solving steps when difficulties or interpersonal conflicts arise. Return to the discussion of shaping behaviors and discuss how to apply this concept to Detective Thinking and Problem Solving. These can be tricky skills for children to learn, so parents may need to do quite a bit of shaping in the beginning when their children are first learning to use them. Ask the parents to describe what they believe shaping would look like for Detective Thinking and Problem Solving. Even using a phrase like "What do you think?" rather than providing reassurance, or "What are some things you could do?" rather than solving problems for the child, can be useful, even if time is not sufficient to go through all Detective Thinking or Problem Solving steps.

Suggested Parent Home Learning Assignment: *Shaping Detective Thinking* and *Problem Solving at Home*

Ask each parent to use Worksheet 15.4 to describe how he or she attempted to shape the use of Detective Thinking and Problem Solving as opposite parenting behaviors to overcontrol and overprotection.

CHAPTER 18

UP-C Session 8: Awareness of Emotional Experiences

E Skill: Experience My Emotions

MATERIALS NEEDED FOR GROUP

- For Each Child Group Session:
    1. Detective CLUES kits for each child
    2. Poker chips
    3. Puzzle
    4. Prize box
    5. Large piece of paper or whiteboard to record children's answers for any group activities
- For Session 8 Only:
    6. Raisins, small candies, pebbles, clay, or putty (depending on which present-moment awareness exercise will be completed)
    7. UP-C Workbook Chapter 8
        a. *Notice It, Say Something about It, Experience It* (Figure 8.1)
        b. *Practicing My Awareness Steps* (Worksheet 8.1)
        c. *Being Aware with My Five Senses* (Worksheet 8.2)
        d. *Present-Moment Awareness Activities* (Figure 8.2)
- For Home Learning:
    8. *Awareness Practice at Home* (Worksheet 8.3)
    9. *Solving the Mystery of Our Emotions: Before, During, and After* (Form 2.1; use the same form started after Session 2)
- Assessments to Be Given at Every Session:
    10. *Weekly Top Problems Tracking Form* (Use the same form started during Session 1 for each child, found in Appendix 11.1 at the end of Chapter 11 of this Therapist Guide)

- For Parent Group Session:
  11. UP-C Workbook Chapter 16
      a. *Notice It, Say Something about It, Experience It* (Figure 16.1)
- For Parent Home Learning:
  12. *Parent Nonjudgmental Awareness Practice at Home* (Worksheet 16.1)
  13. *Emotional Behavior Form—Parent Version* (Form 16.1)

Therapist Preparation

In preparation for this session, you will need to gather materials for the "Using My Five Senses" game such as small candies, pebbles, clay, and/or putty, depending on which present-moment awareness exercise will be completed during session.

Overall Session 8 Goals

The main goal of this session is to introduce the broader goals of the E Skill: Experience My Emotions, as well as practice present-moment awareness and nonjudgmental awareness with children. Awareness and mindfulness strategies presented during this session may be used alone or may be combined with exposure in Sessions 9 and beyond, so they are important strategies to present. However, some children may have difficulty learning more advanced awareness/mindfulness concepts, such as nonjudgmental awareness. Therefore, it is more important to just introduce awareness about the benefits of experiencing emotions (uncomfortable or otherwise) without taking unhelpful actions to lessen or eliminate that experience, and less important to ensure that each child becomes an "expert" at each of the activities taught during this session.

- **Goal 1:** Learn about the "Experience My Emotions" skill.
- **Goal 2:** Teach children about present-moment awareness by playing the "Using My Five Senses" game.
- **Goal 3:** Introduce the idea of nonjudgmental awareness.

Session 8, Goal 1

Learn about the "Experience My Emotions" skill.

While the Group Is Together

As you welcome back the group for the start of the eighth session, circulate and assist parents and children in providing severity ratings for each of their three top problems and continue to praise and encourage children as they work toward their goals. These ratings should be entered on the same *Weekly Top Problems Tracking Form* (Appendix 11.1 at the end of Chapter 11 in this Therapist Guide) begun during Session 1. Also check that each child has completed the home learning assignment. Ask any children who have not completed the home learning assignment to do so next time (or to complete it briefly during the top problems review). For those children who have completed their home learning assignment, distribute one puzzle piece to each. Briefly review content discussed during the previous session and encourage each child to share an aspect of his or her home learning assignment (*Problem Solving at Home*) with the group.

> **Therapist Note**
>
> *Note that exposure therapy concepts are introduced in Sessions 8 and 9 and subsequently practiced in Sessions 9 through 14. Therefore, you may wish to encourage any family who may be stagnating in their top problem ratings by letting them know that many children see significant treatment gains as a result of the behavior change strategies introduced in the sessions to come. As needed during the next several sessions, attend carefully as to whether these behavior change strategies help prompt further improvements in top problem ratings. Revisit this concern in all subsequent sessions and apply Problem Solving steps to further implement or improve treatment skill uptake for any family that does not appear to be showing further improvement during the next few sessions.*

Introduce the "Experience My Emotions" Skill

Introduce children to the goals of this next section of treatment, including learning to pay attention to what is going on in the present moment without thinking about the past or the future, experiencing our emotions without avoiding them or doing something to make them go away, and beginning to approach or face things or situations we have been avoiding in the past because they make us feel scared, sad, angry, or worried. You might do this by saying:

"In the last couple of sessions, we have used our detective brains to come up with good ideas for how to change our minds about something when we fall into a thinking trap and good ideas about how to change our behavior or actions when we are stuck in a tough situation. Today, we are going to work together to learn how to just sit with a strong emotion. This will be the very first step in our new E Skill: Experience My Emotions. Can anyone think of why, if we have an uncomfortable feeling like being very sad, scared, or mad, we might want to just sit with that feeling and see what happens next? It may seem kind of silly, but, for example, if you know for sure that nothing scary is going to happen in your room at night, but you feel scared in your body anyway, what could happen to that scared feeling if you just waited a little bit more time in your room, rather than, let's say, going to mom or dad with your worry?"

Prompt children for ideas about why they might choose to stay in their rooms in this example and wait to see if their scared feeling goes down, reinforcing the idea that this strategy is a good one to use during a tough situation like this, where nothing truly bad is occurring.

Introduction to Emotional Awareness

Next, more formally introduce emotional awareness as a skill used to help children experience their emotions. This can be done by discussing the importance of being aware of and experiencing emotions in the moment without engaging in emotional behaviors. You might wish to say:

"We just talked about emotions you might feel in your room at night. In this group, we have been talking about how everyone experiences strong emotions in all different kinds of situations like this one, and that these emotions can sometimes be very tough to sit with or deal with. Let's look at another example. If you are feeling afraid of something right now—let's say a cat—and you think that I might have a cat next door, your mind might start worrying about whether the cat

will come in here and what it might do. In your body, your heart might start to beat faster or your stomach might feel uncomfortable and you might think about how to get out of here. When you experience emotions like fear in a situation like this one involving a cat, or strong emotions of anger or sadness in other types of situations, you might get overwhelmed and really want to 'do something' to make those uncomfortable feelings go away. For example, in this situation involving feeling afraid of a cat, you might leave the room or the building because the cat could be here.

In both the situation where you might be scared in your room and the one where you might feel afraid of the cat, what do you think would happen if you just sat and felt that strong emotion, the fear in these cases? Remember when we [insert relevant physical activity from Session 4, e.g., ran in place] a few weeks ago? The feelings went away by themselves. If you weren't in danger in your room or while near that cat, is it possible that your uncomfortable feeling would just go away eventually too? [Allow children to further discuss this possibility.] Feelings alone are not harmful, and if we sit with them, they might go down and not feel so strong anymore. In such a case, you can do something more helpful to deal with your room or that cat!"

Review the cycle of avoidance as one thing that gets in the way of being aware. This might be done as follows:

"Think back to your experiences over the past couple weeks, and maybe your whole life! A lot of times, when we feel strong emotions, we try to make them stop as quickly as possible: we run away, stay away from fun things we used to like, fight with friends, avoid the upsetting situation, don't speak in class, go call mom, and so on. In other words, we do anything we can to NOT pay attention to the emotion and to make it go away as quickly as possible. And while these things might make us feel better in the short term, they stop us from learning to experience our emotions and from knowing that there is nothing bad about them.

What happens:

- *If you never speak in school?*
- *If you never go to parties?*
- *If you can never go in and buy something in a store by yourself?*
- *If you never let yourself cry when you feel sad?*
- *If you always start yelling at your friends right away when you get angry?*
- *If you never go outside and play when you're sad?"*

Explain to the children that these kinds of behaviors, although they may seem helpful in the moment, are actually unhelpful to do when they feel strong emotions, may limit the things they can do, and may even stop them from enjoying fun things in their lives. Running away from emotions or from situations that bring them up also stops us from learning that if we just notice that the emotions are there but don't act on them, the emotions will go away on their own.

Session 8, Goal 2

Teach children about present-moment awareness by playing the "Using My Five Senses" game.

Present-Moment Awareness

Instruct children to turn to Figure 8.1: *Notice It, Say Something About It, Experience It.* Use the following script to introduce the steps of present-moment awareness:

> *"Before we start 'sitting with' (or practicing awareness of) our strong emotions, today we are just going to practice noticing, describing, and experiencing the things going on inside us and around us. What we will be doing is paying attention to what is happening in our bodies and our minds, and the sounds and sights and things around us. Noticing, describing, and experiencing in this way is an Emotion Detective skill we call **present-moment awareness**. Again, present-moment awareness is really just a fancy way of saying pay attention to what is happening in the 'here and now.' During all the practices we do today, we are going to be focusing all our attention on one thing at a time and not allowing ourselves to get too distracted by anything else we think or see or hear around us. Can anyone think of times when focusing really hard on one thing could be helpful to you?"*

Allow children to discuss times where paying good attention is useful, like in school while taking a quiz or when an adult is giving an important direction. Ask them what they think would happen in these situations if they tried to pay attention to many things at once. Next, introduce the steps of **noticing it, saying something about it, and experiencing it** to the children, having them follow along using Figure 8.1 from the workbook. Ask the children to use these skills during the upcoming present-moment awareness exercises.

1. **Notice it** (Using their five senses [sight, smell, taste, touch, and hearing] to see what is going on inside their bodies and around them. Focus on only the things they notice right in the present moment!)

2. **Say something about it** (Talking to themselves or writing down what they noticed)
3. **Experience it** (Trying to keep their attention focused on the "here and now" for as long as they can; looking more, listening more, and noticing the things they feel inside their bodies).

Next, lead the children in a present-moment awareness exercise focused on breath awareness, reminding them to practice awareness using all five senses as you instruct them to do the following. Tell the children that this first present-moment awareness exercise is intended to help them practice noticing, saying something about, and experiencing one body sensation only—their breathing. Ask everyone to:

1. *Get into a comfortable position lying on your back or sitting. If you are sitting, keep your back straight and let your shoulders drop.*
2. *Close your eyes if it feels comfortable.*
3. ***Notice*** *your belly, feeling it rise or go out gently as you breathe in and fall or drop back in as you breathe out.*
4. *Notice what is going on around you with your five senses. What do you see, smell, taste, feel, or hear?*
5. *As you breathe, take a second to **Say Something** to yourself about what you just noticed. Keep focusing on each breath as it goes in and out for as long as it lasts. Imagine that each breath in and out is a wave and you are riding the waves of your own breathing.*
6. ***Experience*** *your breathing. If you get distracted, notice what distracted you. Then focus on your breathing again and notice just your belly and the feeling of the breath coming in and out.*
7. *Even if your mind gets distracted from your breath a thousand times, then your "job" is simply to bring it back to your breath every time, no matter what it focuses on.*

Have the children work together following this exercise to complete Worksheet 8.1: *Practicing My Awareness Steps*. In particular, encourage children to work on **noticing** and **describing** with this exercise by saying or writing down (depending on time available) anything they may have sensed with any of their five senses during this practice, even if what they noticed seemed silly or strange. There are no right or wrong answers here, as long as children are sincerely trying to notice what is happening within and around them in the present moment.

Using the "My Five Senses" Games

Next, lead the group as they practice two or three additional present-moment awareness exercises or "using my five senses" games, a few of which are described below. (Additional options are found in Chapter 6 of this Therapist Guide under the heading *Engaging in Present-Moment Awareness Exercises*). The following introduction can be used to orient children to the present moment as you begin each of the present-moment awareness practices below.

> *"We are going to practice some games where we will use all five senses to pay very close attention to something that is here in front of us or happening inside of us right now. If you get distracted during these games, don't worry! It happens to everyone. Just go back to noticing, saying something about, or experiencing what you are doing right now."*

After completing each exercise below (which children can follow along with using Figure 8.2: *Present-Moment Awareness Activities*), ask the children to share any observations they have using Worksheet 8.2: *Being Aware with My Five Senses*. Specifically, query for things they noticed for the first time, any distractions they experienced while practicing these games, and how they brought themselves back to the present moment and experienced what was happening in the "here and now."

Five Senses Game Option 1—What's Around You

Guide the children through the following present-moment awareness exercise, which helps them to focus on what is around them in their present environment:

> *"Look around you. Let your eyes be relaxed, not looking for something or at somewhere because you need to go there. Just look to see what is around you. Let your thoughts slow down as you notice what you see.*
>
> *Start with the big picture: tables, chairs, walls, pictures, doors. Then begin to take in smaller details: your own hands, your fingers, what they're touching. Differing shades of color and light. Maybe one wall of the room you're in right now is in shadow, and another is in full light. Use your other senses, too: do the lights make a buzzing sound? are there cars to be heard passing by? people walking by? Notice it with your senses, your eyes and ears. Now let's focus on what you have/are doing right in front of you. Notice it and say something about it to yourself."*

Five Senses Game Option 2—Exploring a Candy Exercise

Allow the children to select one candy (or other small food item) from a small selection of such, and ask the children to hold it but not eat it yet. Having a small selection of candies in a dish allows you to complete the second awareness practice referenced in this example as well.

"You are an alien from a planet far, far away. Your first day on Earth, you find some candies in a dish. You have never seen candy before. Pick up one of the candies in the dish. Just notice the candy, looking at it carefully as if you had never seen one before. Feel the candy between your fingers and notice its colors. Use your senses of touch and hearing and sight to notice the candy even better. Be aware of any thoughts you might be having about the candy, even if you don't like this candy. Now, re-focus on the candy and lift it to your nose and smell it for a while. Finally, you are going to use your sense of taste by bringing the candy to your lips, being aware of your arm moving your hand to bring it to your mouth and even your mouth and brain feeling excited about eating it (or disgusted by eating it; there are no right or wrong answers here). Take the candy into your mouth and chew it slowly, experiencing the actual taste of the candy. Hold it in your mouth. Pay close attention as you swallow it and it goes down your throat. When you are ready, pick up a different candy and repeat this process again on your own, as if it is now the first candy you have ever seen."

(Note: This exercise is adapted from Williams et al., 2007.)

Five Senses Game Option 3—Pebble Identification Exercise

Collect multiple stones or pebbles with different shapes, sizes, and textures. Have the children close their eyes and each pick one of the pebbles. While their eyes are closed, have them use their other senses to notice and say something about the pebble they picked. After a few minutes, while their eyes are still closed, have the children place their stones back in the pile with the other pebbles. Then ask the children to open their eyes, and with their eyes open and using their other senses, have them identify which pebble was theirs and why. What did they experience about the pebble that allowed them to figure out which was theirs to begin with? This process can be repeated a second time with the group, during which children can pick a different stone. If repeated, did their experience change the second time? Did they focus on more or different things about their pebble/stone than the first time they did it?

Five Senses Game Option 3—Play-Doh Exercise

Have the children each hold and look at a ball of Play-Doh without squeezing it. Have them notice their urges to play with the Play-Doh. Then have them say something about what they notice about the Play-Doh using their senses (but not tasting it!): temperature, smell, feel, shape, color, and so forth. Then have the children experience it by making something out of the Play-Doh.

Session 8, Goal 3

Introduce the idea of nonjudgmental awareness.

Nonjudgmental Awareness

Introduce the concept of nonjudgmental awareness to the children in the following way:

> *"During the present-moment awareness exercises that we just did together, some of you may have had thoughts like 'I feel silly' or 'this is dumb.' We call those thoughts* **judgments,** *and we all have them from time to time. We might also judge our strong emotions and the unhelpful things we did about them as being really negative or bad. For example, we might think it's 'silly' that we felt nervous about answering a question in class or 'bad' that we yelled at our sister or brother or a friend, or we might think it's 'wrong' to feel sad about a scene in a movie we saw because it was 'just a movie' and 'not real life'."*

Gather examples of times when the children judged or said something negative about their emotional experiences. Note that not all children will grasp this concept right away, and be prepared to generate more and more personal examples of judgments one might make about unhelpful behavior during the course of experiencing a strong emotion. Explain that the term **nonjudgmental awareness** (or you could call this detective strategy "NJA" for short) is just a big-sounding group of words that suggests that while we are becoming more aware of our emotions we should try our best not to judge them by calling them "stupid," "bad," or "wrong."

> *"So, what should we do instead? Our goal today is to let ourselves experience any thoughts we might have—no matter what they are—without saying anything bad to ourselves about them, because having an emotion is not a bad thing."*

Here is another way to think about NJA. Using some of the examples generated by the children, you can encourage the children to consider how they would respond to a friend who came to them with the same concerns. Would they say that their friend was "stupid," "wrong," or "bad" for his or her thoughts about these unhelpful behaviors when he or she felt a strong emotion? Or would they tell their friend that it is okay to feel that way—no matter what happened? So, basically, we want the children in group to treat their thoughts the same way they would treat their friend's thoughts about their behavior—with *kindness, respect, and understanding*.

Engaging in Nonjudgmental Awareness Exercises

You can reinforce the concept of NJA with the child group at this point in a couple of different ways:

1. You can do this in a non-emotional way by bringing in a few everyday objects or silly objects (like a toy that is too young for the group's average age) and having the children notice and talk about these objects without judgment. If someone has a judgment, prompt him or her to consider if this is what he or she would say about the object if a friend liked it a lot. Consider both ideas briefly and move on to other ideas the group presents about the objects.

2. To further reinforce the nonjudgmental component of this present-moment awareness practice, you can also conduct a role-play with one of the children or another therapist. You can play the "friend" who is experiencing an emotional situation (perhaps one similar to one of the children's own experiences) and allow the children to assist you with nonjudgmental awareness and offer you kind, respectful, and understanding statements toward "your" feelings in the situation.

3. You can also have the group practice NJA using one of the following two scripts below (Awareness of Thoughts or Awareness of Emotions Exercise).

Awareness of Thoughts

"This is an exercise to practice observing your thoughts and allowing them to flow in and out of your mind without judging or acting upon them. Close your eyes and imagine that you are sitting by a quiet river watching the water flow. Notice how the water quietly moves. It doesn't stop or get stuck; it gently keeps moving along. Take a few moments to watch the water as it flows. Now begin to notice what is in your mind. What are you currently thinking? Gently place that thought onto the river and watch as your thought moves away from you. No matter what pops in your head, simply watch as your thought moves away with the water. If you have

another thought, again place it on the river and watch it flow away. Just watch. If
at some point the water has stopped moving or you become distracted, that's okay.
Just notice that and return to placing each thought in the river and watching
it move away. Continue this exercise for a few minutes and then gently open
your eyes."

Awareness of Emotions Exercise

Prompt the group to think about a time when they felt a strong emotion
this week. This could be something they wrote about in their *Solving the
Mystery of Our Emotions: Before, During, and After* home learning assignment or something they just thought of now. Once everyone has a good
idea of what to focus on, you can state:

"First, put yourself into the present moment by focusing on your breathing. Then,
begin to notice the room around you. Notice things you can see in the room,
the sounds you can hear, any smells. Next, spend a few moments focusing your
attention on feelings in your body. For example, notice the feeling of your body in
the chair or on the floor, and any other feelings as they come and go. Now, turn
your focus to your thoughts as they run through your mind, and the emotions that
you are having. Just notice the experience, without attempting to change or judge
it. When you notice that you are trying to change your thoughts or emotions, or
you notice that you are judging them as good or bad, just notice that and then
bring your focus back to the thought and emotions. Notice the efforts to get rid of
or hold onto certain feelings. Notice how the emotions you are having change, or
how they remain the same."

After completing the practice chosen, ask the group to describe their
impressions of using the NJA skill. Was it helpful to them or unhelpful?
When would be a time that each child might practice this skill in the
next week?

Back Together

As parents return to the group, briefly reinforce the idea that present-
moment awareness practice can be challenging and that we admire everyone for working on this new and important Emotion Detective skill.
As a group, then introduce the home learning assignment on Worksheet
8.3: *Awareness Practice at Home.* Have children and parents work together

while you walk around and help each family try to identify times during the week when present-moment awareness or NJA may be useful for children and their parents to practice. Identify at least one good practice opportunity and ask each parent or child to write this in at the top of the worksheet as a reminder to follow the awareness steps and reflect on their utility this week.

Suggested Home Learning Assignment: *Awareness Practice at Home* and *Solving the Mystery of Our Emotions: Before, During, and After* (with option of assigning ongoing opposite action experiments)

In addition to completing *Awareness Practice at Home* (Worksheet 8.3), children should also add another entry to their *Solving the Mystery of Our Emotions: Before, During, and After* this week.

Overall Parent Session 8 Goals

The main goal of this parent session is to provide a rationale for the importance of *experiencing* emotions rather than avoiding, escaping, or suppressing them. Parents learn about present-moment awareness, a skill that involves noticing and describing what is happening in the present moment without trying to change or get rid of it. Parents practice present-moment awareness of non-emotional and emotional stimuli in session using activities similar to those practiced in the child session. Parents are also introduced to nonjudgmental awareness, a type of present-moment awareness that involves noticing thoughts and emotions in an objective, nonjudgmental way. At the end of this parent session, parents begin creating an *Emotional Behavior Form—Parent Version* (Form 16.1) in preparation for upcoming exposures.

- **Goal 1:** Discuss the importance of learning to experience emotions rather than avoiding them.
- **Goal 2:** Introduce and practice present-moment awareness with the parents.
- **Goal 3:** Introduce and practice nonjudgmental awareness with the parents.
- **Goal 4:** Begin creating an *Emotional Behavior Form—Parent Version* in preparation for upcoming exposures.

Parent Session 8, Goal 1

Discuss the importance of learning to experience emotions rather than avoiding them.

Therapist Note

Remember to begin this session and each subsequent one with a brief check-in (no more than 10 minutes) regarding major changes in child symptoms/functioning over the past week, as well as a review of home learning assignments.

Remind parents that emotions are *normal* (everyone has them), *natural* (they are our body's natural response to, among other things, threatening or upsetting situations), and *not harmful* (in fact, they even help keep us safe or get support from others). Emotions have many benefits, so we wouldn't want to get rid of them. Explain to the parents, however, that many children (and adults too) believe that the solution to struggling with strong emotions is to figure out a way to get rid of them.

In this treatment, we take the opposite stance. Explain that we believe that the goal of our treatment is not to get rid of emotions but rather to minimize distress and impairment that might be associated with them. To do this, *we want to approach strong emotions rather than avoid them, attend to emotions rather than ignore them, and allow ourselves to experience strong emotions rather than suppress them*. Although this approach may at first seem odd, emphasize that it is actually the best long-term approach to reducing the impact that strong emotions have on a child's life. As the parents learned from the cycle of avoidance earlier in treatment, avoidance and other strategies that decrease a strong emotion in the short term are negatively reinforcing. That is, we feel better immediately, so we learn to use the strategy again the next time we feel the emotion. There are several problems with this approach.

Explain to the parents that, as they probably know by now, avoidance often makes us feel worse in the long term and can cause more problems for us. The next time we are in a similar situation, the strong emotions return all over again because we didn't learn to experience them, cope with them, or get through them the first time around. Children's self-efficacy and confidence in their ability to manage their emotions are also impacted. Similarly to avoiding situations that elicit strong emotions, trying to ignore or suppress the physical or cognitive (thinking) parts of an emotional experience also causes problems. These strategies don't make the strong emotions go away—in fact, the strong emotions, thoughts, and body clues often get even stronger, sometimes right away and sometimes a little while later. As time permits, you may wish to elicit some examples of recent child avoidance or similar behaviors from the parents and identify at least one longer-term problem with that behavioral choice.

For these reasons, it is important for children to learn to notice and experience their emotions. Let the parents know that although this may be very uncomfortable at first and will take some practice, doing this will help their child learn that most emotions actually don't last very long if we let them run their course. As a result, their child will become more comfortable with just experiencing emotions as they come up. When emotions are no longer so fear-evoking or distressing, they typically don't last as long either. Paying attention to emotions will also help their child become better at identifying what he or she is feeling and at choosing Emotion Detective skills to help manage the emotions. After all, it is difficult to decide what to do about an emotion if we don't know that we're feeling it in the first place.

Parent Session 8, Goal 2

Introduce and practice present-moment awareness with the parents.

Introduction to Present-Moment Awareness

Explain to the parents that during this session, their child will be learning and practicing a new Emotion Detective skill for experiencing what is happening in the present moment (including his or her present emotions) without doing anything to change what is going on. Here is a sample script for how you might introduce this skill to the parents:

> *"Some of the Emotion Detective skills your child has learned so far—like Detective Thinking and Problem Solving—are ways of reducing the intensity of the emotional experience by either changing the interpretation of the experience or changing the experience itself. However, there will be situations where it might be difficult to use these skills (e.g., if a negative outcome does occur), and there may also be times when your child does use one of the skills but the strong emotion is still there. This is why it is important for your child to learn to sit with an emotion*

and not do anything about it until it goes away. It is unpleasant to have strong emotions and not do anything about them. But, we know that if we just pay attention to these emotions, they will pass.

*Today, your children are learning a skill called **present-moment awareness** that will help them to notice their emotions and to be aware of how long they last and when they pass. Present-moment awareness means fully participating in the 'here and now,' not the future (which hasn't happened yet) or the past (which we can't change). This is much more difficult than it sounds. During the course of their daily lives, many people are often on what we call 'autopilot,' meaning that they are going through the motions of their daily activities without really paying attention to them. When practicing present-moment awareness, we are being fully aware of our surroundings and experiences, including any thoughts, feelings, or action urges that come up.*

When we use present-moment awareness during an emotional experience, we learn that the emotion will pass without hurting us, and we are able to cope with negative emotions without escaping from them. Having this knowledge will increase children's sense of self-efficacy, or their feeling that they can handle or cope with strong emotions more effectively."

Ask the parents to turn to Figure 16.1: *Notice It, Say Something About It, Experience It* in the workbook. Briefly describe each of these skills to the parents, using Figure 16.1 as a guideline. Emphasize the following points about each of the present-moment awareness skills:

1. **Notice it:** Language is an incredible human achievement that sets us apart from other organisms, but it also fundamentally changes our experience of the world and can cause a lot of suffering. Explain to parents that, when we put language to an experience, we change that experience and see it through a particular lens or viewpoint. When we use the present-moment awareness skill of noticing, we are practicing wordlessly noticing our environment or sensations so that we can take in as much as possible about the experience before we begin to interpret it.

2. **Say something about it:** Explain to the parents that this present-moment awareness skill involves *saying* something to ourselves about our experience by trying to stick to the facts and maintain as much objectivity as possible. Children who struggle with strong emotions are often quick to interpret or judge their experiences, and they often take these interpretations or judgments for truth. This can in turn intensify strong emotions.

3. **Experience it:** Explain to the parents that experiencing an activity, situation, or emotion means fully throwing ourselves into it and focusing only on what's happening in the present moment, not the future or the past. Ask parents to think about which of the many things they do during their daily lives they actually allow themselves to fully experience. Emphasize that fully experiencing an activity has an important and positive impact on our happiness and sense of well-being.

After reviewing the *Notice It, Say Something About It, Experience It* skills, explain to the parents that they will be practicing these skills now during session. Choose one or two present-moment awareness exercises (see below) for the parents to practice, and guide them through each one. As you guide parents through the exercises, let them know whether you want them to practice just wordlessly noticing or whether you want them to focus on saying something about the experience to themselves.

Present-Moment Awareness Practice

Choose two or three of the following present-moment awareness exercises to practice with the parents. Scripts and detailed descriptions of these exercises may be found earlier in this chapter:

- Breath Awareness Exercise
- General Present-Moment Awareness Exercise
- Exploring a Candy Exercise
- Pebble Identification Exercise
- Play-Doh Exercise

Discuss the parents' experiences with these exercises. You may wish to use some of the following questions to facilitate this discussion:

- *What was it like when you practiced just noticing without putting words on your experience? Do you think this would be even more challenging in an emotional situation?*
- *Did you notice anything about your experience you had not noticed before or would not have noticed otherwise?*
- *When you were saying something about your experience, what types of things did you say?*
- *Were you able to fully experience the activity? What helped? What made it difficult?*

Parent Session 8, Goal 3

Introduce and practice nonjudgmental awareness with the parents.

Introduction to Nonjudgmental Awareness

Define a **judgment** for the parents as an evaluation of the worth, value, or quality of a particular experience. Judgment words include "good" or "bad," "positive" or "negative," "desirable" or "undesirable." Ask parents if they experienced judgments during any of the present-moment awareness exercises, and ask them to describe those judgments. Emphasize that everyone makes judgments all the time—judgments are part of being human, and negative judgments can even help us to avoid things that are truly dangerous or threatening.

Explain that children who struggle with strong emotions often make more judgments than other people about their emotions and the situations that elicit them. Such children tend to label their emotions as "bad" or "stupid," tell themselves that they shouldn't feel the way they do, or react negatively in other ways to their emotional experiences. These types of judgments can increase children's distress about their emotional experiences, as well as their desire to get rid of the emotions, leading to problematic emotional behaviors.

Tell the parents that their children will be practicing a skill called **nonjudgmental awareness**, which is a type of present-moment awareness that involves noticing and saying something about our experiences in a factual, neutral, and nonjudgmental way. Because judgments often exacerbate our emotional reactions, practicing nonjudgmental awareness of emotions and emotional situations can help reduce the intensity of strong emotions.

Nonjudgmental Awareness Practice

Practice one of the nonjudgmental exercises described earlier in this chapter. Options include:

- Nonjudgmental awareness of an everyday object
- Awareness of Thoughts Exercise
- Awareness of Emotions Exercise

Explain that parents sometimes make judgments about their child's emotions and emotional behaviors as well. These types of judgments can increase parents' frustration with their children and lead to emotional parenting behaviors. Give several examples of judgments parents might make about their children, and solicit additional examples from the parents. As an additional, optional exercise, you might have the parents break up into pairs and take turns first describing one of their child's recent emotional experiences, and then describing the same experience without judgments.

Let the parents know that for home learning, they will be *both* helping their child practice nonjudgmental and present-moment awareness, as well as practicing nonjudgmental awareness themselves.

Parent Session 8, Goal 4

Begin creating an Emotional Behavior Form—Parent Version in preparation for upcoming exposures.

Explain to the parents that in the "E" section of treatment, their children will begin to gradually approach emotional situations that they are currently avoiding or in which they are using problematic emotional behaviors. This is called an **exposure**. Let the parents know that they will learn much more in the next session about why, how, and when their child will be completing exposures during the remainder of treatment. Explain that in preparation for next session's discussion of exposure, we would like parents to begin creating a list of different situations that elicit strong emotions and emotional behaviors from their child.

Ask parents to turn to the *Emotional Behavior Form—Parent Version* (Form 16.1) in the parent workbook. Explain how to complete the form, and ask them to identify at least four or five situations in which their child is currently struggling with strong emotions. Ask parents to also indicate the emotional behavior(s) their child uses in each situation (e.g., avoidance, reassurance-seeking, aggression), as well as the parents' estimate of the intensity of the emotion. Let the parents know that a major focus of the next parent session will be to review this initial *list of emotional behaviors* and add more items to it. If parents are struggling to come up with situations to list on the form, remind them to consider their *Top Problems, Double BDAs* from earlier in treatment, and their child's *BDA* forms.

CHAPTER 19 | UP-C Session 9: Introduction to Emotion Exposure

E Skill: Experience My Emotions

MATERIALS NEEDED FOR GROUP

- For Each Child Group Session:
  1. Detective CLUES kits for each child
  2. Poker chips
  3. Puzzle
  4. Prize box
  5. Large piece of paper or whiteboard to record children's answers for any group activities
- For Session 9 Only:
  6. Videos or songs
  7. UP-C Workbook Chapter 9
     a. *My Emotion Detective Skills!* (Worksheet 9.1)
     b. *Science Experiment Game* (Worksheet 9.2)
     c. *Another Kind of Science Experiment* (Figure 9.1)
     d. *Emotional Behavior Form—Child Version* (Form 9.1)
- For Home Learning:
  8. *Solving the Mystery of Our Emotions: Before, During, and After* (Form 2.1) for an emotion that led to an emotional behavior
- Assessments to Be Given at Every Session:
  9. *Weekly Top Problems Tracking Form* (Use the same form started during Session 1 for each child, found in Appendix 11.1 at the end of Chapter 11 of this Therapist Guide)

- For Parent Group Session:
    10. UP-C Workbook Chapter 16
        a. *Emotion Curve: Avoidance/Escape* (Figure 16.2)
        b. *Emotion Curve: Habituation* (Figure 16.3)
        c. *Emotion Curve: Habituation with Practice* (Figure 16.4)
        d. *Supporting Your Child's Exposures at Home* (Figure 16.5)
        e. *Emotional Behavior Form—Parent Version* (Form 16.2)
- For Parent Home Learning:
    11. *Learning Healthy Emotional Modeling* (Worksheet 16.2)

Therapist Preparation

In preparation for this session, you will need to bring a plastic toy spider or small stuffed animal (e.g., a cat or dog or similar) for a demonstration exposure.

Overall Session 9 Goals

The primary goal of this session is to introduce the concept of a new type of science experiment—one in which children are encouraged to face strong emotions using a variety of exposure techniques—and demonstrate these techniques using a practice situational exposure in session. Prior to introducing exposure, review skills learned to date. During the parent session, you should more comprehensively introduce parents to the concept of situational emotion exposure and also introduce the concept of parental modeling of strong emotions and emotional behaviors, along with appropriate opposite parenting actions for these behaviors.

- **Goal 1:** Review Emotion Detective skills learned to date in the UP-C.
- **Goal 2:** Review the concepts of emotional behaviors and "acting opposite" in preparation for a new type of science experiment called "exposure."
- **Goal 3:** Complete a demonstration of an exposure using a toy or other object.
- **Goal 4:** Work together with children and parents to finalize Emotional Behavior forms.

Session 9, Goal 1

Review Emotion Detective skills learned to date in the UP-C.

While the Group Is Together

As you welcome back the group for the start of the ninth session, circulate and assist parents and children in providing severity ratings for each of their three top problems and continue to praise and encourage children as they work toward their goals. These ratings should be entered on the same *Weekly Top Problems Tracking Form* (Appendix 11.1 at the end of Chapter 11 in this Therapist Guide) begun during Session 1. Also check that each child has completed the home learning assignment. Encourage any children who have not completed the assignment to do so next time (or to complete them briefly during the top problems review). For those children who have completed the assignment, distribute one puzzle piece to each. With the whole group, briefly review content introduced in Session 8 (present-moment awareness and nonjudgmental awareness).

Child Group Alone

Have the group turn to Worksheet 9.1: *My Emotion Detective Skills!* The worksheet provides the opportunity to conduct a game with the entire group to review skills learned in the UP-C to date. These skills (listed in the Skills Bank at the bottom of the worksheet) include the following concepts: Body Scanning, Detective Thinking, Problem Solving, Fun Activities, Identifying Thinking Traps, and Present-Moment Awareness. Earlier in the worksheet is a series of brief vignettes that describe emotional situations that the Emotion Detective characters (Jack, Nina, Suki, and Darrell) are coping with at present. The goal of the worksheet is to write the "ideal" strategy in the box next to each vignette with which it would best fit. The group can work together as a whole to figure out which skill fits with each vignette, with you describing or defining skills again as needed. You can introduce this activity in the following way:

"Today, we are going to learn a new way of using a science experiment to start facing and experiencing our strong emotions, like fear, sadness, and anger. That's a really big goal! And it may take us several sessions to accomplish this goal. So, before we learn more about this new type of science experiment, it might be a good idea to review the Emotion Detective skills we have already learned and tried to use in our own lives. If you look at Worksheet 9.1, you will see that the Emotion Detectives (Jack, Nina, Suki, and Darrell) have been facing some problems, and they need you to help figure out which would be the best skill to help them deal with their current problems. Let's look at the first problem that Jack is facing."

As you go through each vignette, make sure to get at least one child to correctly identify the best strategy and (with your assistance) provide input on the definition and/or an example of that strategy for the problem presented in that vignette.

A key to Worksheet 9.1 is as follows:

- Vignette 1 (Jack)—Body Scanning
- Vignette 2 (Suki)—Problem Solving
- Vignette 3 (Darrell)—Fun Activities
- Vignette 4 (Nina)—Present-Moment Awareness (Detective Thinking might also be appropriate if it was *before* the baseball game; Problem Solving could also be useful in some ways)
- Vignette 5 (Suki)—Identifying Thinking Traps and/or Detective Thinking

As indicated, it is often the case that more than one strategy or a combination of strategies can be utilized to address the problems presented in these vignettes. In other words, there is not always one right answer and other wrong answers to these problems. If a child is thinking critically about how to apply his or her Emotion Detective skills in such situations, then he or she is already on his way to becoming an excellent Emotion Detective!

Session 9, Goal 2
Review the concepts of emotional behaviors and "acting opposite" in preparation for a new type of science experiment called "exposure."

Introduce exposure to the children as another type of therapeutic strategy that involves doing the opposite of what an emotion makes us want to do (by facing or confronting this emotion more directly). You may wish to introduce exposure in the following way:

> *"Over the next couple of weeks, we are going to begin acting opposite of how our emotions make us want to act in different situations that we have stayed away from in the past, often because these situations make us feel strong emotions—like feeling scared, for example. We have a fancy name for the strategy we use when acting opposite in order to face our feelings: **exposure**. Has anyone heard of this term before? Exposure."*

Then, return to the concepts of opposite action and emotional behaviors to help explain the meaning of the term "exposure" and its importance as a new Emotion Detective skill:

> *"There are many possible ways to respond to strong emotions. Sometimes, what we do when we feel a lot of fear, sadness, or anger is find a way to avoid, fight, or escape the thing that is bothering us. And sometimes doing this is a good idea, like if a speeding car is coming at us and we are in danger! For sure, we want to get out of the way of that car. We want to avoid it. But, sometimes, our body and brain trick us a little, and in reality, we are not in real danger when we avoid, do things that might get us in trouble, or escape things. We all use **emotional behaviors** at times to stay safe and help us feel better right away. For example, if you are mad and you yell at your sister, you might feel better for a minute. Or if you are afraid of talking to the new kid at school and you stay home that day from school, you might feel better at first. But, over the long term, you don't learn much when you use emotional behaviors in situations like the one with your sister or meeting new people. The next time you experience that situation, you might be just as upset as the last time it happened because you don't know what to do when these things come up other than try to get away or fight. In other words, when we overuse emotional behaviors while upset, we don't learn what else to do next time we are upset—except keep on using emotional behaviors!*
>
> *To better understand, let's listen to a few stories about Darrell and Suki, who are dealing with some tough situations where 'acting opposite' when faced with tough emotions might be more helpful than using an emotional behavior."*

Emotional Behavior Vignettes

Read the following vignettes to the group to help the children review what it means to use emotional behaviors and what the short- and long-term consequences of using emotional behaviors might be, using Darrell and Suki as examples. Tell children that, after you read a story about Darrell, you will be asking them to answer some questions about what happened and what else he might do next time.

"Darrell has a homework project due on Monday in science and he hasn't been doing well in that class lately. In fact, he's sure he's going to get a bad grade on this assignment too, and it makes him really nervous to think about failing. Every time Darrell's mom reminds him to start working on his science project, he decides he can do it later and he plays a videogame instead. Darrell feels better when he plays videogames. The night before the project is due, he tries to work on it really, really fast, but his worry is very strong, even worse than on the other nights, and he yells to his mom that he isn't going to work on it anymore. Darrell feels like it doesn't matter because he is sure he will fail the assignment anyway."

Then, ask the children to identify the following about the vignette:

"In this example, what was the trigger? What was Darrell's emotional behavior? Did he feel better when he avoided working on his project in the beginning and played a videogame instead (the short term)? What about the night before the test (the long term)? If Darrell wants to try to 'act opposite' of his strong feeling and fear here, what could he do?"

Next, read the following vignette and let the children know that they will similarly be asked to talk about Suki's emotional behavior and how she might act opposite of what her strong feeling is telling her to do:

"Suki has been playing with Nina since they were little. They are good friends. Lately, Suki feels like every time she tries to play with Nina at Nina's house, Nina gets to choose the things they do or play with, and it's making Suki mad. One day, Suki gets so mad at Nina when she feels like she won't listen to her about playing a different game that Suki throws one of Nina's dolls against the wall and the doll breaks. Nina is really sad and, frankly, so is Suki. Nina realizes that she should have given Suki more of a chance to choose what they play at her house, once she talks about it with her mom later. But now Nina isn't sure that she should invite Suki back to her house if Suki is going to break her toys."

Then, ask the children:

"In this example, what was the first trigger for Suki? What was Suki's emotional behavior? Did she feel better when threw the doll (in the short term), even for a second? What about later (in the long term)? How did Suki feel then? Suki may have had a right to be a little mad in this story, but if she were trying to act opposite of her mad feeling, what else could she have done here?"

Re-emphasize to the children that emotional behaviors don't often allow us to learn new things in tough situations like these about how to cope or deal with our strong feelings and that exposure will be one way for us to learn how to sit with these kinds of uncomfortable sensations and make helpful choices going forward:

"Often, when we use an emotional behavior we feel better right away. The problem is that avoiding, escaping, or using angry behaviors when we feel a strong emotion may not allow us to learn anything new about the situations that are making us nervous, angry, or sad. This may prevent us from learning that the situations and/or the emotions we are dealing with may not be dangerous or terrible or that our strong feelings might pass on their own!"

Getting Used to a Strong Emotion

Have the children turn in their workbooks to Figure 9.1: *Another Kind of Science Experiment.* With children following along in the workbook, introduce the idea of using exposure to "get used to" the sensations of a strong emotion (i.e., that the sensations of a strong emotion like fear or anger will habituate or decrease typically over time if a child is not really under threat or in danger). We might call this "a science experiment using exposure":

"It may seem as if the only way to deal with your strong emotions is to use an emotional behavior, as we just discussed. But really, no matter how strong your emotion may be, if you are not in danger, your feelings are likely to go down on their own at some point and you may feel better."

Draw an emotion curve on the board or point to the first one shown in Figure 9.1 and describe that when we feel intense fear or anger, it sometimes feels like these tough emotions will increase forever. It may also be helpful at this point to draw several emotion curves with lower peaks and shorter durations to illustrate "getting used to it over time" and "getting used to it with practice," or identify these additional curves in Figure 9.1. Then walk through the example of Jack and his fear of dogs, as described in Figure 9.1, to illustrate the function of exposure and its potential effects on strong emotions over time and with repeated practice.

Session 9, Goal 3

Complete a demonstration of an exposure using a toy or other object.

Once you review these emotion curves, let the children know that the group will now practice an exposure using the science experiment steps. Have the children turn to Worksheet 9.2: *Science Experiment Game.* You can introduce the rationale for exposure again as follows:

"So, what we have learned from Jack's story [in Figure 9.1] *is that exposure is a way of 'acting opposite' by doing a new type of science experiment. This type of experiment lets us test out how we feel when we face a situation we may be*

avoiding or using another emotional behavior to escape from. The goals when we use exposure are to learn that we can experience whatever emotions come up while in any given situation and that we will still be okay when we do.

We've talked about this idea a lot today, but now we are going to try and actually practice exposure using our science experiment steps. Turn to Worksheet 9.2: Science Experiment Game in your workbook. Let's first just remind ourselves of the five steps that good scientists use when trying to solve a mystery."

Review the science experiment steps on Worksheet 9.2 and introduce the "exposure mystery" to solve. Show the group a toy spider or another toy that might represent a commonly feared animal. Place the toy away from the children and tell them that today's science experiment game is called "exposure to a [name of toy animal]." Ask the group if, in reality, anyone is afraid of [animal]. If one or many children indicate they are, make sure to give them extra responsibility to help come up with the science experiment steps and try them out in session today, expressing and showing empathy to any minor distress. Have the children fill out Worksheet 9.2 with the activity they will be doing on top (where it says "The science experiment we are doing is") by writing "exposure/getting closer to a [name of toy animal]." You can then say the following:

"Now that we know what our mystery is, let's start with a question. One question might be, if I were afraid of [toy animal], how can I get used to this feeling? As a group, let's write down some guesses about how we could get used to this feeling and see what happens to it over time. Does anyone have ideas? What can we do to get used to being around [toy animal]?"

Solicit a number of ideas about how to approach (versus avoid) the toy animal. As time permits, place the ideas in order from *easiest to hardest to do* on the board.

Then, have them fill out steps 1 and 2 on Worksheet 9.2 with a question about what might happen (step 1; e.g., "What will happen when I pet the dog?") and their "best guess" of what might happen after the first step (step 2; e.g., "It won't be as scary as I thought. The dog will stay calm"). Encourage children to take turns trying successively harder and harder steps and observe how it goes. Have children write observations on Worksheet 9.2 (step 3; e.g., "It wasn't so scary. The dog seems nice") and draw conclusions (step 4; e.g., "I got used to it. My guess was right that it would not be scary"). Finally, using information gathered during this initial experiment, discuss what would happen if we tried the experiment again, and write that down under step 5 on the worksheet (e.g., "It might get even easier with practice"). Refer back to the last emotion curve in Figure 9.1 as needed and ask the group what would happen if we practiced facing our fear of this (toy animal) over time. Would it get easier or harder? Hint: Easier!

Back Together

Session 9, Goal 4

Work together with children and parents to finalize Emotional Behavior forms.

Building Emotional Behavior Forms

Work with the children and parents together to refine the *Emotional Behavior Form—Parent Version* (Form 16.1) that the parents have been working on during this session and the previous one. First, explain that the *Emotional Behavior* forms that parents created for their children will help for planning other science experiments in which the children will be facing feelings and doing (exposure) exercises, both at home and during upcoming sessions. Instruct the children to turn to Form 9.1: *Emotional Behavior Form—Child Version* in their workbooks and take a look at this blank form as well as their parent's completed form (Form 16.1) within the workbook. For each item on the form provided by the parent, have the child and parent discuss whether to add this item to Form 9.1 to be worked on during treatment. Have children provide their own emotion ratings and contribute ideas about other emotional behaviors they may use in each situation. The child will likely have additional items to add to the form at this point, and you should obtain information about the situation, emotional behaviors, and emotional intensity for these additional items as well and have the child add them to the child's form. This procedure might include asking the children the following questions about their *Emotional Behavior Form—Child Version*:

Referencing their parent form:

- Are these your most feared/avoided/upsetting situations?
- Should we add things?

- Should we take some things off?
- Which are most important things to do/least important things to do first (prioritizing)?

Questions to consider when helping children to generate additional items:

- What activities do you want to do but often avoid?
- What situations make you feel the most anxious or scared? Do you stay away from any of those situations? How often?
- What do you do when you are feeling sad and have no energy?
- What situations make you most angry? What do you do when you are feeling angry?
- Do you ever do things when you are upset that you regret (or wish you didn't do) later?

Therapist Note

Some children may be upset or reluctant to share ratings or discuss items generated by their parents. Emphasize to families that this is a collaborative activity and that the child definitely gets a vote in what types of exposure/facing feelings exercises are done. Mention that you have already gotten their parents' opinions about things to work on and that you really want the children's opinions about anything they want to add or change. However, if children strongly resist creating the child version of this form, do not require them to do so at this time.

Suggested Home Learning Assignment: *Solving the Mystery of Our Emotions: Before, During, and After* (with option of assigning ongoing opposite action experiments)

Have the children add another entry to their *Solving the Mystery of Our Emotions: Before, During, and After*. This week, instruct them to try to choose a situation when they used an emotional behavior (e.g., avoided or acted aggressively in response to an emotion). Parents may need to help choose an appropriate situation. Then, have parents and children discuss whether the "after" part might have been different if they had instead acted opposite of how their emotion made them want to act. What would happen right away if they had acted differently? What about in the long run?

The main goal of this parent session is to familiarize parents with situational emotion exposure, a different type of science experiment for acting opposite of what emotions tell their child to do. Exposures form the foundation of Sessions 9 through 14 of this treatment and are one of its most important active ingredients. Therefore, it is essential for parents to develop a strong grasp of exposure principles so that they can help implement exposures with their child at home, reinforce their child appropriately for completing exposures, and continue to encourage exposure practice after treatment ends.

- **Goal 1:** Introduce parents to the concept of situational emotion exposure, a different type of science experiment.
- **Goal 2:** Explain the parent's role in practicing exposures at home.
- **Goal 3:** Introduce parents to the emotional parenting behavior of excessive modeling of intense emotions and avoidance and its opposite parenting behavior, healthy emotional modeling.
- **Goal 4:** Continue to develop the *Emotional Behavior Form* in preparation for upcoming exposures.

Parent Session 9 Content (Divided by Goals)

Parent Session 9, Goal 1

Introduce parents to the concept of situational emotion exposure, a different type of science experiment.

> **Therapist Note**
> *Remember to begin this session and each subsequent one with a brief check-in (no more than 10 minutes) regarding major changes in child symptoms/functioning over the past week, as well as a review of home learning assignments.*

Situational Emotion Exposure as Another Type of Science Experiment

Begin the discussion of situational emotion exposure by letting the parents know that today they will be learning about another type of science experiment for emotions. Remind parents that so far in treatment, their children have practiced several different types of experiments to see what happens when they do the opposite of what their emotion is telling them to do in a situation. Review these different types of experiments with the parents, including:

- **Acting Opposite Science Experiments (Session 3):** seeing what happens when we do the opposite of the behavior that our emotions want us to do
- **Sensational Exposures (Session 4):** seeing what happens when we experience a strong physical sensation and don't do anything to get rid of it
- **Present-Moment and Nonjudgmental Awareness Exercises (Session 8):** seeing what happens when we use our present-moment awareness skills and nonjudgmental awareness skills to just notice our emotions and experiences, without doing anything about them.

Explain to the parents that all of these different types of science experiments (or exposures) have helped their children begin to change the way they approach strong emotions. Instead of immediately trying to escape emotions or do something to make emotions go away, their children have been learning to just notice and sit with the emotion, without acting on it. However, up to this point in treatment, the children have been primarily practicing this new approach toward emotions in situations that come up naturally in day-to-day life. Explain to the parents that, beginning next week, in a very gradual manner, their children will begin to purposely approach and stick with situations that bring up strong emotions for them. This is called a *situational emotion exposure.* Completing a **situational emotion exposure** means engaging in a situation in which the child experiences an uncomfortable emotion—including fear, anxiety, sadness, or anger—without avoiding the situation or using another type of emotional behavior.

Explain to the parents how situational emotion exposures proceed according to the steps of a science experiment. As with other types of experiments discussed previously in this treatment, the child will begin situational emotion exposures by defining the experimental task (or the exposure task) with the help of you and/or the parent. The child will then identify his or her initial guesses (or hypotheses) about what will happen in that experiment and evaluate these guesses to determine if they are realistic (using Detective Questioning and Detective Thinking). The child will then monitor the progress and outcomes of the experiment through use of good awareness skills throughout the exposure. In the end, the results of the experiment should be compared to the child's initial guesses about what might happen.

How and Why Situational Emotion Exposures Work

Explain to the parents what typically happens when their child approaches or considers approaching a situation that brings up strong emotions, including anxiety, fear, anger, or sadness. Their child likely experiences high levels of emotion and a strong physiological response (e.g., increased heart rate, change in body temperature, muscle tension). In addition to experiencing these strong physiological sensations, children may focus on beliefs that the situation is threatening or dangerous, unfair in some way, or beyond their ability to cope effectively. As a result, children may try to avoid the situation outright, or use other emotional behaviors to immediately try to reduce the emotion they are feeling. Children typically feel much better in the short term after using these behaviors, but their high level of emotion in the situation and their maladaptive response are reinforced.

Suggest to the parents that, if their children begin to face situations that elicit strong emotions without avoiding them or engaging in any emotional behaviors to lessen their experience of them, their strong emotions will start to feel less intense over time. This happens, in part, because of something called *habituation*.

Explain that **habituation** involves purposely allowing an intense emotional response to occur when presented with a feared or upsetting situation, without trying to get out of that situation, resulting in the response becoming less intense over time. Encourage the parents to turn to Figure 16.2: *Emotion Curve: Avoidance/Escape*. Explain that the curve represents the intensity of their child's emotion over time. Referring to the curve, explain that the rapid descent after the peak of the curve has probably been happening as a result of avoidance or use of other emotional behaviors that may quickly reduce the intensity of an emotion. However, explain that avoidance and other emotional behaviors prevent their child from learning that reduction in emotion will eventually occur as a result of staying in the situation and that negative consequences will generally not result from staying in a situation instead of avoiding (other than simply feeling uncomfortable). Ask the parents to turn their attention Figure 16.3: *Emotion Curve: Habituation* as you illustrate this point.

Let the parents know that when their child begins to approach uncomfortable situations that he or she has previously avoided or in which she or he has used problematic emotional behaviors, the child's discomfort in those situations may not reduce all the way. Emphasize that this is a *completely normal response*, and that the child may even feel some discomfort the entire time he or she is in the situation. Even if the child's anxiety does not fully reduce, the next time he or she approaches the situation or one like it, it will likely not be quite as uncomfortable or anxiety-provoking. Explain to the parents that this is sometimes referred to as **between-session habituation**, and ask them to turn to Figure 16.4: *Emotion Curve: Habituation with Practice* to illustrate this point.

Inform the parents that another reason why exposure works so well is that when a child repeatedly faces situations that cause strong or uncomfortable emotions, he or she may realize that his or her first interpretation (i.e., thinking trap) of what might happen is not true—or, if it is true, the outcome is not as terrible as the child anticipated. This phenomenon is sometimes referred to as **belief disconfirmation**. As the child continues to approach the uncomfortable situation, he or she gathers new and more helpful evidence of what is most likely to happen in the situation. For example, children may learn that they are able to survive the uncomfortable situation, that the worst possible outcome did not occur or was not actually that bad, or that strong emotions become more tolerable as one gets used to experiencing them. As a result, the child will become more confident in his or her ability to cope with difficult situations.

Parent Session 9, Goal 2
Explain the parent's role in practicing exposures at home.

Inform the parents that toward the end of today's parent session, they will be working with their child's therapist to fill in the *Emotional Behavior Form—Child Version*. Their child will also provide input on the parent form during together time at the end of this session, and parents will finalize the *Emotional Behavior Form—Parent Version* over the next week. Then, beginning next session, their child will begin to practice situational emotion exposures both during session and at home. Emphasize that parent involvement is crucial to the success of their child's exposures. Most children do not *want* to do exposures, at least initially, due to the uncomfortable feelings exposures elicit. It is therefore important for parents to be highly involved in choosing an appropriate exposure; planning when, where, and how to complete it; and encouraging and cheerleading their child before, during, and after the exposure. Children benefit most from this treatment when parents are involved in conducting exposures each week during treatment and after treatment terminates.

Explain to the parents that they will receive a lot of support in conducting exposures at home. Parents will be able to witness therapists conduct a group exposure with the children during the next session, and they will also have opportunities to observe therapists model steps for conducting exposures during future sessions. Parents will also have opportunities to receive live feedback on conducting exposures during session, and therapists will help parents plan exposures to do at home each week.

Ask parents to turn to Figure 16.5: *Supporting Your Child's Exposures at Home*. Review this figure with the parents, ensuring comprehension of each point.

Parent Session 9, Goal 3

Introduce parents to the emotional parenting behavior of excessive modeling of intense emotions and avoidance and its opposite parenting behavior, healthy emotional modeling

---

Therapist Note

Be mindful of your time in this parent session. If there is insufficient time to cover all material, you may wish to cover Goal 3 in a future meeting and move on to Goal 4.

Emotional Parenting Behavior: Excessive Modeling of Intense Emotions and Avoidance

Explain to the parents that as their children begin to approach distressing situations without using emotional behaviors, it is important for the parents to think about how they as parents typically respond to situations and emotions that they themselves find distressing. Many parents who participate in this treatment may have a propensity to experience strong or uncontrollable emotions themselves; we know from research that difficulties with anxiety, depression, or intense emotions have a genetic basis. Explain to the parents that even if they have never been diagnosed with a clinical disorder per se, some of them may tend to use avoidance behaviors, safety behaviors, or other emotional behaviors that can be easily perceived as "the norm" in their household. Although everyone uses emotional behaviors occasionally, parents who use certain emotional behaviors frequently or consistently may inadvertently teach their child to use the same emotional behaviors. This is sometimes referred to as *modeling*.

Modeling refers to learning a behavior by watching someone else *model* or demonstrate that behavior. Ask parents to identify skills and behaviors they themselves have learned via modeling. Based on their answers, highlight the range of different behaviors and skills we learn through this process (e.g., learning a dance, learning norms and expectations for behavior in meetings). Point out that one important way children learn is by observing how the significant people in their lives (particularly their parents) think and act. Therefore, by excessively expressing strong emotions, voicing distorted thinking, and engaging in emotional behaviors in front of their children, parents may be inadvertently teaching their children to respond to emotions in the way they themselves do.

Therapist Note

As you present this material, keep in mind that many parents are unaware of their own engagement in emotional behaviors and, if they are aware, may tend to normalize or minimize them.

Opposite Parenting Behavior: Healthy Emotional Modeling

When addressing modeling as an emotional behavior, it is important to remind parents that they are certainly allowed, expected, and even encouraged to have their own emotional experiences! Remind them that the purpose of this treatment is not to get rid of emotions but to learn when we are reacting to our emotions in a way that is not helpful and to change some of the emotional behaviors we are using. Emotions are of course normal, natural, and not harmful for parents as well as for children.

Encourage parents to reflect on emotional behaviors they might have used over the past several weeks, and ask them to consider what their child might have learned about the situation by observing the parents' emotional responses. For many parents, just building awareness of the relationship between their own emotional expressions and behaviors and their child's may be enough for the parents to begin modeling different responses. Additionally, Worksheet 16.2: *Learning Healthy Emotional Modeling* includes three steps for parents to use in order to practice modeling healthier expressions and regulation of their emotions in front of their child. Review each of these steps with the parents. For their home learning assignment this week, parents will use the bottom half of this worksheet to identify an area in which they may be modeling unhelpful emotional behaviors for their child and to practice healthier emotional modeling.

Parent Session 9, Goal 4

Continue to develop the Emotional Behavior Form in preparation for upcoming exposures.

In the large parent group or in smaller groups of parents (depending upon the number of therapists available), review each parent's initial attempt to create an *Emotional Behavior Form—Parent Version* for exposures. As you review and help the parents revise each item, keep the following questions in mind:

- **Are the items on the form appropriate targets for *this* treatment model?** Occasionally, parents will place items on the form that they would like their children to do or do more consistently but that do not necessarily elicit strong emotions. For example, "do the dishes each night" would not be an appropriate item if it is not associated with a strong emotional response.
- **Are the items on the form concrete and well operationalized?** In order to design effective exposure exercises, it is important for each item to be as specific, concrete, and well operationalized as possible. For example, if a parent has listed "going to school" as an activity that causes her child significant distress, ask the parent what different aspects of school seem to provoke anxiety. Is separation from the parent difficult? Is walking through the halls a source of anxiety? Does the child become very distressed when it is time to take a test? By asking specific questions, you can begin to hone in on the primary source of distress and find ways to simulate the situation in session or at home.
- **Do the items on the form range in difficulty?** A good rule of thumb is that some items on the form should be low difficulty, some medium difficulty, and others high difficulty.

After assisting parents in revising the items already on their form, you may wish to draw upon your knowledge of each child and family to suggest additional items. By the end of this session, each parent should have a near-complete *Emotional Behavior Form—Parent Version*. An extra copy is also provided (Form 16.2).

CHAPTER 20

UP-C Session 10: Facing Our Emotions—Part 1

E Skill: Experience My Emotions

MATERIALS NEEDED FOR GROUP

- For Each Child Group Session:
  1. Detective CLUES kits for each child
  2. Poker chips
  3. Puzzle
  4. Prize box
  5. Large piece of paper or whiteboard to record children's answers for any group activities
- For Session 10 Only:
  6. Copy of most recently updated version of *Emotional Behavior Form—Child Version* (Form 9.1) that children and parents completed together during the last session
  7. UP-C Workbook Chapter 10
     a. *Types of Science Experiments* (Figure 10.1)
     b. *Safety Behaviors* (Figure 10.2)
     c. *Facing Strong Emotions Together Experiment* (Worksheet 10.1)
     d. *The Emotion Thermometer* (Figure 10.3)
- For Home Learning:
  8. *My Emotion Ladder for Home Learning* (Form 10.1)
  9. *Solving the Mystery of Our Emotions: Before, During, and After* (Form 2.1; use the same form started after Session 2)

- Assessments to be Given at Every Session:
  10. *Weekly Top Problems Tracking Form* (Use the same form started during Session 1 for each child, found in Appendix 11.1 at the end of Chapter 11 of this Therapist Guide)
- For Parent Group Session:
  11. UP-C Workbook Chapter 16
      a. *Exposure Examples for Different Problem Areas* (Table 16.2)
      b. *How to Use Opposite Parenting Behaviors to Support Exposures* (Table 16.3)
      c. *Emotion Ladder* (Form 16.3)
      d. *Sample Emotional Behavior Form* (Figure 16.6)
      e. *Sample Emotion Ladder* (Figure 16.7)
- For Parent Home Learning:
  12. *Using Opposite Parenting Behaviors to Support Exposures at Home* (Worksheet 16.3)

Therapist Preparation

In preparation for this session, you will need to gather together and bring any necessary materials for the in-session group exposure. These materials will vary depending upon the type of group exposure you choose and may include pencils and paper to record short speeches for a public speaking exposure or a brief skit or a book for the children to read aloud.

Overall Session 10 Goals

The main purposes of this session are to review situational emotion exposures (presented to children as experiments for facing emotions and getting used to them) and to allow the children to complete their first situational emotion exposure in the group context. There are many options for group exposures, so be creative! The best group exposures are ones that are relevant in some way to all the participants but are not too emotionally intense for any one child. At the end of the session, children may complete the group exposure (or demonstrate some aspect of it) with parents present, as appropriate. The session concludes with initial planning for a first at-home exposure.

- **Goal 1:** Review the concept of using science experiments to face strong emotions.
- **Goal 2:** Introduce the idea of safety behaviors and subtle avoidance behaviors (e.g., distraction).
- **Goal 3:** Practice a science experiment to face strong emotions as a group (sample situational emotion exposure).
- **Goal 4:** Make plans for future science experiments for facing strong emotions (individualized situational emotion exposures).

Session 10 Content (Divided by Goals)

Session 10, Goal 1

Review the concept of using science experiments to face strong emotions.

While the Group Is Together

As you welcome back the group for the start of the tenth session, circulate and assist parents and children in providing severity ratings for each of their three top problems and continue to praise and encourage children as they work toward their goals. These ratings should be entered on the same *Weekly Top Problems Tracking Form* (Appendix 11.1 at the end of Chapter 11 in this Therapist Guide) begun during Session 1. Also check that each child has completed the home learning assignment. Ask any children who have not completed the home learning assignment to do so next time (or to complete it briefly during the top problems review). For those children who have completed their home learning assignment, distribute one puzzle piece to each. Briefly review content discussed during the previous session, being sure to revisit the ideas of using science experiments to face emotions and "getting used to it with practice." Encourage each child to share an aspect of his or her home learning assignment (*Solving the Mystery of Our Emotions: Before, During, and After* in which an emotional behavior occurred) with the group.

Review Different Science Experiments Learned in Emotion Detectives

Have the children open their workbooks to Figure 10.1: *Types of Science Experiments*. With the children following along in their workbooks, review the definition of science experiments. Then remind the children of some of the different types of science experiments they have practiced thus far:

- Opposite action: When we do the opposite of what our emotion wants us to do (e.g., practicing doing something fun when we feel down or sad)
- Facing our body clues: When we make ourselves feel body clues on purpose (e.g., by doing things like running around or holding our breath) and watch those feelings as they change over time
- Facing our strong emotions/exposure: When we approach and stick with a situation that makes us feel strong emotions and makes us want to use unhelpful behaviors.

Next, review the definition of an **exposure** (e.g., a science experiment in which we face our strong emotions) in more detail. Discuss how exposures can help to reduce strong emotions both the first time we practice approaching a difficult situation and when we face our emotions in the situation again and again over time. Exposures can initially be quite scary or anxiety-provoking for children, so it is important to communicate that the children will be practicing exposure safely and that they will have choices about the types of exposures they will complete for future in-session and at-home science experiments:

> *"We are going to continue our science experiments for facing our emotions today. Remember when we discussed the idea of exposure? Exposures are when we do things (such as approaching the toy animal little by little, like we did in the last session) that we know may cause us to feel strong emotions. However, if we work on noticing those emotions and experiencing them rather than doing something to feel better right away, we may find that we can deal with the emotions and that they lessen over time. It's kind of like your strong emotions are waves in the ocean during these science experiments or exposures. We are going to notice the waves as they go up and then eventually go back down. We are also going to notice how these emotions start to lessen the more we practice experiencing them, like waves that get smaller and smaller as they approach the shore.*

*When we face our emotions using exposures and get used to these emotions over time, we will always consider your **safety** and your **choices**. Your safety is important to all of us and we will never ask you to do an exposure or a science experiment where you are truly unsafe. You might feel silly or strange or even another stronger emotion when you face your emotions, but we will not put you in danger. We will also consider your choices. Beginning with today's session, you will always have a voice in what kinds of things you work on practicing in your own science experiments. And, the experiments that one person does in the group may be different from things that other children in group do, although today we will all be doing the same exposure or science experiment. The important thing to remember here is that you have a say in which experiments we will do both in session and at home and that these experiments will be safe."*

Session 10, Goal 2

Introduce the idea of safety behaviors and subtle avoidance behaviors (e.g., distraction).

Have the children turn to Figure 10.2: *Safety Behaviors* in their workbooks. Using this figure as a guide, introduce **safety behaviors** (subtle avoidance behaviors children use or objects/people they bring with them to feel safer in emotional situations). Discuss the objects, people, and behaviors that children sometimes use to help them get through difficult or fearful situations. This can be done as follows:

"Before we start our facing our emotions experiment for today, let's talk about some things that some kids do to make themselves feel better during exposures. Sometimes we might be having a strong emotion or feeling about something but be able to face our emotions or do our exposure, as long as we have a special thing or person around. For example, when I was young I had a pink blanket, and it kept me safe. I carried my blanket with me EVERYWHERE, and thought I wasn't safe without it. It was kind of like a magic blanket that could always keep me safe. I used to be VERY afraid of getting a shot. I wouldn't even want to go to the doctor if I thought I might need to get a shot. Unless I had my blanket. If I had my blanket, I could tuck my head inside it, and smell home and everything safe, and then it was okay for me to get the shot, even if it might hurt for a second. Sometimes, I didn't even notice that it hurt at all. But, if I ever forgot my blanket, suddenly I was very, very scared about going to the doctor again. Although my blanket (or thing I bring along to make me feel safe) made it possible for me to do things I was otherwise afraid of, and it wasn't the worst thing in the world for me to take it with me when I needed a shot, you could also say that I didn't know if the shot was really that bad —even without my blanket. I kind of distracted

myself with the blanket and used it to protect me. When I grew up and had to give my blanket up, it was hard for me to get shots at first. I was still very scared. But, eventually I realized that, with or without my blanket, it just hurt for a tiny second and then it was over with, and my fear started to come down.

Do you bring along any things or people in your life that make you feel safe when you are having a strong emotion? Do you have anything you do to feel safer? Take a look at Figure 10.2 and raise your hand or put a check next to the things you do to make you feel safe when you are feeling strong emotions."

Help the group brainstorm other examples of safety behaviors and subtle avoidance behaviors, such as:

- Distracting ourselves by singing a song in our head or keeping busy with something
- Keeping a water bottle, cell phone, or other object (like a blanket) with us at all times
- Bringing someone with us everywhere
- Asking our mom or dad lots of questions ("Will it be alright?" "What will happen?")
- Focusing on our breathing rather than the scary situation.

Follow this brainstorming session by asking the children to identify their own safety behaviors/subtle avoidance behaviors and keep note of any relevant safety or subtle avoidance behaviors that may need to be faded from subsequent exposures. This might be explained to children as follows:

"When you practice facing your emotions, it is very important that you keep an eye out for possible safety behaviors. There may be things you do—like looking away, distracting yourself with something, or pretending the situation isn't happening— that keep you from fully experiencing the exposure. You need to pay attention, and try hard to experience all of your emotions, even though it might feel hard or uncomfortable."

Session 10, Goal 3

Practice a science experiment to face strong emotions as a group (sample situational emotion exposure).

The group science experiment to face strong emotions (i.e., group exposure) can be anything that would be beneficial to the majority of the children in the group and should generally be something that, overall, would be among the least intense items on the children's *Emotional Behavior Forms*. In other words, try to pick an exposure that will elicit some distress without being so difficult that it will cause anyone to become overwhelmed or try to escape. Often we recommend a gentle exposure to a social threat (e.g., having the children all walk around with funny hats or wearing face paint in an office building where others may see them, asking strangers for a pen, or performing something in front of their parents). We find that these types of exposures typically elicit some level of emotion for most children and are relatively easy to personalize. However, we have also implemented group exposures to a wide array of triggers, including shots, Halloween costumes, or mild darkness exposures, depending on the common themes presented across group members' *Emotional Behavior Forms*. You may also choose to break the larger group into two smaller groups and conduct two separate group exposures, if it seems more personalized. Ultimately, the goal is to elicit a small amount of anxiety to teach the purpose, function, and utility of exposures.

Introducing and Implementing a Sample Group Public Speaking Exposure

This section provides a description of a public speaking exercise as one option for group exposure. Note that the same basic steps outlined below can be applied to other group exposures, such as the ones discussed above.

Explain to the children that some people get nervous, scared, or embarrassed about speaking in front of a group, or they may even feel sad or angry when these types of public speaking situations occur. Tell the group that for the first **facing strong emotions/exposure experiment** today, each member of the group will practice saying something in front of all the parents, therapists, and other children. Then, provide each group member with a question and ask each group member to prepare an answer to the question to present in front of the larger group. Questions may include:

- What do you want to be when you grow up?
- What would you do as the president of the United States?
- Who in the world would you most like to meet, and why?
- What is your favorite vacation and why?

Alternative options for a public speaking exposure include having the children perform a short skit, tell a story, or read aloud about a silly object or funny thing the body can do. Regardless of the public speaking exposure chosen, each child should present his or her answer or reading to the group (total of about 1 minute per child). Explain to each of the children what their role will be during the group exposure. You may choose to adjust the difficulty of these roles either upward or downward based on each child's anticipated level of emotional distress during the exposure.

Have the group open their workbooks to Worksheet 10.1: *Facing Strong Emotions Together Experiment* and follow along as you go through each step of the exposure activity:

1. **Start with a Question.** First, have the group members write down the exposure activity chosen by you and the question that they will complete and answer as a group (e.g., "Will my anxiety level change on the Emotion Thermometer as I read my questions aloud?").

2. **Make a Guess.** Then, as a group, come up with a "best guess" of what might happen during the activity and write this down under number 2 on Worksheet 10.1 (e.g., "I will be afraid that I will mess up and my palms might get sweaty"). Before the exposure, it may be helpful to assist the children in some brief Detective Thinking about the upcoming exposure and/or practice using a brief awareness/mindfulness exercise. You can encourage the children to use present-moment awareness, body scanning, or nonjudgmental awareness techniques throughout the exposure as well to increase their focus on the experience of any strong emotions that occur during the exposure.

3. **Try Out the Experiment.** During the activity, you should ask children how strong their emotions are on Figure 10.3: *The Emotion Thermometer,* before, during, and right after the exposure. It may make most sense to continue to use the 0-to-8 scale introduced in previous sessions, but some children may prefer to modify this scale by using a larger range of numbers. Alternatively, you may prefer to have younger children who have difficulty with a numerical rating system rate their emotions as "cold," "cool," "warm," and "hot."

4. **Watch How It Goes.** After the activity, have the children share how it went for them and write down anything they noticed under number 4 on Worksheet 10.1. Specifically, probe children about whether it went how they guessed it might or turned out differently.

5. **Try My Experiment Again.** Ask children what they think would happen to their emotions if the exposure were repeated, and have them write down how it might go under number 5 on Worksheet 10.1.

> **Therapist Note**
>
> *The goal of exposures is to actually elicit at least a small amount of fear. This can be difficult for you to watch; however, it is a necessary part of the process. Remember that all strong emotions will reduce in their intensity eventually. If someone has a particularly strong reaction or tries/threatens to leave the room, it can be helpful to offer some alternatives or let the child know that he or she has choices that allow him her to still participate in the exposure, but lessen the intensity (e.g., if a child refuses to talk during the public speaking exposure even after encouragement, you may give her the opportunity to talk away from the group or even by herself in the room). You can also work with the child who is having a particularly difficult time to more formally break down the steps in the activity chosen as needed to demonstrate how one can gradually approach or deal with the strong emotions that the activity may elicit and promote a sense of confidence. You might say, "Step 1 is read one question in front of the group, Step 2 is read a whole paragraph in front of the group, and Step 3 is make up a few sentences to share with the group," and have the child who is having difficulty choose where he or she wants to start with the exposure practice. The ultimate goal is for the child who is having a particularly tough time to experience success in this initial exposure and feel as though he or she has faced a strong emotion today successfully.*

Back Together

Session 10, Goal 4

Make plans for future science experiments for facing strong emotions (individualized situational emotion exposures).

Complete Emotion Ladder

When the group is back together, have the children work with their parents and therapist to complete Form 10.1: *My Emotion Ladder for Home Learning* from the workbook. Form 10.1 allows you to help parents and children to break down larger goals for facing emotions into smaller, more manageable exposure steps to approach at home. A sample completed form has been provided for reference within the parent section of the workbook (Figure 16.7). Each step on Form 10.1 represents one aspect or step of an exposure (or response prevention, as needed) activity, and each subsequent (higher) step on the ladder builds on the one before (below) it, eventually leading to a larger exposure goal at the top of the ladder. Thus, by "climbing up" the Emotion Ladder on Form 10.1, children are facing stronger and stronger emotions, with the eventual goal of conquering the most difficult "goal" situation at the top of the page. Form 10.1 can be described as follows:

> *"Work with your parent and therapist to decide your first goal for facing strong emotions at home this week for home learning. Then, break down that goal into smaller steps and write each step down on Form 10.1: My Emotion Ladder for Home Learning. This emotion ladder will help you work on facing tough emotions in baby steps or a little at a time, so that you can feel confident about some smaller steps toward facing strong emotions before trying more challenging steps. Remember, you should start with facing things that are a little bit easier before trying the harder stuff, since facing emotions often gets easier with practice! Since being brave and facing emotions is hard work, you will also be getting rewards for facing tough emotions and for not using unhelpful emotional behaviors (like avoiding, escaping, or becoming aggressive) when you do."*

Completing this form will facilitate at-home exposures. Using Form 10.1, assist parents and children with breaking down at least one individual item on the *Emotional Behavior Form—Child Version* (Form 9.1) into concrete, manageable steps. For example, if a child has "Pet a slimy toad" on the *Emotional Behavior Form*, this larger goal might be broken down into concrete steps such as "Stand 5 feet away from slimy toad," "Stand right next to slimy toad without touching it," "Touch slimy toad's back for 1 second," "Hold slimy toad in hand for 5 seconds," and so forth. Encourage the parents and children to choose an item lower down on the *Emotional Behavior Form—Child Version*. Next, circulate around the room and assist parents and children in identifying one or two "baby steps" for this low-intensity item on their *Emotional Behavior Form—Child Version* to work on for an at-home exposure this week. In determining which item to work on and any smaller exposure steps that will be attempted, consider the following:

1. Parent(s) and children should collaboratively agree to the chosen exposure steps.
2. Try to identify when, where, and how the exposure will be completed for home learning.

3. Discuss potential rewards for successful completion of the home learning exposure.

> **Therapist Note**
>
> *Keep in mind that some children may be sensitive to any discussion of baby steps identified for exposures. You (or the child's parents) may need to change, add, or adjust steps on the child's ladder during the course of future exposures, and thus a review of only a few initial steps on the child's Emotion Ladder may be sufficient, particularly for a more reactive or emotionally intense child.*

Review Pragmatic Considerations for Session 11 Exposure

The first in vivo exposure will take place during the next session, and this next session is typically held at a community location (often a local shopping center, grocery store, or similar). Before ending today's group, select a meeting place and time with group members, if you are following this plan, and encourage the parents to schedule a little extra time to find parking to ensure that the exposure starts on time. If you want the children to have any items/money, make sure to let the parents know in advance, as well as the purpose of those items (e.g., to purchase rewards or aid in the planned exposure).

> **Suggested Home Learning Assignment:** *My Emotion Ladder for Home Learning* and *Solving the Mystery of Our Emotions: Before, During, and After*
>
> In addition to completing one or two steps on *My Emotion Ladder for Home Learning* (Form 10.1), children should also add another entry to their *Solving the Mystery of Our Emotions: Before, During, and After* this week.

Overall Parent Session 10 Goals

The main goal of this parent session is to prepare parents for facilitating and supporting exposures. Review the concept of exposure and discuss applications of exposure to various problem areas or concerns. Introduce the concept of safety behaviors, and encourage the parents to identify any safety behaviors their children may be using and to make a plan for eliminating these. Also, explain to the parents about how they can put all their opposite parenting behaviors to good use in order to support their child before, during, and after exposures.

- **Goal 1:** Review the concept of a situational emotion exposure and discuss applications of exposure to different symptom presentations.
- **Goal 2:** Introduce and discuss the concept of safety behaviors.
- **Goal 3:** Explain how parents can use all of their opposite parenting behaviors to support their child's exposures.
- **Goal 4:** Introduce the *Emotion Ladder* for exposures and assist parents in finalizing *Emotional Behavior Forms*.

Parent Session 10 Content (Divided by Goals)

Parent Session 10, Goal 1

Review the concept of a situational emotion exposure and discuss applications of exposure to different symptom presentations.

> **Therapist Note**
> *Remember to begin this session and each subsequent one with a brief check-in regarding major changes in child symptoms/functioning over the past week, as well as a review of home learning assignments.*

Review of Situational Emotion Exposures

Briefly review the concept of a **situational emotion exposure**, which involves engaging in a situation that elicits distressing emotions—including fear, anxiety, sadness, or anger—without avoiding the situation or using another type of emotional behavior. Explain to parents that situational emotion exposures will be introduced to the children as science experiments for facing their emotions. Use Table 20.1 to remind parents of the different reasons why therapists and researchers think exposures are so effective. It may also be helpful for you yourself to review the explanation of exposure in Session 9 prior to this session.

Applying Exposure to Different Symptom Presentations

Exposure therapy was originally developed as a behavioral approach to treating fear and anxiety disorders, such as specific phobias or social anxiety disorder. Many therapists and parents who know about exposures may

Table 20.1 Why Does Exposure Work?

Habituation	Children experience a reduction in the level of their strong emotion the longer they stay in the situation.
Between-Session Habituation (i.e., Habituation with Practice)	Each time children repeat a similar exposure, they experience less intense emotions and their emotions reduce more quickly.
Belief Disconfirmation	Children learn that their initial beliefs about the situation and what might happen if they approach it are untrue.
Distress Tolerance	Children learn that they are able to tolerate or get through a situation without using unhelpful emotional behaviors.

think about exposure to fear situations specifically, but in this treatment, we advocate the benefits of exposure for a wide range of emotions and situations that bring up strong emotions. It may be helpful to communicate this background to parents as you see fit, especially if you believe that they hold certain expectations about exposure therapy from prior reading or experience. Emphasize that, in this treatment, you will work very carefully to tailor exposures to their child's particular emotional concerns.

Explain to the parents that the main goal of exposure is to experience the emotion that comes up in a difficult situation—regardless of whether the emotion is anxiety, anger, sadness, guilt, or something else—and to stay in the situation without avoiding or using other unhelpful emotional behaviors in an effort to reduce the emotion. Explain that, although we often focus on avoidance in this treatment, the emotional behaviors that some children struggle with may not always appear to be avoidant in nature. For example, a child who is angry or frustrated may yell, slam doors, snap at family members, throw a tantrum, or become physically aggressive. To most parents these seem like the opposite of avoidant behaviors, and in some ways they are. However, many children act out in these ways *because they find it difficult or uncomfortable to sit with and tolerate their anger* without doing anything to act on it, so they avoid doing so by acting out. We want to teach children to be able to experience anger or frustration without acting on it immediately, and then to choose a more effective behavior once the anger and frustration begin to reduce.

It is often helpful for parents to see examples of different types of exposures for certain symptoms or problem areas. Ask the parents to turn to Table 16.2: *Exposure Examples for Different Problem Areas* in the parent section of the workbook. Review the different examples of exposures with the parents, and address any questions that arise about how to apply certain types of exposures to their own child.

One type of exposure listed in Table 16.2 under "Obsessions and Compulsions" that may be important to review with the parents is **exposure and response prevention**, the type of exposure most helpful for obsessive-compulsive disorder symptoms. In exposure and response prevention, children are exposed to certain intrusive thoughts (i.e., obsessions) or situations that elicit obsessions, and they are asked to refrain from performing the repetitive behaviors or mental rituals (i.e., compulsions) they would typically perform. If it is too difficult for the child to refrain from performing the behavior entirely, he or she might be asked to delay performing the behavior for a certain period of time or try to "mess with" the compulsion in some way (e.g., doing things in a different order or only some aspect of a compulsion). Walk the parents through the examples of exposure and response prevention in Table 16.2, and provide additional examples if necessary.

Parent Session 10, Goal 2
Introduce and discuss the concept of safety behaviors.

Introduce parents to the concept of **safety behaviors**, which are objects, people, or behaviors a child relies on to feel safe in a situation that brings up strong emotions. Safety behaviors may help to temporarily reduce a child's level of emotion in certain situations as a result of classical conditioning procedures. Although you do not necessarily need to explain classical conditioning to parents, it may be helpful to briefly explain the reason why safety behaviors reduce strong emotions. Their children have learned from prior experiences to associate a particular object, behavior, or person with safety because nothing bad happened to them the last time they were in a difficult situation if the object or person was present or if that behavior was used. In other words, they have become signals of safety.

Safety behaviors also distract children from their strong emotions and prevent them from being fully aware of the present moment. As a result, they fail to attend to information that the situation is safe or that nothing bad is happening. Because they miss this new and corrective information, they are unable to use it as evidence against their initial hypotheses about what might happen in the situation.

Point out to the parents that safety behaviors are common, even among adults. Ask the parents to volunteer examples of safety behaviors they have used as an adult. Some common safety behaviors include:

- Keeping your phone out in social situations to use if you feel uncomfortable or awkward
- Relying on a friend to accompany you to a social event
- Feeling safe at home when your spouse is there, but worrying about your family's safety when your spouse is away on a trip.

After parents have reflected upon their own safety behaviors, ask them to identify any safety behaviors their child relies upon in situations that bring up strong emotions. Encourage them to consider both people and objects their child might rely on to feel safe, as well as subtle avoidance behaviors their child might use to cognitively avoid or distract from the situation. Safety behaviors can run the gamut, but common ones used by children with emotional disorders are:

- Carrying a stuffed animal around when feeling anxious or sad
- Relying on a parent to attend birthday parties, school, or other situations
- Avoiding eye contact when talking to new people
- Asking for excessive reassurance before entering an emotional situation
- Using headphones in unstructured social situations or frustrating situations
- Carrying a snack and/or water bottle around at all times
- Using mental rituals to distract from emotional situations (e.g., repeating a phrase, counting to a high number).

Discuss with the parents whether they believe there are any benefits to using safety behaviors. Acknowledge that (a) many of these behaviors can be typical and/or temporarily helpful and (b) sometimes, at higher levels of emotion, use of safety behaviors allows children to approach and stick with situations they would otherwise avoid, which can make them helpful under certain conditions. However, safety behaviors may also be problematic. Children often believe that they are unable to approach or cope with situations without using the safety behavior, or that a situation is only safe because they use the safety behavior. Then, when they have to approach the situation without the safety behavior, strong emotions and urges to use emotional behaviors return.

Explain to the parents that, ultimately, the goal is for their children to approach and stick with emotional situations without using safety behaviors. Sometimes, safety behaviors can be eliminated fairly easily during the natural course of an exposure. For example, if a child carries around a water bottle to feel safe, you might practice doing exposures without the water bottle. At other times, safety behaviors are quite difficult to eliminate because children may have significant difficulty approaching a situation without them. If the latter situation occurs, explain that therapists and parents may wish to allow children to continue using the safety behavior until the exposure becomes easier (i.e., until children habituate and/ or learn to tolerate the distress), and then phase the safety behavior out. Encourage parents to consider how phasing out a safety behavior can be an exposure "step" on Forms 16.3 (parent emotion ladders) and 10.1 (child emotion ladders) they will work on with their children later in this session.

Parent Session 10, Goal 3

Explain how parents can use all of their opposite parenting behaviors to support their child's exposures.

At this point in treatment, parents have become more aware of their use of four different emotional parenting behaviors that research suggests may be unhelpful or less helpful in managing their child's strong emotions. Remind parents of the four opposite parenting behaviors they have learned to counter these emotional parenting behaviors (expressing empathy, healthy independence-granting, consistent use of praise and discipline, and healthy emotional modeling), and, as time permits, encourage them to briefly discuss the ways in which they have begun using these opposite parenting behaviors at home.

Situational emotion exposures provide an excellent opportunity for parents to practice using all four opposite parenting behaviors. Ask the parents to share ideas for how they might use their opposite parenting behaviors to support their child's exposures. Then, share the following suggestions with the parents for each opposite parenting behavior. It may be helpful for parents to turn to Table 16.3: *How to Use Opposite Parenting Behaviors to Support Exposures* in the parent workbook as you review this material.

- **Expressing Empathy**: Exposures bring up strong, uncomfortable emotions and can be quite challenging! Remind parents to use their expressing empathy steps before and/or during their child's exposures, and review the steps as needed. Expressing empathy can be particularly beneficial when parents are feeling frustrated by their child's difficulty approaching an exposure, attempts at negotiation, or refusal to follow through with an exposure.

- **Consistent Use of Reinforcement and Discipline**: Remind parents of the importance of reinforcing their child after each and every exposure with praise and/or a reward. Let parents know that, at the end of this session, they will be working with their child to identify rewards for completing an at-home exposure and exposures in session next week. When parents and children identify and plan an appropriate exposure, it is also important to consistently follow through with exposure completion.

- **Healthy Independence-Granting**: Exposures typically result in the child experiencing some amount of distress or strong emotion, and it can be difficult for parents to allow their child to experience that emotion and complete the exposure. Parents may be tempted to step in and help or rescue their child from the situation. Although it may sometimes be necessary for parents to step in and reduce the difficulty of exposure if a child is experiencing excessive distress, most of the time it is best for parents to express empathy for their child's struggles but wait until the emotion reduces and the child is able to complete the exposure on his or her own.

- **Healthy Emotional Modeling**: At times, parents may share some of the same fears or worries as their child. They may become frustrated by some of the same situations or disgusted by some of the same objects. There may also be times where parents find certain exposures silly or embarrassing. Let parents know that it is okay to feel this way (after all, we're trying to take a nonjudgmental stance toward emotions in this treatment). However, it is important that parents not model unhelpful emotions or emotional behaviors during their child's exposures. If parents are concerned about their ability to support certain exposures due to their own strong emotions, encourage them to address their concerns with you.

Parent Session 10, Goal 4
Introduce the Emotion Ladder for exposures and assist parents in finalizing Emotional Behavior Forms.

By now, families should have a relatively complete *Emotional Behavior Form—Child Version* with a number of situations that evoke strong emotions and the emotional behaviors children use in those situations. However, in order to actually begin exposures, it is often helpful to develop a step-by-step plan for working on each situation listed on the form. In our experience, many of the situations on an *Emotional Behavior Form* can actually be broken down into a number of different exposures, each of which build upon one another and help children reach their ultimate goal of reducing their strong emotions and emotional behaviors in the situation. This is where *Emotion Ladders* come in handy.

Direct parents to the *Emotion Ladder* (Form 16.3). Explain that they and their child will choose one situation from the *Emotional Behavior Form—Child Version* when they reunite in a few moments, and they will then use the *My Emotion Ladder for Home Learning* (Form 10.1 in the child workbook) to identify a number of smaller, more approachable steps toward completing the larger goal of facing the emotional situation without using emotional behaviors. Before reuniting with the children, assist parents in finalizing their *Emotional Behavior Form—Child Version* as necessary (therapists should have copies available for use in the parent session). To prepare for individualized situational emotion exposures in the next session, you may also wish to assist parents in creating an *Emotion Ladder* (Form 16.3) for one of the lower-level items on the *Emotional Behavior Form—Child Version*.

Many parents find it helpful to review an example of a completed *Emotional Behavior Form* and *Emotion Ladder*. Direct parents to the *Sample Emotional Behavior Form* (Figure 16.6) and the *Sample Emotion Ladder* (Figure 16.7), the latter of which illustrates a series of gradual exposure steps for the bottom situation on the *Sample Emotional Behavior Form*.

Suggested Parent Home Learning Assignment: *Using Opposite Parenting Behaviors to Support Exposures at Home*

For this week's home learning assignment, parents will be assisting their child in completing an exposure (ideally one of lower difficulty for the child). During together time at the end of this session, parents and children will work with the therapists to identify an appropriate exposure to complete at home. Parents should attempt to use each of the four opposite parenting behaviors during their child's exposure, and they should indicate how they used them on Worksheet 16.3: *Using Opposite Parenting Behaviors to Support Exposures at Home.*

E Skill: Experience My Emotions

MATERIALS NEEDED FOR GROUP

- For Each Child Group Session:
    1. Detective CLUES kits for each child
    2. Poker chips
    3. Puzzle
    4. Prize box
    5. Large piece of paper or whiteboard to record children's answers for any group activities
- For Sessions 11 through 14 Only:
    6. Each child's completed *Emotional Behavior Form—Child Version* (Form 9.1)
    7. Copy of each parent's completed *Emotion Ladder* (Form 16.3)
    8. UP-C Workbook Chapter 11
        a. *Facing Strong Emotions Together—Review* (Figure 11.1)
        b. *The Emotion Thermometer* (Figure 11.2)
        c. *My Emotion Ladder for Session 11* (Form 11.1)
        d. *My Emotion Ladder for Session 12* (Form 11.2)
        e. *My Emotion Ladder for Session 13* (Form 11.3)
        f. *My Emotion Ladder for Session 14* (Form 11.4)
- For Home Learning:
    9. Taking at least one step on *My Emotion Ladder* or on *Emotional Behavior Form—Child Version* between sessions (Form 11.1, 11.2, 11.3, or 11.4 depending on session)

10. *Solving the Mystery of Our Emotions: Before, During, and After* (Form 2.1) for an emotion that led to an emotional behavior between sessions

■ Assessments to Be Given at Every Session:

11. *Weekly Top Problems Tracking Form* (Use the same form started during Session 1 for each child, found in Appendix 11.1 at the end of Chapter 11 of this Therapist Guide)

■ For Parent Group Session:

12. UP-C Workbook Chapter 16
    a. *Emotional Behavior Form—Updated Parent Version* (Form 16.5)

■ For Parent Home Learning:

13. *Situational Emotion Exposure Tracking Form* (Form 16.4)

Therapist Preparation

In Sessions 11 through 14 of the UP-C, therapists conduct personalized situational emotion exposures with child group members individually or in small groups. *There is no formal parent group for these sessions.* Additionally, unlike previous chapters, which more explicitly outline step-by-step instructions for conducting sessions, this chapter is framed as more of a guide for you in conducting situational emotion exposures with children and parents. Since goals of situational emotion exposure practice depend heavily on the needs of individual children and their families, procedures outlined for these sessions are flexible in nature and client-dependent. Procedurally, all therapists assist with child situational emotion exposure activities. Materials for each situational emotion exposure session depend on the situational emotion exposures planned for group members. Therefore, it is vital that you have a strong indication of the particular situational emotion exposure exercises planned for each session.

> **Therapist Note**
> *For therapists less familiar with exposure therapy, please review Chapter 7 of this Therapist Guide, which discusses the rationale and procedures for conducting situational emotion exposures in the UP-A. You may also wish to consult the parent workbook material for Sessions 11 through 14 before*

finalizing exposure plans for these sessions. Together, these materials provide extensive guidance on how to select situational emotion exposures for children, as well as common pitfalls and modifications that each therapist should be familiar with to optimize situational emotion exposures in these UP-C sessions.

Overall Sessions 11 Through 14 Goals

The goal of these sessions is to have each child complete several successful situational emotion exposures that reflect increasingly challenging items on his or her *Emotional Behavior Form—Child Version*. Initial situational emotion exposures in Session 11 allow the child to become accustomed to situational emotion exposures, as well as exposure planning, and allow therapists to assess children's responses to various emotion triggers. Sessions 12 through 14 provide extensive time to further challenge children and parents as they attempt increasingly difficult items from their *Emotional Behavior Form—Child Version*. Although there is no formal parent group for these sessions, parents should be directed to review workbook and home learning exercises in the companion materials for these sessions. At a minimum, you should meet with each child and parent together at the end of each session to prepare *Emotion Ladders* as needed and plan for situational emotion exposures at home. Parents may also be recruited to assist with child situational emotion exposures during session as appropriate to *Emotional Behavior Form* content.

- **Goal 1:** Plan and execute initial situational emotion exposure in Session 11.
- **Goal 2:** Plan and execute additional situational emotion exposure activities in Sessions 12 through 14.

Sessions 11 Through 14 Content (Divided by Goals)

Sessions 11 Through 14, Goal 1
Plan and execute initial situational emotion exposure in Session 11.

> **Therapist Note**
>
> *For those doing the UP-C as a group, you may conduct all Session 11 situational emotion exposures at a common community location, such as a shopping center or grocery store, if feasible, with each individual child or small group of children completing therapist-assisted situational emotion exposures within the same location. Aside from the pragmatic benefits of conducting all of the children's situational emotion exposure activities in one location, additional benefits of this "common location plan" are for group members and their parents to support one another during initial situational emotion exposures and provide a single venue for shared decision-making during these activities. **However, a common community location is not completely necessary to build such support during Session 11, if such a plan is not possible or preferred by you.** Thus, these initial situational emotion exposures can be personalized and attempted in other ways (e.g., with individual children/small groups doing separate situational emotion exposure work in different locations or within the primary therapy setting). This flexibility reflects an understanding that the demands of particular therapy settings may limit the amount of "off-site" situational emotion exposure that can be accomplished with the group. However, for purposes of illustration, Goal 1 (below) describes how to conduct the initial situational emotion exposure within a common community location.*

While the Group Is Together

If the location of the initial planned situational emotion exposure for Session 11 allows for it, circulate and assist parents and children in providing severity ratings for each of their three top problems and continue to praise and encourage children as they work toward their goals. These ratings should be entered on the same *Weekly Top Problems Tracking Form* (Appendix 11.1 at the end of Chapter 11 in this Therapist Guide) begun during Session 1. Also check that each child has completed his or her home learning assignment. Encourage any children who have not completed the assignment to do so next time (or to complete it briefly during the top problems review). For those children who have completed the assignment, distribute one puzzle piece to each. If this session is occurring in a community location, you may choose to distribute puzzle pieces during the next session taking place at the clinic instead.

Situational Emotion Exposure Preparation

Next, as you begin Session 11, orient families to situational emotion exposure plans as a group, if possible. Individual therapists can also prepare families for situational emotion exposures independently as needed (e.g., if families arrive at different times or no private space exists for a group meeting at the exposure location). Either way, briefly review the following with each family.

Conducting Situational Emotion Exposures

Review the Rationale for Exposures

Have families turn to Figure 11.1 in the workbook, *Facing Strong Emotions Together—Review*. This review should take no more than 5 minutes and may be introduced as follows:

> *"Just as a reminder: when a situation makes us feel scared, angry, worried, or sad, we often want to get away from that situation because of the uncomfortable feelings that it brings up. Today, just like Emotion Detectives Jack and Nina, we will be facing some of those uncomfortable emotions together here at* [insert name of exposure location]. *Some of us may feel a little nervous or not know exactly what to expect today, so before we begin our situational emotion exposure practice, we will review the Emotional Behavior Form—Child Version together and discuss what options we have for practicing facing a strong emotion today. We can even create an Emotion Ladder to get a better sense of how to break down whatever situational emotion exposure we choose together into smaller, more manageable steps. Whatever we choose to do, we should remember that this is just an experiment and like any good Emotion Detective, we want to pay attention and really notice how it goes today. We can use Jack's Steps to Facing Strong Emotions on Figure 11.1 (once we've picked out what we might do today!) to check our guesses about what could happen and see if our experiences match our guesses or not! For example, our strong emotions might go up in some of the situations we choose today and, if so, we should use all of our awareness skills to notice what happens. It might not be too bad after all! Also remember that the more we practice these situational emotion exposures, the easier they will likely become over time."*

Select the First Situational Emotion Exposure Activity

As mentioned in the "Therapist Preparation" section above, it is strongly recommended that you already have an idea of what situational emotion exposures are *feasible* and *reasonable* given the setting of exposure practice and what is *appropriate* to each child's *Emotional Behavior Form—Child Version*. In almost all cases, you should choose Session 11 situational emotion exposures from the lesser- to moderate-intensity items on the *Emotional Behavior Form—Child Version* of each child *to start*.

Often, there are subsets of children within each treatment group that may be divided into smaller groups (of two or three children) with similar plans for situational emotion exposure activities. For example, if two children both have fears of embarrassment or frustration after losing, one therapist can plan to work with both children at the same time on their situational emotion exposure activities for that day. Small-group situational emotion exposures often have the benefit of providing extra encouragement and support to children as they see other children succeed. It is not uncommon to see children in these small groups provide praise to each other for their hard work, but you should consider the composition of such groups carefully in advance to ensure that they are to the therapeutic benefit of all children involved.

Table 21.1 provides options that you may wish to consider when choosing situational emotion exposures, although you should not consider yourself limited by the options presented in this table in terms of efforts to create effective situational emotion exposure opportunities for each child's individual needs.

Prepare the Children and Parents

If the child(ren) appear very hesitant or nervous, return *to Jack's Steps to Facing Strong Emotions* on Figure 11.1 and discuss the child(ren)'s guesses about what might happen before departing. Try to minimize parent and therapist provision of excessive reassurance or any communications that might suggest the child is in danger of anything other than *feeling uncomfortable*. Instead, review the principles outlined within *Jack's Steps to Facing Strong Emotions* while emphasizing the idea of just noticing, saying something about, and experiencing any uncomfortable sensations or worry thoughts the child(ren) may experience, as needed. Detective Thinking strategies are excellent to use here to reappraise any worry thoughts that arise *ahead* of the situational emotion exposure (as opposed to *during* the situational emotion exposure, when we would generally encourage use of awareness strategies instead of Detective Thinking steps).

Before, during, and after the situational emotion exposure, check in with the child regarding his or her emotional intensity or temperature, using

Table 21.1 Common Situational Emotion Exposure Ideas for Different Problem Areas

Obsessions/Compulsions	Social Fears	Worries	Sadness	Anger/Frustration
Delaying a compulsion for increasingly long lengths of time (e.g., 3 minutes, then 5 minutes, then 10 minutes)	Doing something embarrassing in public (e.g., wearing a silly hat, going to buy something but not having enough money)	Making a mistake or messing something up (e.g., schoolwork) on purpose	Doing fun activities even when not feeling motivated	Practice tolerating losing at a game (e.g., a board game, Tic-Tac-Toe)
Sitting with an obsession for increasingly long lengths of time (e.g., 3 minutes, then 5 minutes, then 10 minutes)	Reading/speaking in front of a group of people (can often increase this in duration or in number of participants to make more difficult)	Doing something that might upset or disappoint someone else	Talking about an achievement and practice focusing on the positive rather than negative details	Having a mock argument with someone and staying calm
Not doing a compulsion at all	Having a conversation with someone (can often increase this in duration or in number of participants to make more difficult)	Thinking about or doing something that brings up worries and not asking for reassurance from parents or therapist	Working on consistent performance of self-care activities	Playing with a toy or game that a sibling wants to play with and staying calm
Changing a compulsion in some way in order to avoid doing it exactly how OCD wants (e.g., counting to a different number, handwashing in a different way, checking in a different order)	Stopping a new person to ask a question or ask for directions	Using a narrative or story to facilitate exposure to worry-related situations	Watching a funny video when feeling sad or down	Repeatedly performing a very boring task
Decreasing frequency of a compulsion (e.g., handwashing only three times per day)	Sitting in silence with someone for a specific length of time without saying anything	Watching a video or listening to a song that evokes worry content	Keeping to a scheduled activity even when tired or wishing to withdraw	Tolerating an unfair situation or being asked to perform an impossible task

Figure 11.2: *The Emotion Thermometer*. Use the child's ratings as a guide to see how the experiment went and assess whether he or she should repeat the activity or proceed with other steps or situational emotion exposures. If a child continues to report very high emotion levels after the situational emotion exposure is over, or if you noted significant behavioral signs of

distress, you may wish to repeat the situational emotion exposure one or more times. If the situational emotion exposure provokes low levels of distress, you may choose to repeat it once just to ensure it was being completed without subtle avoidance behaviors, like distraction, or you may add sensational exposures to increase the intensity of the activity, as discussed below. Your confidence that the child will succeed in his or her initial situational emotion exposure activity should not waver throughout this discussion.

As an option, you can use Form 11.1: *My Emotion Ladder for Session 11* to break down additional selected situational emotion exposure activities into smaller, more manageable steps, particularly if a child is having a challenge conceptualizing how a more feared exposure could start with a smaller, easier-to-handle "baby step." *However, for most children, it will not be necessary to write down steps on a physical Emotion Ladder at all*; rather, plans for situational emotion exposure practice can be established via a discussion that proceeds from the initial situational emotion exposure activity onward. For example, after completing an initial situational emotion exposure activity involving staying in a crowded store where someone might get sick for 3 minutes (e.g., for a child with contamination concerns or fears about vomiting), you could ask the child to reflect on how challenging or easy this was for him or her using *The Emotion Thermometer* (Figure 11.2) ratings and what the next step might be, rather than writing these down in advance. By not committing to all steps on paper in advance, you may also find that you have more flexibility to adapt steps to the amount of distress or difficulty experienced by the child in vivo or in the moment.

Have the Parents Wait in a Nearby Location

Once basic exposure activity plans have been discussed and you are ready to proceed to the first exposure setting, have the parents go and wait in a nearby location. Establish how parents will remain in contact with you; whether money or other means are needed for any potential rewards following brave behavior; and, at a minimum, what time parents should return to review situational emotion exposure progress. In general, the parents should be available to witness or briefly participate in one or more situational emotion exposures toward the end of the session, if possible.

Conducting Situational Emotion Exposures

While conducting situational emotion exposures with individual group members or small groups of children, keep in mind the following general principles and details. Again, therapists are encouraged to review both Chapter 7 of the UP-A and the parent workbook materials for these sessions to familiarize themselves with common challenges and adjustments that may need to be made as they proceed through initial situational emotion exposures and those to follow in Sessions 12 through 14.

Ease of Putting the Task Together

In general, it is helpful to have between 60 and 70 minutes available for initial situational emotion exposures during Session 11 and those to follow in Sessions 12 through 14. This should allow time for multiple situational emotion exposure tasks. Try to take advantage of successes with initial, lesser-intensity situational emotion exposure items to build momentum for trying more difficult tasks. This will require some forethought so that the child can move quickly from one task to another, but you also may need to adjust planned steps depending upon the child's response to situational emotion exposure tasks. Time should be reserved at the end of each exposure to briefly process the child's responses to the situational emotion exposure experiment, to re-rate the intensity of the activity using *The Emotion Thermometer* (Figure 11.2), and to use Emotion Detective skills to reduce any unhelpful post-event processing or negative thinking about the experiment that may occur. If, for example, you note that a child is very worried that others may be thinking negative thoughts about him after doing an embarrassing situational emotion exposure task, encourage the child to use Detective Thinking or nonjudgmental awareness skills to address these concerns. This should not be a lengthy processing of the exposure, but it should not be forgotten because of timing or pragmatic concerns either.

Difficulty of the Task

As noted above, the therapist should generally start with tasks that are of low to moderate intensity. The initial task must be difficult enough for the child to experience a strong emotion, but not so intense that the child is likely to attempt to escape or fully avoid the situational emotion exposure. Research on situational emotion exposure intensity suggests that as therapists progress by making situational emotion exposures increasingly naturalistic (e.g., like the contexts in which a child's strong emotions normally occur outside of session) and even unexpected at times (e.g., a feared dog happens to appear as you walk down the street with the child client, so you decide to ask if you can pet it), this can promote longer-term recall of information about the safety of the situation or object.

Note that a situational emotion exposure task may often turn out to be either easier or more difficult than you or the child think it will be. Therefore, you may want to enter each situational emotion exposure task with ideas about how to quickly adjust the difficulty of the task to make it harder or easier, depending upon the child's ratings on *The Emotion Thermometer* (Figure 11.2). Typically, the goal is for the child to succeed, *briefly* process the situational emotion exposure, and move on to a more difficult, related task. If a child is spending an inordinate amount of time approaching a situation, experiencing high anticipatory anxiety, and demonstrating significant avoidance behaviors, you may want to adjust the difficulty of the task slightly and work up to the more difficult exposure in a slower, step-by-step fashion.

Duration of the Task

A situational emotion exposure should generally proceed until a child is able to observe that he or she is safe or that he or she can tolerate the strong emotion without doing anything to act on it or reduce it. Ideally, some level of reduction in the child's emotional intensity ratings will occur. However, it should be noted that the most recent research suggests that significant within-session habituation (i.e., a significant reduction in the level of emotional intensity) may not be essential for overall, longer-term improvement to occur. That being said, there are several challenges to ending a situational emotion exposure task when emotional intensity is too high with children. If you terminate a task while the anxiety level is still very high, the experience may be counterproductive because:

- The child may remember the task as difficult or become unduly frustrated with not having mastered it.

- The child may continue to believe he or she has to escape for the emotional intensity to lessen.
- The child may be reluctant to return to sessions or approach similar situations in the future.

Therefore, look for and explicitly point out small successes of any sort during a particularly challenging situational emotion exposure, even if the child and you end up compromising to lessen the intensity of the situational emotion exposure slightly. This helps end the session on a positive note and increases the child's level of positive emotion as he or she completes situational emotion exposure tasks for the day.

Tasks that are too brief for emotional intensity to lessen significantly in a single try (e.g., asking a stranger for the time) should be done repeatedly in quick succession until the intensity ratings decrease and/or the child's ability to tolerate the situational emotion exposure task increases (e.g., asking multiple people for the time, right in a row). With situational emotion exposures like these, emphasize reduction in emotion ratings from the first situational emotion exposure attempt to the fourth or the fifth attempt.

Inclusion of Sensational Exposures

It is important for the child to experience a fair amount of emotional intensity when completing situational emotion exposures. If the child does not find the tasks sufficiently distressing, you may want to incorporate sensational exposures (e.g., holding breath, running in place, shaking head side to side) before or during the situational emotion exposure to heighten the physical feelings of anxiety and thereby intensify the situational emotion exposure. This may promote habituation within the situational emotion exposure more quickly, if that is your goal at the time.

Rewards

Make sure you reward your Emotion Detective for his or her hard work. Small rewards (e.g., high fives, verbal praise) are appropriate after the completion of each situational emotion exposure. Remember, this is a very difficult day for the child, and we want to show him or her how proud we are! A slightly larger reward (e.g., an ice-cream cone, a treat from a local store, or a small prize) may be appropriate at the end of the session, if the parent agrees.

Back Together

The group (or individual families) meets back together at a predetermined location. As noted below, time should be reserved to review or practice the "bravery showcase" with the parents, and therapists should convey a high degree of praise and excitement for successes. Even if the child was not successful in achieving all planned situational emotion exposures, an effort should be made to encourage the child and parents that they made positive steps toward reducing unwanted emotional distress today and that further practice at home should help cement the lessons learned. Work with families to then identify which item from the *Emotional Behavior Form—Child Version* or Form 11.1: *My Emotion Ladder for Session 11* (if using this with the particular child) will make for good home learning practice.

Bravery Showcase

It is often appropriate to end the situational emotion exposure session by having a "bravery showcase" for parents. This is when the children repeat a task that they have previously accomplished successfully, this time in front of their parents or with a parent leading the situational emotion exposure itself. This allows the parents to witness how situational emotion exposures are conducted, how rewards and praise are delivered, and how their child can be successful at something that causes the child anxiety or discomfort. Doing a situational emotion exposure with the parent present or allowing the parent to lead a situational emotion exposure is especially important when you have concerns about the parent's ability to cope with his or her own distress or to manage the child's distress in home learning situational emotion exposures, or simply when you need to give the parent more feedback about how to conduct a situational emotion exposure effectively through increased direct instruction.

Sessions 11 Through 14, Goal 2

Plan and execute additional situational emotion exposure activities in Sessions 12 through 14.

The goals for Sessions 12 through 14 are similar in nature to those of Session 11. Each group within this interval proceeds like the first, but with increasingly challenging situational emotion exposures planned from the children's *Emotional Behavior Form—Child Version* and/or *My Emotion Ladder* (either Form 11.1, 11.2, 11.3, or 11.4 in the workbook, depending on how many emotion ladders the child has used thus far for situational emotion exposure practice). It is not necessary to meet at a community location for each subsequent situational emotion exposure; rather, you should consider the demands of your practice setting, the types of situational emotion exposures planned, and time/transportation constraints of each individual family when determining the location of these situational emotion exposures.

As noted, additional *Emotion Ladders* (Forms 11.2–11.4) are available in the child section of the workbook for use during session or home learning situational emotion exposures through Session 14.

Therapist Note

Session 15—the final session of this treatment and Chapter 22 in this Therapist Guide—includes several worksheets for parents to complete during session. These worksheets focus on reviewing and assessing mastery of skills learned by both child and parent during the UP-C program (Worksheets 17.1 and 17.2) and on creating a post-treatment progress plan (Worksheet 17.3). If parents are not involved in Session 14 situational exposures, you may wish to assign them all or portions of Worksheets 17.1 and 17.2 to complete during Session 14. These worksheets can also be assigned for additional home learning. There may be several advantages of asking parents to begin these worksheets ahead of Session 15, including providing parents additional time to consider their and their child's current skill level and freeing up time in Session 15 for creating a more detailed post-treatment progress plan and celebrating accomplishments.

Prior to parents' departure (if applicable), ask parents to bring snacks or other materials needed for the final celebratory session (see Chapter 22 in this Therapist Guide for more information).

Suggested Home Learning Assignment: *My Emotion Ladder* **for Sessions 11 Through 14, respectively; and** *Solving the Mystery of Our Emotions: Before, During, and After*

Instruct parents and children to work together over the coming week to help children be brave and take at least one step (ideally two or three steps) on *My Emotion Ladder* (Forms 11.1–11.4) or on their *Emotional Behavior Form—Child Version* if they are not using *My Emotion Ladder* for situational emotion exposures. Also, have the children add another entry to their *Solving the Mystery of Our Emotions: Before, During, and After*.

CHAPTER 22

UP-C Session 15: Wrap-up and Relapse Prevention

S Skill: Stay Healthy and Happy

MATERIALS NEEDED FOR GROUP

- For Each Child Group Session:
  1. Detective CLUES kits for each child
  2. Poker chips
  3. Puzzle
  4. Prize box
  5. Large piece of paper or whiteboard to record children's answers for any group activities
- For Session 15 Only:
  6. Party supplies (e.g., snacks, drinks for children and parents)
  7. E and S Badges
  8. *Top Problems Progress Forms* (Appendix 22.1 at the end of this chapter)
  9. UP-C Workbook Chapter 12
     a. *My Emotion Detective Tool Kit* (Figure 12.1)
     b. *Taking Stock of All I've Accomplished* (Worksheet 12.1)
     c. *Becoming My Own Therapist!* (Worksheet 12.2)
     d. *Emotion Detective Completion Certificate* (Worksheet 12.3)
- Assessments to Be Given at Every Session:
  10. *Weekly Top Problems Tracking Form* (Use the same form started during Session 1 for each child, found in Appendix 11.1 at the end of Chapter 11 of this Therapist Guide)
- For Parent Group Session:
  11. UP-C Workbook Chapter 17
     a. *Emotion Detective Skills (CLUES)* (Table 17.1)

b. *Reviewing Your Child's Emotion Detective Skills* (Worksheet 17.1)

c. *Reviewing Your Opposite Parenting Behaviors* (Worksheet 17.2)

d. *Supporting Your Emotion Detective After Treatment* (Worksheet 17.3)

e. *Lapse Versus Relapse* (Table 17.2)

▪ For Parent Home Learning:

12. Implement plan from Worksheet 17.3: *Supporting Your Emotion Detective After Treatment*

Therapist Preparation

In preparation for this session, you may wish to bring special snacks and drinks or other celebratory supplies (e.g., party decorations or balloons, child-appropriate party music, prizes for child group members) for the end-of-therapy celebration/graduation, or ask parents, in advance, to contribute these for this session. You will also need to bring the children's final two CLUES badges (E and S) to distribute at the end of this session. Prior to session, make copies of *Top Problems Progress Forms* (found in Appendix 22.1 at the end of this chapter) for each family. Fill in these *Top Problems Progress Forms* for each family to demonstrate change in top problems during the course of the UP-C treatment to parents (and children, if appropriate) using top problem ratings gathered weekly in the *Weekly Top Problems Tracking Form*. As noted at the end of Chapter 21, you may wish to request that parents complete Worksheets 17.1 and 17.2 from the workbook in advance of this session in order to review perceptions of progress toward treatment goals efficiently.

Overall Session 15 Goals

The goals of this session are to review skills learned during the UP-C group and the progress that each child has made, as well as to help transition each family to using their Emotion Detective skills more independently after treatment is over. At the end of the session, the children will receive their final two CLUES badges to celebrate completion of the final sections of treatment. Parents, children, and therapists all participate together as a group in this end-of-treatment celebration of each child's progress.

- **Goal 1:** Review Emotion Detective skills learned in the UP-C program.
- **Goal 2:** Plan for facing strong emotions in the future.
- **Goal 3:** Celebrate progress made in treatment program.

Session 15 Content (Divided by Goals)

Session 15, Goal 1

Review Emotion Detective skills learned in the UP-C program.

While the Group Is Together

As you welcome back the group for this final session, circulate and assist parents and children in providing severity ratings for each of their three top problems and continue to praise and encourage children on their accomplishments in the UP-C. These ratings should be entered on the same *Weekly Top Problems Tracking Form* (Appendix 11.1 at the end of Chapter 11 in this Therapist Guide) begun during Session 1 and added as final points on the *Top Problems Progress Forms* (Appendix 22.1 at the end of this chapter), to be utilized (with parents alone) in this session. These completed forms can be shared with children as well, should you and the parents decide this makes sense (i.e., if progress has been made that the child might feel proud to see and/or if the child is cognitively able to understand these graphs). Also check that each child has completed his or her home learning assignment. For those children who have completed the assignment, distribute one puzzle piece to each. Ensure that all puzzle pieces have now been distributed; if they have not, distribute extra puzzle pieces for home learning completion or for other behaviors early in this session, as children will be completing their puzzle together in this session.

> **Therapist Note**
>
> *The child-alone portion of group should look and feel like a celebration of achievements from the start, although you will be reviewing UP-C content throughout this time. You can provide treat-like snacks or ask parents to provide these in advance. You may also wish to play child-appropriate music and/or hang party decorations in the room to create a celebratory mood. Intermittent breaks in content review may provide a good moment for group dancing, singing, prizes for excellent responding to queries in session, or just snacking, as appropriate and feasible, to retain a party atmosphere throughout session.*

Review of Treatment

Review major treatment skills with the children. For each skill, briefly review important content as well as a few of the memorable activities associated with that skill. This can be accomplished by first directing children to open their workbooks to Figure 12.1: *My Emotion Detective Tool Kit.* You may wish to have children volunteer to read portions of the worksheet aloud or have a therapist direct review of this material. You can refer to Table 22.1: *Emotion Detective Tool Kit* (replicated within Figure 12.1 in the child workbook) as a guide and review each skill (left column) and the fun activities (completed during sessions) used to learn it (right column). After reviewing all of the skills, have the children volunteer to share with the group which skills or activities were their favorite and which skills have been most helpful to them throughout treatment. Reinforce the idea that different children may benefit from different Emotion Detective skills during the course of this treatment and that this is to be expected. No matter which skills benefited an individual child the most or are most memorable to him or her, remind children that they are all on their way to becoming true Emotion Detectives, just like Jack and Nina.

Session 15, Goal 2

Plan for facing strong emotions in the future.

Table 22.1 Emotion Detective Tool Kit

Skill	Fun Activities
C Skill: Consider How I Feel Explain that the content for this skill covered the three parts of an emotion: feelings, thoughts, and behaviours.	True and False Alarm The Emotion Thermometer Acting Opposite Experiments Emotion and Activity Diary Finding Body Clues How to Body Scan
L Skill: Look at My Thoughts Note that the content for this skill covered thinking traps, which are shortcuts or automatic ways of thinking about a situation. Review that thinking traps often lead us to make negative or unrealistic conclusions about a situation without having evidence that something bad is happening, so we practiced being Emotion Detectives to start questioning those thoughts.	Thinking Trap Characters Flexible Thinking
U Skill: Use Detective Thinking and Problem Solving Explain that the content for this skill covered using Detective Thinking to solve thinking traps. We also worked on Problem Solving and problems that can come up with other people.	Mystery Game Detective Thinking Problem Solving
E Skill: Experience My Emotions Note that the content for this skill was facing strong emotions	Notice It, Say Something About It, Experience It Present-Moment and Nonjudgmental Awareness Facing Strong Emotions

S: Stay Healthy and Happy

Remind the children that emotions are normal, natural, and not harmful, and that they will continue to experience strong or uncomfortable emotions from time to time after this treatment. As discussed in previous sessions, the purpose of this treatment is not to get rid of emotions that bother us, but to learn some different Emotion Detective skills for managing emotions in helpful ways (versus less helpful or unhelpful ways), so that they don't bother us or get in the way so much of doing the things we wish to do each day. Let the children know that they can now use all of the above skills to deal with feeling scared, sad, angry, worried, and so on, in more helpful ways. Identify that this has been hard work for each child and that you are proud of their efforts thus far!

Then, *consider leading a discussion* about when the most important times to use Emotion Detective skills might be for each child. First, ask the children to volunteer examples of some different times or situations when the Emotion Detective skills just reviewed would be helpful to use. Examples might include having a fight with a friend, getting teased or picked on, answering a question in class, not being chosen for an honor or award, feeling sad when a pet dies, or being removed from a sports game. Remind the children that sometimes it is most helpful to use their skills before they are even in an emotional situation (e.g., Detective Thinking), sometimes it is most helpful to use their skills during an emotional situation (e.g., some acting opposite techniques, body scanning and other awareness techniques), and other times it is most helpful for them to use their skills after an emotional situation (e.g., Problem Solving).

Relapse Prevention

Review the following worksheets from the child workbook: *Taking Stock of All I've Accomplished* (Worksheet 12.1) and *Becoming My Own Therapist!* (Worksheet 12.2). For Worksheet 12.1, make sure to provide children with some time to brainstorm different accomplishments they are proud of having achieved during treatment. This may follow logically and easily from the Emotion Detective skill review or require additional thought to help children identify new or more helpful behaviors or ways of thinking adopted during treatment. After brainstorming, allow children time to share one thing they are most proud of working on or accomplishing during treatment, and make sure to provide further praise to each child.

Worksheet 12.2 is designed to help the children consider how they might transition from having a therapist coach them through using their Emotion Detective skills in difficult situations or when experiencing strong emotions to taking increased ownership of coaching themselves through these situations, with the assistance of their parents. Explain to the children that now that treatment is ending, as fully-fledged Emotion Detectives, they are ready to become their own therapist too. Ask the children to brainstorm how their therapists have helped them to approach and stick with difficult situations. Examples might include:

- Coming up with a plan or an experiment to practice facing strong emotions
- Reminding them to use their Emotion Detective skills
- Checking in during sessions to make sure children followed their plan
- Providing encouragement when things got difficult
- Praising or rewarding them for their hard work.

Ask children to discuss how they can begin to take on all these therapist roles, with the help of their parents.

Then, use the *Becoming My Own Therapist!* worksheet to assist children with identifying up to five things or situations they still need to work on after treatment ends. Encourage the children to consider their top problems and their *Emotional Behavior Form—Child Version* to identify areas of continued difficulty, as needed. You may also wish to help children consider what would be the next step for some of the experiments and exposures they successfully completed during treatment. After children have identified approximately five things or situations to work on, assist them in devising a plan for how to work on these situations and which skills they can use.

Therapist Note

Remind the children of the importance of checking in with their parents and discussing their emotions!

Session 15, Goal 3

Celebrate progress made in the treatment program.

Celebrate the End of Treatment

Have all the children dump out the puzzle pieces that they have accumulated during treatment, and have them put the puzzle together. If possible, make sure that you have distributed all puzzle pieces by the time children reach this activity. However, you can encourage them to try to guess the prize associated with the puzzle even if they haven't received all of the puzzle pieces.

Celebrate with cookies (or some other snack), drinks, and music! Typically, this celebration will feature an item identified in the puzzle they just completed (e.g., cookies, party decorations).

Back Together

When the parents return, have each parent share with the group the one thing that they are most proud of their child having accomplished. The rest of the group applauds and provides support for each of the children after the parent shares. Some parents may also wish to share their child's *Top Problems Progress Forms* with the child at this time as well, particularly if this form suggests excellent accomplishments in treatment. Then, fill out Worksheet 12:3: *Emotion Detective Completion Certificate* in each child's workbook to indicate that the child has now graduated from the UP-C Emotion Detectives program.

This final session concludes with a continuation of the party that began during the child group, with celebration being the main goal of any remaining time. At the end of session, hand out E and S badges and congratulate each child on learning ALL of his or her CLUES and becoming a fully-fledged Emotion Detective!

Overall Parent Session 15 Goals

The main goals of this final session are to review skills learned to date, to review each child's progress to date, and to help parents create a plan for sustaining progress after treatment. Begin by reviewing both Emotion Detective skills and opposite parenting behaviors learned over the course of treatment. Invite the parents to share their perceptions of their child's progress, both during exposures and during treatment more generally. Help parents identify areas for continued progress and assist them with developing a plan for sustaining progress and making further gains after treatment. At the end of session, parents learn the difference between lapses and relapses and identify the clues that might indicate that a return to treatment is necessary.

- **Goal 1:** Review Emotion Detective skills and opposite parenting behaviors.
- **Goal 2:** Discuss and celebrate each child's progress.
- **Goal 3:** Create a plan for sustaining and furthering progress after treatment.
- **Goal 4:** Distinguish lapses from relapses and help parents recognize warning signs of a relapse.

Parent Session 15 Content (Divided by Goals)

Parent Session 15, Goal 1

Review Emotion Detective skills and opposite parenting behaviors.

Therapist Note

Unlike in previous sessions, there is no need to conduct a formal check-in or review of home learning assignments. Both a final check-in and a review of recent exposures are built in to the overall session goals

---

Emotion Detective Skills Review

Direct parents to Table 17.1: *Emotion Detective Skills (CLUES)* in the parent workbook. Using this table as a guide, review each of the important concepts/skills the children (and parents) have learned over the course of this treatment. As you review each concept/skill, encourage parents to use the spaces provided in Worksheet 17.1: *Reviewing Your Child's Emotion Detective Skills* to write down the situations in which their child currently uses each skill and rate the effectiveness of their child's use of the skill, if this has not been completed in advance of this session.

Ask each parent to briefly discuss which skills their child currently appears to be using consistently and effectively, as well as which skills they believe their child requires further practice with in order to master. You may choose to provide feedback regarding your own observations and perceptions of each child's current skill level. Emphasize the importance of continuing to practice Emotion Detective skills in a variety of settings and situations after treatment ends.

Opposite Parenting Behaviors Review

Using Worksheet 17.2: *Reviewing Your Opposite Parenting Behaviors* in the parent section of the workbook, review each of the opposite parenting behaviors listed (as well as their corresponding emotional behaviors). During this conversation, ask parents to use this worksheet to briefly indicate situations in which they are effectively using each of the opposite parenting behaviors, as well as situations in which they could use these parenting behaviors more often (if this has not been completed previous to this session). If time permits, you may choose to have parents share examples of situations in which they believe they need to practice more frequent or more consistent use of opposite parenting behaviors. Explain that self-assessments like these are important, as they allow parents to check in with themselves about how effectively they are using certain skills. Encourage the parents to continue to practice all opposite parenting behaviors after the end of treatment, particularly in situations where skills use is currently occurring less frequently or effectively.

Parent Session 15, Goal 2

Discuss and celebrate each child's progress.

Progress Review

Encourage each parent to briefly discuss his or her child's progress, particularly since the beginning of the "E" skill, but also over the course of treatment more generally. You may wish to use the following questions to guide this discussion:

- What changes have you observed in your child's emotions and behaviors?
- What situations is your child now more willing to approach and tolerate?
- Are there certain emotions your child experiences less often? Ones your child experiences more often?
- Have you noticed changes in your child's reaction to negative emotions (e.g., sadness, anxiety, and anger)?
- Do you notice differences in the way your child thinks about emotional situations?

Highlight progress that you as the therapist have noticed in each child, particularly if any parents appear discouraged about their child's current level of symptoms and functioning. Review the pattern of changes in child and parent top problems ratings as seen in the completed *Top Problems Progress Forms*. Normalize the fact that most children still have emotions and behaviors they need to work on at the end of treatment. Determine with each family whether to share this *Top Problems Progress Forms* with individual child clients when the groups reunite. This is a personal decision for each family, dependent on progress, anticipated child understanding of the progress-monitoring graph, and parent comfort with his or her child viewing this graph. Explain to the parents, regardless of whether they share the *Top Problems Progress Forms* with their child, that later in this session they will be able to identify areas of continued difficulty and creating a plan to continue to work on these areas after treatment.

Celebrating Progress

Explain to the parents that when they reunite with their children at the end of the session, they will participate in a group celebration. During this group celebration, all parents will be asked to share what they are most proud of their child for accomplishing during treatment. It may be helpful to ask the parents what they plan to share during the celebration in order to ensure that they are planning to share helpful, supportive, and accurate statements of their child's progress.

Parent Session 15, Goal 3

Create a plan for sustaining and furthering progress after treatment.

Identifying Areas for Further Progress

Ask parents to turn to Worksheet 17.3: *Supporting Your Emotion Detective After Treatment*. Discuss the fact that, right now, their child likely has built up a significant amount of momentum as a result of completing situational emotion exposures both in session and at home for the past five or so weeks. Hopefully, these exposures will have helped the children begin to develop a habit of approaching and/or sticking with tough or emotional situations without using unhelpful emotional behaviors. In order to help the children, sustain this habit, as well as continue practicing their Emotion Detective skills, parents will be identifying three goals for their child to work on after treatment concludes. These goals may involve additional exposures, but they may also involve using Emotion Detective skills more often or in different types of situations. You should also emphasize that, although the children may have successfully completed particular exposures in the clinic or with you, it may be helpful to practice these same exposures in different situations or in the child's natural environment.

Assist parents with identifying three goals for their child to work on after treatment. Consulting the *Top Problems Progress Forms* or the most recent version of the *Emotional Behavior Form* may be of help in identifying these goals.

Creating a Post-Treatment Progress Plan

Using the bottom of Worksheet 17.3: *Supporting Your Emotion Detective After Treatment*, help each parent identify five steps for achieving one of the goals on the top portion of the worksheet. You should also assist the parents in identifying skills their child can use to complete each step, as well as opposite parenting behaviors they can use to support their child.

Parent Session 15, Goal 4
Distinguish lapses from relapses and help parents recognize warning signs of a relapse.

Lapses Versus Relapses

Express your hope that each child will continue to make progress after treatment ends, and that there will not be cause for any of the children to return to treatment. However, emphasize that even children who are very successful with this program will experience temporary setbacks after treatment is over. These setbacks may occur for a variety of reasons, but some common ones are:

- The child did not have an opportunity to work on all of his or her problem areas during this treatment
- The child has to learn to use Emotion Detective skills in a brand-new situation he or she has never experienced before
- The child is under additional stress or is having to cope with an acutely stressful situation.

Explain that, in these types of situations, it is perfectly normal for children to experience temporarily increased feelings of anxiety, sadness, anger, or some other emotions. Children may also revert to using unhelpful emotional behaviors they have not used in a long while, or may begin using certain emotional behaviors more often. Temporary increases in the intensity or frequency of negative emotions and in the use of unhelpful emotional behaviors may be considered a **lapse**. Parents can help children navigate these types of situations by helping their child identify his or her emotions, reminding him or her of the different Emotion Detective skills he or she could use in the situation, and helping their child choose and practice appropriate skills.

Distinguish a lapse from a **relapse**, which is a sustained period of increased emotional intensity and engagement in problematic emotional behaviors such as avoidance, escape, aggression, and withdrawal. Ask parents to turn to Table 17.2: *Lapse Versus Relapse*, which contains helpful descriptions for distinguishing a temporary lapse from a more sustained relapse. Explain to the parents that they can use this table in the future if they are ever concerned about their child's symptoms or functioning and are wondering if it is time to bring their child back to treatment. The more their child's symptoms fit into the "relapse" rather than the "lapse" column, the more a return to treatment may be indicated. Encourage parents to also volunteer more personalized examples of signs that their child might be experiencing a relapse and may need to return to treatment.

Before you reunite with the children, positively reinforce parents for their hard work and dedication to this treatment!

Suggested Parent Home Learning Assignment:

Although there is no formal home learning assignment, parents should work on implementing their plan from Worksheet 17.3: *Supporting Your Emotion Detective After Treatment*.

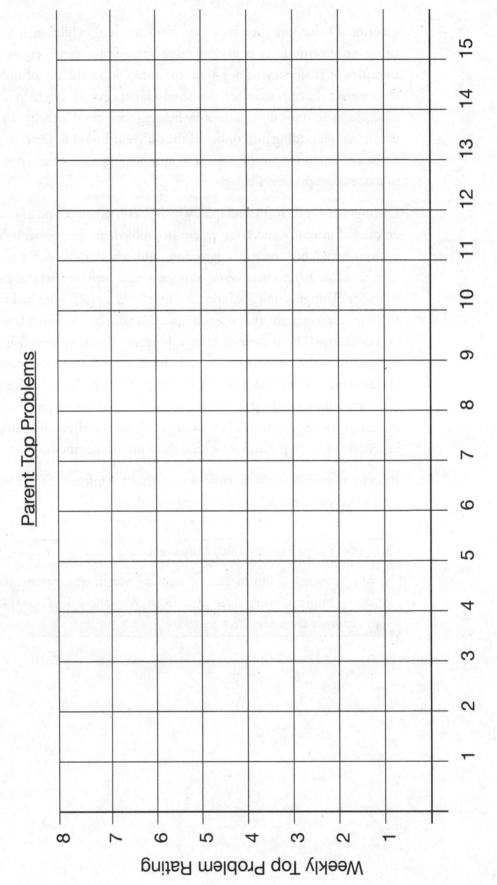

Appendix 22.1: Top Problems Progress Forms

Parent Top Problems

Weekly Top Problem Rating

Session of Treatment

Child Top Problems

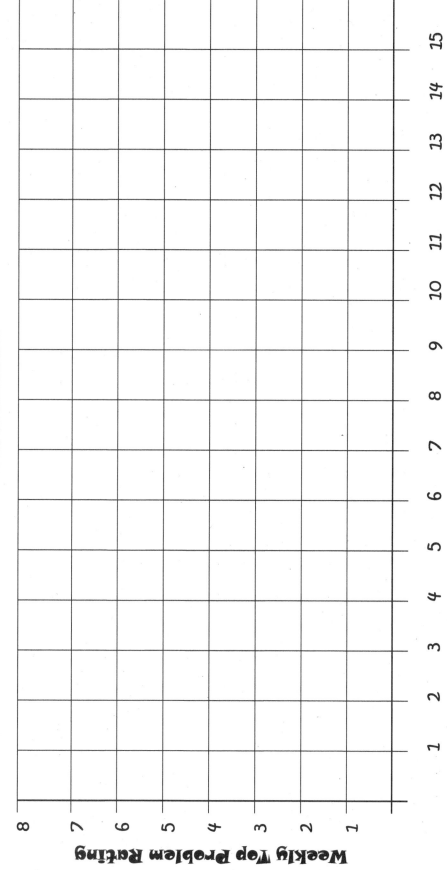

Weekly Top Problem Rating

8 7 6 5 4 3 2 1

Session of Treatment

1 2 3 4 5 6 7 8 9 10 11 12 13 14 15

Variations and Adaptations

CHAPTER 23

UP-A Group and UP-C Individual Therapy Variations, Other Adaptations

Considerations for Adapting UP-A and UP-C for Use with Different Populations

Flexibility of the Unified Protocols

One of the clear advantages of a transdiagnostic, unified approach to treating emotional disorders in children and adolescents is its flexibility and adaptability. Because this treatment targets a common set of underlying features of emotional disorders (e.g., high levels of intense emotions, distress reactions to intense emotions, unhelpful behavioral choices when experiencing intense emotions, and so forth), the skills detailed in these treatments are applicable to any disorder or problem area sharing these core features. These include anxiety and depressive disorders and also obsessive-compulsive (OC) spectrum disorders, tic disorders, stress-related disorders, somatic symptom disorders, and potentially even some eating disorders. However, the flexibility of this model often raises questions for therapists about whether and how to adapt these treatments for a wide range of emotional disorder presentations and clinical settings.

In this chapter, we review some of the most common modifications that may be needed for using the UP-C and UP-A under different conditions and with different types of symptom presentations. Although the UP-A is presented in an individual treatment format and the UP-C within a group treatment format in this manual, both treatments can certainly be delivered in either individual or group therapy formats. Accordingly, we provide suggestions in this chapter for delivering the UP-A in a group therapy format and the UP-C in an individual therapy format, based on our own clinical experiences and on our experiences supervising and consulting with other clinicians and researchers. While these experiences have provided us with a wealth of information about how to adapt these treatments for different formats, we present these suggestions with the caveat that, as of the publication of this Therapist Guide, efficacy data exist only for individual-format UP-A and group-format UP-C.

We also recognize that certain classes of disorders may share the same core features of emotional disorders discussed in this Therapist Guide but may differ slightly with respect to some underlying features or efficacious treatment strategies. For example, psychoeducation for OC-spectrum presentations could be altered slightly to account for the ego-dystonic and intrusive nature of OC symptoms (e.g., by externalizing them or giving them a silly name that indicates that they are "external" to the child's own beliefs and intentions; March & Mulle, 1998), while exposure procedures may require slight modifications to accommodate exposure and response prevention. We provide suggestions in this chapter for modifications that may be helpful in treating children and adolescents with OC-spectrum disorders, stress-related disorders, and Tourette's/tic disorders with these protocols.

Finally, although we recommend using all 8 UP-A treatment modules and all 15 UP-C treatment sessions when first delivering these treatments, certain types of cases may call for increased flexibility in the delivery and timing of core treatment components. There may be some types of cases where you wish to spend more time than is recommended on certain treatment modules or components, and other cases where you may wish to eliminate certain modules or components entirely. In this chapter, we provide additional guidance for altering the structure and content of treatment in such ways.

Utilization of the UP-A in a Group Therapy Format

Although written as an individual therapy approach, the UP-A could certainly be delivered in a group format similar to the format of the UP-C, either with or without significant parent involvement. Many adolescents enjoy the support, understanding, and camaraderie of other adolescents struggling with similar concerns to themselves. Similarly, parents, who are often frustrated and demoralized by parenting an emotional adolescent, may also enjoy an opportunity to share their struggles and triumphs in the group setting. However, some significant modifications to the UP-A

Therapist Guide and workbook materials are required to deliver this treatment to a group of adolescent clients and their parents.

If using the UP-A in a group setting, therapists should **follow the general timeline of content delivery seen in the UP-C**, with an additional motivational enhancement (UP-A Module 1) session preceding this content, making for a total of 16 recommended sessions, utilizing this structure:

- Sessions 2 and 3 would focus on emotion education material from UP-A Module 2.
- Session 4 would focus on opposite action and behavioral experiments for sadness from UP-A Module 3.
- Session 5 (UP-A Module 4) would include an abbreviated discussion of physical sensations associated with strong emotions, body scanning, and brief sensational exposure practice.
- Sessions 6 and 7 would include an introduction to flexible thinking and cognitive reappraisal (UP-A Module 5), while Session 8 would focus on problem-solving skills, also from UP-A Module 5.
- Session 9 would introduce adolescents to present-moment awareness and nonjudgmental awareness materials, whereas in Session 10 they would practice these skills further in the context of generalized emotion exposures all from UP-A Module 6.
- Sessions 11 through 15 would include increasingly challenging situational emotion exposures from UP-A Module 7, followed by relapse prevention activities from UP-A Module 8 in Session 16.

A shorter group could be achieved by lessening the number of situational exposure–focused sessions or eliminating the initial motivational enhancement session. However, it is unlikely that all UP-A content could be delivered in fewer than 12 to 14 sessions overall.

When planning to use the UP-A in a group, consider whether and to what degree **parent involvement** will be incorporated. When using the UP-A as an individual therapy, significant parent involvement is optional and the UP-A parent module (Module-P; Chapter 9 in this Therapist Guide) is used as needed to target particular concerns and emotional parenting behaviors. In a group setting, if sufficient therapists are available, a concurrent parent group can be organized, even using the UP-C parent session materials and workbook to support weekly content delivery. Although meant to accompany the child-directed content from the UP-C more specifically, this content is largely applicable to and appropriate for parents of adolescent clients and could be utilized in a similar structure to the UP-C groups (e.g., meet with adolescents and parents together first, followed by adolescent and parent group alone time and then reconvening for review of home learning assignments briefly at the end of each session). Alternatively, parents may be incorporated more briefly at the beginning and end of each UP-A group session to review progress to date and home learning assignments. In this case, existing UP-A module summary forms can also be utilized to support communication about session content for a slightly extended adolescent–parent review time, when appropriate. It can be useful to have the adolescents help "teach" the parents UP-A skills learned in this shared module summary form during review time to foster further collaboration within families.

There are relatively few materials that require modification if using the UP-A in a group environment. The **structure of each session** itself will be more fixed in a group setting than in an individual therapy context, which means that you may need to consider the pacing and extent of materials to be presented in each session ahead of time, to allow for sufficient time to review content intended. Since we have not formally tested the UP-A in a group setting, the amount of time needed per session to achieve all content specified is not clear, although approximately 90 minutes per group (similar to the UP-C) is likely to be sufficient. In addition, you may need to consider the **pacing and frequency of home learning assignments** given the more structured weekly session format of a group. For example, although no home learning assignment is given for UP-A Module 1, you may wish to initiate a focus on weekly home learning practice by moving the *Before, During, and After* form into this initial session from Module 2 and teaching adolescents how to begin tracking their emotional experiences prior to more formal emotion education in Session 2. Other home learning practices may need to be simplified or reduced as needed to ensure that the group is not overly burdened by too many home learning assignments weekly.

Finally, similar to the UP-C, therapists conducting the UP-A in a group may need to consider the diagnostic diversity of adolescent clients when planning how and with whom adolescents will perform **situational emotion exposures** from Module 7. In the UP-C, therapists work with children in smaller, often more diagnostically homogenous subgroups to engage in similar exposure activities, allowing the children to provide one another with support and empathy as they progress through a range of emotion-evoking scenarios. We generally recommend that therapists conducting the UP-A in a group format follow this same general subgroup structure when planning situational emotion exposures, considering not only diagnostic similarities but also the number of therapists available to forge subgroups and ideal subgroupings of adolescents that can effectively support one another in a positive and kind manner.

Utilization of the UP-C in an Individual Therapy Format

Although the UP-C is presented within a group format in this Therapist Guide, the treatment can easily be modified for use as an individual therapy for children. The UP-C was originally designed as a group treatment for several reasons. First, the group treatment format facilitates the presentation of material in a fun, engaging, and developmentally appropriate manner for children (e.g., using craft projects and games to teach the children skills). Second, participating in a group therapy easily allows for naturalistic exposures for children with certain types of emotional concerns. For example, within a group therapy program, children who struggle with social worries must interact with a group of other children, which could help them face related emotions in group and learn to deal with these social concerns effectively. Similarly, children who have difficulty speaking in front of others (a symptom of selective mutism) are naturally given many opportunities to deal with their distress over speaking with various peers and adults within the group. Individuals experiencing separation worries are also provided with naturalistic exposure opportunities within the context of group therapy in that such children can practice coping with being separated from their parents during children-only sessions. Finally, within a group format, parents have ample opportunity to learn both Emotion Detective (CLUES) skills and parenting skills in parent-only sessions, which occur as part of the group therapy program.

Despite the fact that there are obvious reasons to conduct the UP-C in a group setting, this is not always possible due to recruitment issues, therapist availability, client preferences, or other reasons. In such cases, the UP-C is quite easily adapted for use with an individual child and his or her family. Prior to implementing the UP-C as an individual therapy, please see guidelines outlined below. We provide an overview of some of the more significant modifications you would likely need to make to deliver this treatment as an individual therapy, but please note that this list is not exhaustive and other modifications may be made, as needed.

1. **Parent Involvement.** Unless you plan to conduct two full sessions weekly (one primarily for the child and one primarily for the parent), the presentation of parent material will need to be abbreviated in an individual therapy context. We have typically accomplished this by spending approximately 30 to 40 minutes with the child, 5 minutes with child and parent reviewing session content and home learning assignments, and then 10 to 15 minutes with the parent alone. This suggested session structure will not provide ample time for parents to learn and master all UP-C parent content in session, so it is even more important when using an individual treatment format to develop a clear case conceptualization of parenting factors that may be contributing to the child client's symptoms and emotional distress. Once you choose the most relevant skills and parenting strategies from the parent sections of the treatment to review in more detail with the parents in session, you can then provide parents with the remaining parent workbook materials to review on their own, encouraging them to address—with you—any questions or concerns regarding the materials that they may have.

   The level of parent involvement in treatment, as well as the relative amount of session time you choose to devote to the child and parent components of this treatment, may also depend on the age and attention span of the child. For example, more parent-alone time and parent involvement may be important for younger children who have more difficulty implementing skills independently (therefore requiring more parent support), and also might have more difficulty sustaining attention in session compared to an older child.

2. **Group Activities.** While some activities require little modification for use with one individual child (e.g., Acting Opposite Experiments, Detective Thinking Practice, Problem Solving Practice, Practicing My Awareness Steps), other activities may need to be modified in minor or major ways for an individual therapy format (e.g., True Alarm/False Alarm Game, Mystery Game, Problem Solving Game). For example, instead of completing these in an activity-based, experiential format, you might choose to explain them more didactically to the child client. You may also participate in these activities as another "group member," providing suggestions and ideas. Another option is to invite the child's parents, siblings, or other family members in for a session or two in order to participate in the group activity.

3. **Length of Sessions.** When conducting the UP-C as an individual therapy, session length may be limited to 50 to 60 minutes, once

per week, as this is more typical of most clinical treatment settings. Although group sessions are typically 90 minutes long, the presentation of material typically takes less time with an individual child, as activities and sharing of ideas typically proceeds much more quickly with one child compared to a group of children. One exception to this rule would be if you would like to increase parent involvement (as mentioned above), in which case you may consider extending the length of sessions.

4. **Use of Reinforcement.** We strongly recommend using frequent and consistent reinforcement for brave, on-task, and prosocial behaviors in individual therapy sessions, much as you would in a UP-C group therapy session. Individual therapy clients can also create and decorate CLUES kits during the first session to store tokens and CLUES badges. You may reward your individual client with tokens (e.g., poker chips) for desired behaviors during your individual therapy sessions and allow your child client to exchange these tokens for prizes. We typically choose to eliminate the use of puzzle pieces as reinforcements for home learning completion in an individual therapy format due to practical constraints, although other reinforcements or tokens may be used instead.

5. **Modification of Materials.** When you are conducting the UP-C with one child, you may find that he or she does not require as much emphasis on certain skills and perhaps more on others. This is to be expected and is okay! Every child experiencing an emotional disorder is different, and often some skills are more applicable to one child's symptom presentation than to another's. One luxury of conducting the UP-C individually is that you can spend more time emphasizing skills that seem to be effective for the specific child you are working with, or that are more challenging for the child to master, and less time emphasizing others.

Tips for Modifying the UP-A and UP-C for Specific Disorders

While the application of the UP-A and the UP-C to most anxiety and depressive disorders is quite straightforward, the components of these emotion-focused treatments can easily be modified slightly to effectively target symptoms of related emotional disorders such as OC-spectrum disorders (e.g., OCD), tic disorders, and trauma or stress-related disorders (e.g., PTSD, acute stress disorder, some adjustment disorders), among others. See Table 23.1: *Modifying the UP-A and UP-C for Specific Disorders*

Table 23.1 Modifying the UP-A and UP-C for Specific Disorders

Module in UP-A/ Emotion Detective (CLUES) Skill in UP-C	Obsessive-Compulsive and Related Disorders (OCD and OC-Related Disorders)	Tic and Related Impulse Control Disorders (Tourette's Disorder, Tic Disorder)	Trauma- and Stress-Related Disorders (PTSD, Acute Stress Disorder, Adjustment Disorder)
Module 2: Getting to Know Your Emotions and Behaviors **(C Skill Session 2)**	**Make emotion education more OC-specific by:** - Emphasizing the externalization of OC symptoms - Providing additional psychoeducation on the neurological basis of OC symptoms - Defining obsessions as thoughts and compulsions as emotional behaviors - Discussing the cycle of obsessions and compulsions as one type of cycle of emotional behaviors (e.g., performing compulsions to avoid or escape from obsessions)	*Note that individuals participating in treatment with tic disorders are more appropriate candidates for the UP-A or UP-C if they also have additional emotional disorders/symptoms. Emotion education materials are geared toward these symptoms rather than tics.* **However, emotion education materials in the C skill/Module 2 can be applied to tics in the following way:** - The trigger is the urge to tic or anything that triggers tic (e.g., sitting in class, taking a test, watching TV, reading). - Body clues are urges to perform the tic. - Emotional behavior is the tic.	*Note that individuals with trauma and stress-related disorders have many of the same types of emotional experiences and reactions to them as individuals with anxiety or depressive disorders. Triggers, however, may be different (e.g., while an individual with social anxiety disorder may have an emotional experience in response to a social trigger, those with PTSD-like symptoms may have an emotional experience in response to a trauma trigger).* **Make emotion education more trauma- or stress-specific by:** - Still breaking emotional experiences into their component parts (thoughts, feelings, behaviors, consequences). - Working to normalize and empathize with emotions of guilt or shame, as children and adolescents who have experienced trauma are more likely to experience high levels of these emotions, especially when recalling or ruminating about traumatic or stressful experiences.

Table 23.1 Continued

Module in UP-A/ Emotion Detective (CLUES) Skill in UP-C	Obsessive-Compulsive and Related Disorders (OCD and OC-Related Disorders)	Tic and Related Impulse Control Disorders (Tourette's Disorder, Tic Disorder)	Trauma- and Stress-Related Disorders (PTSD, Acute Stress Disorder, Adjustment Disorder)
Module 3: Introduction to Emotion-Focused Behavioral Experiments **(C Skill Session 3)**	- Introduce one opposite action as "bossing back" OC thoughts (acknowledging them but knowing we do not need to do what the emotion or uncomfortable feeling tells us to do). - Conduct opposite action experiments using simple Exposure/Response Prevention (E/RP) exercises (e.g., assist the child or adolescent in completing a behavioral experiment to see what happens if, instead of washing his or her hands right after the child or adolescent touches the door, he or she washes them in 15 minutes). - You might also choose to begin exposure early in these cases in order to provide more E/RP practice. This would require early use of Module 7 (E Skill Session 9) materials.	- Introduce one opposite action as not performing tic (also known as "habit reversal") in response to the urge to perform a tic. - Conduct opposite action experiments using simple habit reversal exercises (e.g., introducing competing responses such as incompatible motor movements following urge to perform a tic).	- While triggers of emotional experiences might differ from those of a child or adolescent without a trauma history, the idea of acting opposite to how this emotional experience makes one want to act is essentially the same.
Module 5: Being Flexible in Your Thinking **(L Skill Session 5 & U Skill Session 6)**	- These children and adolescents are more likely to fall into the "Magical Thinking" thinking trap in UP-A Module 5. You might consider incorporating this thinking trap into UP-C Session 5 for these children.	N/A	N/A

(continued)

Table 23.1 Continued

Module in UP-A/ Emotion Detective (CLUES) Skill in UP-C	Obsessive-Compulsive and Related Disorders (OCD and OC-Related Disorders)	Tic and Related Impulse Control Disorders (Tourette's Disorder, Tic Disorder)	Trauma- and Stress-Related Disorders (PTSD, Acute Stress Disorder, Adjustment Disorder)
	- Obsessive thinking is much less conducive to cognitive restructuring, as it tends to be rigid, inflexible, and difficult to challenge with evidence. Module 7 (E Skill section) of treatment might be more effective than Detective Thinking for these types of thoughts.		
Module 7: Situational Emotion Exposure **(E Skill Sessions 9-14)**	- Situational emotion exposures should target, at least partially, obsessions/compulsions via E/RP exercises within and between sessions. - Home learning practice is especially important here as these behaviors are quite resistant to change. E/RP must be practiced frequently and consistently in multiple settings.	- Consider incorporating more habit reversal techniques here, such as introducing additional competing responses or applying previously effective competing responses in new settings. - Remaining situational exposure practice should focus on other emotional problems experienced by the child/adolescent.	- Since you will most likely not be able to (and would never want to) expose children and adolescents to the situations that traumatized them in the first place, consider incorporating a trauma narrative, which can be considered a type of imaginal exposure. A trauma narrative involves creating a general story of what happened to the individual and gradually building upon the story by incorporating more and more detail and emotion. - Exposure practice can take longer with these individuals, as they may require very gradual exposure to trauma triggers or details of the traumatic event.

for tips on how and when during treatment you *might* consider modifying these treatments to target issues specific to these types of disorders. However, please keep in mind that the UP-C and the UP-A are likely sufficient in their unmodified format for a range of emotional disorders and that such variations are not required for success.

We certainly recognize that the suggestions we have provided in this chapter are not exhaustive, and additional or different modifications may be required to optimize this treatment's applicability to a particular context or symptom presentation. This is of course not unique to the UP-C/UP-A and is true of all evidence-based treatments. Overall, we recommend taking the approach that has sometimes been referred to as "flexibility within fidelity" (Kendall & Beidas, 2007) in modifying treatments for your unique clients and treatment settings. In other words, we suggest using your case conceptualization and/or setting constraints to personalize this treatment model, while still adhering to its underlying core principles.

References

Albano, A. M., Clarke, G., Heimberg R. G., & Kendall, P. C. (1998). *Emotion management training*. Unpublished manual.

Ammerman, R. T., Bellack, A. S., Van Hasselt, V. B., Ellard, K. K., Deckersbach, T., Sylvia, L. G., & Barlow, D. H. (2012). Transdiagnostic treatment of bipolar disorder and comorbid anxiety with the unified protocol. *Behavior Modification, 36*(4), 482–508. doi:10.1177/0145445512451272

Angold, A., Costello, E. J., & Erkanli, A. (1999). Comorbidity. *Journal of Child Psychology and Psychiatry, 40*, 57–87. doi:10.1111/1469-7610.00424

Barlow, D. H., Ellard, K. K., Sauer-Zavala, S., Bullis, J. R., & Carl, J. R. (2014a). The origins of neuroticism. *Perspectives on Psychological Science, 9*(5), 481–496. doi:10.1177/1745691614544528

Barlow, D. H., Farchione, T. J., Bullis, J. R., Gallagher, M. W., Murray-Latin, H., Sauer-Zavala, S., . . . Cassiello-Robbins, C. (2017). The Unified Protocol for Transdiagnostic Treatment of Emotional Disorders compared with diagnosis-specific protocols for anxiety disorders: A randomized clinical trial. *JAMA Psychiatry*. doi:10.1001/jamapsychiatry.2017.2164.

Barlow, D. H., Farchione, T. J., Fairholme, C. P., Ellard, K. K., Boisseau, C. L., Allen, L. B., & Ehrenreich-May, J. (2011). *Unified Protocol for Transdiagnostic Treatment of Emotional Disorders: Therapist guide*. New York: Oxford University Press.

Barlow, D. H., & Kennedy, K. A. (2016). New approaches to diagnosis and treatment in anxiety and related emotional disorders: A focus on temperament. *Canadian Psychology/Psychologie Canadienne, 57*(1), 8–20. doi:10.1037/cap0000039

Barlow, D. H., Sauer-Zavala, S., Carl, J. R., Bullis, J. R., & Ellard, K. K. (2014b). The nature, diagnosis, and treatment of neuroticism: Back to the future. *Clinical Psychological Science, 2*(3), 344–365.

Bentley, K. H. (2017). Applying the unified protocol transdiagnostic treatment to nonsuicidal self-injury and co-occurring emotional disorders: A case illustration. *Journal of Clinical Psychology*. doi:10.1002/jclp.22452

Bentley, K. H., Nock, M., Sauer-Zavala, S., Gorman, B., & Barlow, D. H. (2017). A functional analysis of two transdiagnostic, emotion-focused interventions on nonsuicidal self-injury. *Journal of Consulting and Clinical Psychology*. doi: 10.1037/ccp0000205.

Boomsma, D. I., Van Beijsterveldt, C. E. M., & Hudziak, J. J. (2005). Genetic and environmental influences on anxious/depression during childhood: A study from the Netherlands Twin Register. *Genes, Brain and Behavior, 4*(8), 466–481. doi:10.1111/j.1601-183X.2005.00141.x

Boswell, J. F., Anderson, L. M., & Barlow, D. H. (2014). An idiographic analysis of change processes in the unified transdiagnostic treatment of depression. *Journal of Consulting and Clinical Psychology, 82*(6), 1060–1071. doi:10.1037/a0037403

Brady, E. U., & Kendall, P. C. (1992). Comorbidity of anxiety and depression in children and adolescents. *Psychological Bulletin, 111*(2), 244–255. doi:10.1037/0033-2909.111.2.24

Bullis, J. R., Fortune, M. R., Farchione, T. J., & Barlow, D. H. (2014). A preliminary investigation of the long-term outcome of the unified protocol for transdiagnostic treatment of emotional disorders. *Comprehensive Psychiatry*, *55*(8), 1920–1927. doi:http://doi.org/10.1016/j.comppsych.2014.07.016

Bullis, J. R., Sauer-Zavala, S., Bentley, K. H., Thompson-Hollands, J., Carl, J. R., & Barlow, D. H. (2015). The Unified Protocol for Transdiagnostic Treatment of Emotional Disorders: Preliminary exploration of effectiveness for group delivery. *Behavior Modification*, *39*(2), 295–321. doi:10.1177/0145445514553094

Conklin, L. R., Cassiello-Robbins, C., Brake, C. A., Sauer-Zavala, S., Farchione, T. J., Ciraulo, D. A., & Barlow, D. H. (2015). Relationships among adaptive and maladaptive emotion regulation strategies and psychopathology during the treatment of comorbid anxiety and alcohol use disorders. *Behaviour Research and Therapy*, *73*, 124–130. doi:http://doi.org/10.1016/j.brat.2015.08.

Cummings, C. M., Caporino, N. E., & Kendall, P. C. (2014). Comorbidity of anxiety and depression in children and adolescents: 20 years after. *Psychological Bulletin*, *140*(3), 816–845. doi:10.1037/a0034733

Drake, K. L., & Ginsburg, G. S. (2012). Family factors in the development, treatment, and prevention of childhood anxiety disorders. *Clinical Child and Family Psychology Review*, *15*(2), 144–162. doi:10.1007/s10567-011-0109-0

Ehrenreich, J. T., Goldstein, C. R., Wright, L. R., & Barlow, D. H. (2009). Development of a unified protocol for the treatment of emotional disorders in youth. *Child & Family Behavior Therapy*, *31*(1), 20–37.

Ehrenreich-May, J., & Bilek, E. L. (2011). Universal prevention of anxiety and depression in a recreational camp setting: An initial open trial. *Child and Youth Care Forum*, *40*(6), 435–455. doi: 10.1007/s10566-011-9148-4

Ehrenreich-May, J., & Bilek, E. L. (2012). The development of a transdiagnostic cognitive behavioral group intervention for childhood anxiety disorders and co-occurring depression symptoms. *Cognitive and Behavioral Practice*, *19*(1), 41–55. doi:10.1016/j.cbpra.2011.02.003

Ehrenreich-May, J., Bilek, E. L., Queen, A. H., Remmes, C. A., & Marciel, K. (2013). The unified protocols for the treatment of emotional disorders in childhood and adolescence. In J. Ehrenreich-May & B. Chu (Eds.), *Transdiagnostic mechanisms and treatment of youth psychopathology*. New York: Guilford Press.

Ehrenreich-May, J., Rosenfield, D., Queen, A. H., Kennedy, S. M., Remmes, C. S., & Barlow, D. H. (2017). An initial waitlist-controlled trial of the unified protocol for the treatment of emotional disorders in adolescents. *Journal of Anxiety Disorders*, *46*, 46–55. doi:http://doi.org/10.1016/j.janxdis.2016.10.006

Eley, T. C., Bolton, D., O'Connor, T. G., Perrin, S., Smith, P., & Plomin, R. (2003). A twin study of anxiety-related behaviours in pre-school children. *Journal of Child Psychology and Psychiatry*, *44*, 945–960.

Ellard, K. K., Deckersbach, T., Sylvia, L. G., Nierenberg, A. A., & Barlow, D. H. (2012). Transdiagnostic treatment of bipolar disorder and comorbid anxiety with the Unified Protocol: A clinical replication series. *Behavior Modification*, *36*, 482–508.

Farchione, T. J., & Barlow, D. H. (Eds.). (2017). *Applications of the Unified Protocol for Transdiagnostic Treatment of Emotional Disorders*. New York: Oxford University Press.

Farchione, T. J., Fairholme, C. P., Ellard, K. K., Boisseau, C. L., Thompson-Hollands, J., Carl, J. R., Barlow, D. H. (2012). Unified Protocol for Transdiagnostic Treatment of Emotional Disorders: A Randomized Controlled Trial. *Behavior Therapy*, *43*(3), 666–678. http://doi.org/10.1016/j.beth.2012.01.001

Ginsburg, G. S., Siqueland, L., Masia-Warner, C., & Hedtke, K. A. (2004). Anxiety disorders in children: Family matters. *Cognitive and Behavioral Practice*, *11*(1), 28–43. doi:http://doi.org/10.1016/S1077-7229(04)80005-1

Keenan, K., & Hipwell, A. E. (2005) Preadolescent clues to understanding depression in girls. *Clinical Child and Family Psychology Review*, *8*(2), 89. doi:10.1007/s10567-005-4750-3

Kendall, P. C., & Beidas, R. S. (2007). Smoothing the trail for dissemination of evidence-based practices for youth: Flexibility within fidelity. *Professional Psychology: Research & Practice*, *38*(1), 13–20. doi:10.1037/0735-7028.38.1.13

Kennedy, S. M., Bilek, E. L., & Ehrenreich-May, J. (2017). A randomized controlled pilot trial of the Unified Protocol for Transdiagnostic Treatment of Emotional Disorders in Children.

Leahy, R. L. (2003). *Roadblocks in cognitive-behavioral therapy: Transforming challenges into opportunities for change.* New York: Guilford Press.

Leyfer, O., Gallo, K. P., Cooper-Vince, C., & Pincus, D. B. (2013). Patterns and predictors of comorbidity of DSM-IV anxiety disorders in a clinical sample of children and adolescents. *Journal of Anxiety Disorders*, *27*(3), 306–311. doi:http://doi.org/10.1016/j.janxdis.2013.01.010

Linehan, M. M. (2015). *DBT skills training manual* (2nd ed.). New York: Guilford Press.

Lopez, M. E., Stoddard, J. A., Noorollah, A., Zerbi, G., Payne, L. A., Hitchcock, C. A., . . . Ray, D. B. (2015). Examining the efficacy of the unified protocol for transdiagnostic treatment of emotional disorders in the treatment of individuals with borderline personality disorder. *Cognitive and Behavioral Practice*, *22*(4), 522–533. doi:10.1016/j.cbpra.2014.06.006

March, J. S., & Mulle, K. (1998). *OCD in children and adolescents: A cognitive-behavioral treatment manual.* New York: Guilford Press.

Marchette, L., & Weisz, J. R. (2017). Practitioner review: Empirical evolution of youth psychotherapy toward transdiagnostic approaches. *Journal of Child Psychology and Psychiatry.* doi:10.1111/jcpp.12747

Middeldorp, C. M., Cath, D. C., Van Dyck, R., & Boomsma, D. I. (2005). The co-morbidity of anxiety and depression in the perspective of genetic epidemiology. A review of twin and family studies. *Psychological Medicine*, *35*(5), 611–624. doi:10.1017/s003329170400412x

Miller, W. R., & Rollnick, S. (2002). *Motivational interviewing: Preparing people for change* (2nd ed.). New York: Guilford Press.

Queen, A.H., Barlow, D.H., & Ehrenreich-May, J. (2014). The trajectories of adolescent anxiety and depressive symptoms over the course of a transdiagnostic treatment. *Journal of Anxiety Disorders*, *28*(6), 511–521. doi: 10.1016/j.janxdis.2014.05.007

Sauer-Zavala, S., Boswell, J. F., Gallagher, M. W., Bentley, K. H., Ametaj, A., & Barlow, D. H. (2012). The role of negative affectivity and negative reactivity to emotions in predicting outcomes in the unified protocol for the transdiagnostic treatment of emotional disorders. *Behaviour Research and Therapy*, *50*(9), 551–557. doi:10.1016/j.brat.2012.05.005

Sobell, L. C., & Sobell, M. B. (2003). Using motivational interviewing techniques to talk with clients about their alcohol use. *Cognitive and Behavioral Practice*, *10*(3), 214–221. doi:10.1016/S1077-7229(03)80033-0

Trosper, S. E., Buzzella, B. A., Bennett, S. M., & Ehrenreich, J. T. (2009). Emotion regulation in youth with emotional disorders: Implications for a unified treatment approach. *Clinical Child and Family Psychology Review, 12,* 234–254.

Weisz, J. R., Chorpita, B. F., Frye, A., Ng, M. Y., Lau, N., Bearman, S. K., & Hoagwood, K. E. (2011). Youth top problems: Using idiographic, consumer-guided assessment to identify treatment needs and to track change during psychotherapy. *Journal of Consulting and Clinical Psychology, 79*(3), 369–380. doi:10.1037/a0023307

Wilamowska, Z. A., Thompson-Hollands, J., Fairholme, C. P., Ellard, K. K., Farchione, T. J., & Barlow, D. H. (2010), Conceptual background, development, and preliminary data from the unified protocol for transdiagnostic treatment of emotional disorders. *Depression and Anxiety, 27,* 882–890. doi:10.1002/da.20735

Williams, J. M., Teasdale, J., Segal, Z., & Kabat-Zinn, J. (2007). *The mindful way through depression: Freeing yourself from chronic unhappiness.* New York: Guilford Press.

Jill Ehrenreich-May, PhD, is the Director of the Child and Adolescent Mood and Anxiety Treatment (CAMAT) program and Associate Professor in the Child Division of the Department of Psychology at the University of Miami. In addition to the development and evaluation of evidence-based treatment approaches for anxiety and depressive disorders in youth, she is particularly interested in clinician training and the dissemination and implementation of effective treatments in environments that maximize their impact and benefit for children. Her current research has been supported by grants from the National Institute of Mental Health and the Children's Trust.

Sarah M. Kennedy, PhD, is a postdoctoral fellow at Children's Hospital Colorado, where she provides clinical services and conducts research on transdiagnostic approaches to assessment and treatment of emotional disorders in youth. She has published numerous book chapters and articles on the etiology and treatment of emotional disorders in children and adolescents.

Jamie A. Sherman, MS, is a doctoral candidate in the child clinical psychology program at the University of Miami. Clinically, she is interested in providing effective treatment for youth with a variety of anxiety and mood concerns. Her research focuses on the development and evaluation of evidence-supported treatments for pediatric mood and anxiety disorders.

Emily L. Bilek, PhD, is a Clinical Assistant Professor at the University of Michigan in the Department of Psychiatry. Her research interests include the investigation of treatment mechanisms and treatment enhancement for cognitive behavioral therapies, and treatment deployment and dissemination.

Brian A. Buzzella, PhD, ABPP, is currently Director of the VA San Diego's Family Mental Health Program and H. S. Clinical Assistant Professor of Psychiatry at the University of California San Diego.

Shannon M. Bennett, PhD, is an Assistant Professor of Psychology in Clinical Psychiatry at Weill Cornell Medicine, and is the Director of Psychology for the Division of Child and Adolescent Psychiatry. Dr. Bennett serves as the Co-Director of the Pediatric OCD, Anxiety, and Tic Disorders Program at Weill Cornell Medicine and is the Site Clinical Director of the New York Presbyterian Hospital Youth Anxiety Center. Dr. Bennett currently leads a research and clinical program serving children, adolescents, and young adults with anxiety and related disorders.

David H. Barlow, PhD, ABPP, is Professor of Psychiatry and Psychology Emeritus at Boston University and the Founder and Director of the Center for Anxiety and Related Disorders, Emeritus. He has received numerous awards and has published over 600 articles and chapters and over 80 books, and his research has been continuously funded by the National Institutes of Health for over 45 years. He is editor- in- chief for the Treatments *That Work* series of therapist manuals and patient workbooks for Oxford University Press.